Assessing the Health Status of Older Adults

Elena M. Andresen, PhD, completed her doctorate in epidemiology at the University of Washington, Seattle, in 1991. She was an Assistant Professor in the Department of Community and Preventive Medicine at the University of Rochester School of Medicine and Dentistry from 1991 to 1996 and is currently Associate Professor of Epidemiology in the Department of Community Health at the School of Public Health at Saint Louis University. Dr. Andresen's contributions to this book stem from her work at the University of Washington as part of the Center for Health Promotion for Older Adults (funded by the Centers for Disease Control and Prevention) as well as research at the University of Rochester. Dr. Andresen is a chronic diseases epidemiologist with research interests in diabetes and cardiovascular diseases as well as an interest in outcomes research, especially in the measurement of health-related quality of life and health status. Her current research at Saint Louis University includes a special interest project on the validity of health-related quality of life and function-disability measures funded by the Centers for Disease Control and Prevention.

Barbara M. Rothenberg, MPA, MA, is Director of Quality Assessment with the Rochester Health Commission in Rochester, New York, and is developing a strategy for measuring the quality of and access to health care on a communitywide basis. As a researcher with the Health Services Research Core of the Rochester Area Pepper Center, she collaborated with Dr. Andresen on several studies of the use of the SF-36 and the Sickness Impact Profile among older adults and developed a cost-effectiveness analysis of a smoking cessation intervention, also among older adults. She has also played a key role in technology assessments and in analyses of large Medicare claims databases. She received a master's of public affairs from the Woodrow Wilson School of Public and International Affairs at Princeton University and a master's degree in Political Science from Stanford University.

James G. Zimmer, MD, DTPH (London), is Associate Chair of the Department of Community and Preventive Medicine at the University of Rochester School of Medicine and Dentistry. His primary research activities are in health services research on aging and long-term care. He has done a number of studies of utilization and quality assessment in nursing homes and has been Director of the Health Services Research Core of the Rochester Area Pepper Center over the past five years. He has also been research director of several randomized controlled trials of community-based long-term-care interventions, including a physician-led home care team, two models of case management, a geriatric evaluation clinic, and a health maintenance tracking system for the prevention of chronic disease. He is currently research director of randomized controlled trials of an expanded system of medical care for acute episodes in nursing homes and of case management and consumer-directed care for high risk patients in primary care practices. He received an M.D. from Yale University and a Diploma in Tropical Public Health from the London School of Hygiene.

Assessing the Health Status of Older Adults

Elena Andresen, PhD
Barbara Rothenberg, MPA, MA
James G. Zimmer, MD

Editors

 Springer Publishing Company

Springer Publishing Company, Inc.
536 Broadway
New York, NY 10012-3955

Cover design by: Margaret Dunin
Acquisitions Editor: Bill Tucker
Production Editor: Susan Gamer

97 98 99 00 01 / 5 4 3 2 1

Library of Congress Cataloging-in-Publication Data

Assessing the health status of older adults / Elena Andresen, Barbara Rothenberg, James
  G. Zimmer, editors.
    p. cm.
  Includes bibliographical references and indexes.
  ISBN 0-8261-9780-9
  1. Aged—Diseases—Diagnosis. 2. Medical screening. 3. Health status
indicators. I. Andresen, Elena. II. Rothenberg, Barbara, M.P.A. III. Zimmer,
James, G.
  [DNLM: 1. Geriatric Assessment. 2. Health Status Indicators—in old age.
WT 30 A846 1997]
RC953.A87 1997
618.97'075—dc21
DNLM/DLC
for Library of Congress   97-20430
                                       CIP

Printed in the United States of America

Contents

Contributors

Elena M. Andresen
Associate Professor of Epidemiology
Department of Community Health
School of Public Health
St. Louis University
St. Louis, Missouri

Lesley H. Curtis
Associate Provost
University of Rochester
Rochester, New York

Robin E. Henderson, PhD
Assistant Professor, Physical
   Medicine / Rehabilitation and
   Psychiatry
University of Rochester School of
   Medicine and Dentistry
Monroe Community Hospital
Rochester, New York

Jurgis Karuza, PhD
Visiting Professor of Medicine,
   University of Rochester School of
   Medicine and Dentistry
Medical Administration
Monroe Community Hospital
Rochester, New York

Paul R. Katz, MD
Associate Professor
Department of Medicine, University
   of Rochester School of Medicine
   and Dentistry

Medicine Director, Monroe
   Community Hospital
Rochester, New York

Cathleen Mooney, RN, MS
Associate
Department of Community and
   Preventive Medicine
University of Rochester School of
   Medicine and Dentistry
Rochester, New York

Deborah J. Ossip-Klein, PhD
Research Associate Professor
Department of Community and
   Preventive Medicine
University of Rochester School of
   Medicine and Dentistry
Monroe Community Hospital
Rochester, New York

Barbara M. Rothenberg, MPA, MA
Director of Quality Assessment
Rochester Health Commission
Rochester, New York

James G. Zimmer, MD
Associate Professor
Department of Community and
   Preventive Medicine
University of Rochester School of
   Medicine and Dentistry
Rochester, New York

Acknowledgments

Preparation of this volume was supported in part by the Rochester Area Pepper Center (NIA Grant No. 5 P60 AG10463). Deborah Ossip-Klein's work on chapter 5 was supported in part by the Department of Veterans Affairs Health Services Research and Development Service Developmental Project DEV 92-005.

We would like to acknowledge the assistance of Nancy Bowley, RN, who was involved in the planning phases of this project and who compiled some of the initial reference lists for the chapters; Judith Baggs, RN, PhD, for her insightful comments on the discussion of APACHE in Chapter 3; and Valerie Bruemmer, MD, for her assistance in selecting the instruments discussed in chapter 1. We would also like to thank Briana Chen, Caryn Graff, Pamela Polashenski, and Allison Warner for bibliographic assistance, and Connie French and Helen Weeks for assistance in preparing the manuscript.

Introduction

Elena M. Andresen

RATIONALE, PURPOSE, AND ORGANIZATION

This book is intended for gerontological and clinical researchers, educators, and students. It will also prove useful for clinicians as they increasingly find themselves faced with a bewildering menu of choices for categorizing and classifying the health of their older patients. This book reviews five topics in health status measurement and suggests how to choose among competing instruments for different settings and uses.

Researchers have long sought mechanisms for measuring the health of groups or entire populations. According to the definition of the World Health Organization, *health* is not only the absence of disease; rather, it encompasses complete mental, physical, and social well-being. Consequently, clinicians and researchers need to measure different health states that incorporate aspects beyond the diagnoses of disease and even the severity of disease. Health status, then, is a multidimensional measure for characterizing older adults that is meant to augment or even replace classifications based only on diagnoses, clinical exams, and tests. Increasingly, the measurement of health status is being promoted in research, clinical, and institutional settings. Some researchers have considerable experience with the terminology, methods, and uses of the instruments described in this book. We hope to reach the wider audience of professionals who are relatively uninitiated.

The measurement of older adults' health status is a complex area. It requires researchers and clinicians to understand the benefits and limitations of available instruments and to choose measurement tools according to the needs of each study and their selected population. This book will assist investigators in making intelligent choices and will provide useful information for clinicians, educators, and students. The authors of the five chapters seek to provide the reader with state-of-the-science knowledge for specific content areas relating to the health of older adults. Whenever possible, the authors make recommendations for selecting specific instruments, although these recommendations may be limited by evidence (or lack of evidence) among some populations or groups.

The purpose of this book is threefold. First, we provide a review of selected methods for measuring five areas of health among older adults:

1. Physical and functional assessment
2. General multidimensional health status assessment
3. Measures of disease severity and comorbidity
4. Screening for cognition or mental status
5. Screening for depression

Second, we provide, in annotated bibliographies, the developmental and research literature on selected health status measures. Third, we provide references to results of other selected comparative research on the application of these measures among older adults. In addition, each chapter provides a summary and straightforward guide, a "jump start" to understanding how to measure the health status of older adults.

To provide a useful summary of each topic, the authors have been selective in their choice of instruments. There is a bewildering array of comparable and competing ways to measure each topic or content area. We attempt to provide competent, but not exhaustive, suggestions and alternatives. Consequently, some measures may not be included. The book provides a starting place for decisions about selecting and understanding health status instruments and covers some of those most widely used. For topics with a broad application (e.g., screening for depression), one or more instruments have been chosen specifically because they were useful across the age spectrum. These instruments will allow researchers and others to consider how a particular area of health is (or is not) affected by increasing age without having to use an arbitrary age cutoff. For example, in an application concerning women, a researcher might define *older adults* as those age 50 and older, because this is an approximate biological age for categorizing women in terms of menopause. Another study might define *older adults* in terms of eligibility for Medicare (age 65). A third study might consider changes in health among all adults age 18 and older.

The chapters include a critical overview and summary of the literature. For some topics, other useful reviews are available, and the reader is directed to them for more detail or alternative views. For example, some of the topics covered in this book are reviewed in the 1994 volume of the *Annual Review of Gerontology and Geriatrics* (Lawton & Teresi, 1994).

Each chapter also includes an annotated, alphabetical bibliography of the key literature regarding the development, testing, and use of these instruments. Each annotated bibliography is subdivided into two sections: (1) development and methods and (2) applications. The first section gives readers the best basic development references for each instrument, plus reviews of studies that have established key limitations or strengths of the instrument as applied to older adults. For some well-established instruments—for example, the Center for Epidemiologic Studies Depression Scale (CES-D)—there are also discussions of abbreviated versions of the scale or discussions of alternative scales. When there are such alternatives, the literature that describes them is also given if it pertains to older adults.

The second section of the annotated bibliographies provides a selected list of studies applying the instrument. Some measurement tools have long histories and literally hundreds of potential references. The criteria for selecting published examples, given many choices, were that they provide examples of large, well-conducted, and recent studies that concentrate on results in adults aged 65 and older or on patient populations with diseases typical of older ages: for example, stroke, arthritis, and hip fracture. In addition, when many good studies were available, examples were chosen from research based in the United States rather than in other countries. Important examples, references, and associated materials, such as reviews, books, and other measurement tools, are also cited without annotation in a more comprehensive list at the end of each chapter. If a reference has been annotated, it is marked with an asterisk (*) in the reference list and in the overview.

THE COMPLEXITY OF HEALTH STATUS MEASUREMENT

Clinical, epidemiological, and health services research on the health of older adults depends, in part, on measuring different health states to distinguish among individuals. Some research has focused on mortality, incident disease, or a loss of physical function that puts older adults in a dependent role (Boult, Kane, Lewis, Boult, & McCaffrey, 1994; Camacho, Strawbridge, Cohen, & Kaplan, 1993; Foley et al., 1990). As the definition of *health* has expanded, so has the need to distinguish among more finely defined and multidimensional states of health. Measurement of physical functioning is only one domain of measuring health status, which usually includes other domains, such as social and mental health and their roles.

Physical function is still a vital part of assessing institutionalized or frail older adults, and the Activities of Daily Living Scale (ADL) and the Instrumental Activities of Daily Living Scale (IADL) are the questionnaires most commonly used (Deniston & Jette, 1980; Fillenbaum & Smyer, 1981; Grauer & Birnbom, 1975; Katz, Downs, Cash, & Grotz, 1970; Kovar & Lawton, 1994; Kuriansky & Gurland, 1976; Lawton & Brody, 1969; Plutchik et al., 1970). These instruments specifically measure the functional status of older, institutionalized, or disabled persons. Items on the ADL include basic self-maintenance tasks that a person needs to perform daily, such as grooming, transferring to and from bed, and walking. On the IADL, items address activities that require a higher level of functioning or tasks that require the use of an "instrument." Instrumental activities, thus, include using a telephone, doing the laundry, and using public transportation.

Chapter 1 gives a review of ADL and IADL scales and performance-based functional assessment tools. These assessments are all useful and continue to be used to predict dependency and screen for individuals' ability to perform self-care tasks. For example, use of home health care services increased with both increasing ADLs and IADLs among older adults surveyed in the National Health Interview Survey Supplement on Aging (Fredman, Droger, & Rabin, 1992). It is important to note also that the number of individuals who are unable to perform ADLs does increase with age. The National Health and Nutrition Examination Survey (NHANES) found that both men and women aged 65 to 74 had more difficulty with all of the ADL items than those aged 55 to 64. Some of the increases were quite dramatic: For example, 12.1% of men aged 55 to 64 reported at least some difficulty with dressing and grooming; by ages 65 to 74, the figure rose to 21.2% (Foley et al., 1990). An Australian study found that as many as 14% of those aged 65 to 74 may have some problem with daily activities; and this increased to a prevalence of 52% for those over 80 (Maddox, 1981). However, ADLs are not particularly useful in assessing most older adults living in the community, who are about 95% of the population aged 65 and older (Van Nostrand, 1993). The expansion of the ADL scales to include so-called instrumental items allows the assessment of older persons who have a higher level of functioning. Nonetheless, community-dwelling older adults, by and large, will not demonstrate even medium levels of dysfunction on these scales. Many individuals receive scores of zero (no measurable dysfunction), presenting the problem of a "ceiling" effect: That is, most individuals will not be distinguishable from one another, because their health is too "good" to be assessed by the measurement tool. In addition, neither the ADL nor the IADL scales measure other important health domains such as social and mental health, mental status, and well-being. Performance tests of function also tend to be limited to frail older adults and do not include a broadly defined measure of health status. However, they offer other advantages, such as their objectivity and their relevance to the daily tasks these individuals need to perform. Three examples are discussed in detail in Chapter 1: the Timed Manual Performance test (*Williams & Hadler, 1981; *Williams, Hadler, & Earp, 1982), the Get Up and Go test (*Mathias, Nayak, & Isaacs, 1985; *Podsiadlo & Richardson, 1991), and the 6-minute-walk test (*Butland, Pang, Gross, Woodcock, & Geddes, 1982; *Guyatt, Sullivan, & Thompson, 1985).

---

*As explained above, the asterisk indicates that a reference is annotated.

An emphasis on measures of illness and disability among older adults such as the ADL/IADL scales ignores the reality that these are not relevant for the majority of patients that most clinicians see in their practices. To offer advice and encouragement to healthier patients about promoting health, measures that are useful in showing change in a positive direction are required. This need formed part of the motivation for the development of multidimensional measures of health status. Furthermore, ADL/IADL scales overlap with other comprehensive measures of health status and may not provide additional information when used in tandem. The Sickness Impact Profile (SIP), for example, contains scales measuring health-related limitations in the areas of personal care, ambulation, and home maintenance.

Chapter 2 concentrates on three multidimensional instruments. The oldest measure reviewed in Chapter 2, the Sickness Impact Profile (SIP), has been used broadly for older adults and patient groups; the newest, the Short Form 36, or SF-36, has had more limited testing among older adults. The most complex instrument covered in Chapter 2 is the Quality of Well-Being (QWB) Scale. The multidimensional health measures presented in Chapter 2 will not automatically solve the ceiling problem of measurement described for ADL and IADL scales. It is still possible for a scale to yield a very compressed range of scores if the scale defines *positive health* as a state that is simply free of symptoms and detrimental conditions and does not include measurement of positive health states. For example, the SIP yields an average score of 4% or less for community-dwelling persons (*Bergner, Bobbitt, Carter, & Gilson, 1981), because it measures increasingly *declining* health status on a scale where a positive state (no symptoms) is scored zero. The SF-36 may have an advantage in the measurement of positive health status because it contains a broader range of health and measures domains like "vitality." But it is not clear that the SF-36 has an advantage for older adults with disabilities, whose scores may cluster at the lower end of the scale for a "floor" effect. In other words, their health status is too poor compared with a general population, and the SF-36 may not distinguish among meaningful, personally and clinically relevant differences in health status. It will be clear to the reader that no one type of measure should be applied in every population, and Chapters 1 and 2 provide recommendations for selecting the most appropriate measure. Relevant discussions of theoretical structures and measures of functional and general health are offered by Teresi and Holmes (1994), Lawton and Lawrence (1994), and George (1994). It should also be noted that not all authors consider these multidimensional health status instruments as representing a state-of-the-science appropriate for assessing older adults (George, 1994).

Chapter 3 completes our discussion of general health status by introducing methods of measuring severity of disease or comorbid conditions. Like the measures of general health status discussed in Chapter 2, these adjustment methods have been spurred by the need for comparisons among individuals, groups, or institutions to understand different patterns of outcomes and potential interventions to improve them. All of these measures are intended to control for "legitimate" variability among individuals that is independent of the process being examined (e.g., the care provided by a hospital or physician or a specific type of procedure or treatment). The purpose is to distinguish between the impact of a process or treatment and the effect of the individual's underlying characteristics before treatment. Unlike general health status questionnaires, the measures of severity of illness incorporate information about specific medical diagnoses, conditions, and levels of severity. The authors identify a variety of computer programs and chart-based methods and summarize the utility, advantages, and disadvantages of the various techniques. These measures have been applied in different settings, including health services research, clinical studies, and hospital-based quality improvement programs. These techniques are now widespread and are gaining importance in policy and decision making about systems of health care. We can expect that changes in the American health care system will rely on current and future refinements of severity adjustment methods to monitor, and perhaps even to market, various health care options.

Multidimensional instruments, like the SIP and SF-36, also contain an abbreviated summary of mental health status. However, for some clinical and research purposes, a more specific measure may be required. Chapters 4 and 5 review the measurement of cognitive function and depressive symptoms among older adults.

Chapter 4 summarizes the increasing problem—that is, increasing in terms of numbers of individuals affected—of organic mental disorders and examines methods of screening older adults for these disorders. The authors thoroughly review the most favored tool, the Mini-Mental State Examination (MMSE). They discuss a variety of potential caveats about its use with ethnic subgroups and with persons of lower educational attainment. Because of the number of important methodological studies, the authors have chosen to offer a lengthy annotated bibliography section on development and testing and fewer entries on applications; however, a good selection of research using the MMSE is listed among the references. Chapter 4 also discusses the problem of underdiagnosis, particularly of mild or early dementia, and examines alternative screening methods. These include approaches to assessing individuals who have lost verbal ability and an intriguing new performance screening method, the "clock test," as well as the application of psychiatric and behavioral scales to screening for dementia. The important issue of distinguishing dementia from depression is addressed as well.

Clinical depression is best diagnosed by specialists using very specific and thorough questionnaires and procedures. But for general clinical surveillance, case-finding, and broad-based research on general populations, depressive symptoms may be measured more easily using self-administered questionnaires. Depressive symptoms are a common mental health problem and have a complex relationship to increasing age, especially as individuals respond to stressful life events, including loss of loved ones and deteriorating health. Chapter 5 reviews three questionnaires commonly used to screen for depressive symptoms: the Center for Epidemiologic Studies Depression (CES-D) Scale, the Geriatric Depression Scale (GDS), and the Beck Depression Inventory (BDI). Two of these screening questionnaires were selected because they are used across the age span; all three also have significant track records in research on older adults. Clinical use of depression screening tools is still lagging. The future of screening instruments as clinical tools, either to measure specific components of health like depression or to measure general health status, is discussed below.

SELECTING A MEASURE

This book would be brief if there were a single universally applicable tool for measuring all important aspects of health status among older adults. But as workers in the mechanical and skilled trades know, one needs the right tool for the job. Before selecting a measurement tool, readers should investigate (1) whether the measure was developed for their specific population or use, or has been successfully tested and applied to it; and (2) whether the tool has practical utility and has undergone rigorous testing using appropriate psychometric methods.

Common to all processes comparing competing measurement tools is an understanding of the target group of interest in this book: older adults. Everyone would agree that a questionnaire used to assess mood or stress among college students would be poorly applied to older adults in nursing homes without considerable testing in the new population. However, some survey tools that have been tested broadly across age groups may still offer only limited information about their specific utility for older adults. Measurement instruments should have known track records for the specific application needs of a researcher or clinician. Surprisingly, some of the most obvious and practical problems of applying measures to older adults are often left out of the literature on development and testing. For example, is there a literacy barrier, a cultural barrier, or a sensory barrier in the use of a particular self-administered survey? Are many older adults ''put off'' by certain questions because of typical social conventions or their own experiences? Most surveys have some scoring algorithm to use in case of missing questions. But is there a pattern to these missing items suggesting a problem with acceptability or understanding? When these and other applications problems have been addressed by the literature, they are noted. For example, as described in Chapter 5, the Center for Epidemiological Studies Depression (CES-D) survey began as a research survey for the general population, but it has an impressive testing and applications record with older adults. For a more thorough review of the issues of research methods with older adults, three books are especially recommended: Lawton and Herzog, 1989; Lawton and Teresi, 1994; and Wallace and Woolson, 1992.

Understanding the practical application of health status measures is vital to making a selection from competing potential instruments. If one wishes to measure the physical function of clinic patients while they are waiting for appointments, would it be practical to use specially trained technicians and apply one of the performance-based measures described in Chapter 1? In a nursing home, are nurses, aides, or other surrogates able to provide accurate information about the limitations of residents with severe dementia? More subtle practical issues are also important. For example, some researchers may need to consider using a large-print version of a questionnaire or installing special volume-enhancing equipment for a survey by telephone. Some situations may require a selection of appropriate subjects for research or patients for further testing in stages. For example, when a survey requires older adults to provide information directly about their habits, feelings, or perceptions, it may be necessary to precede the survey with a screening for cognitive function (see examples in Chapter 4) or to ask for a professional judgment from the person's clinical health care provider. If a particular measure has been extensively used with insured, white older adults in urban health maintenance organizations, how does it fare when applied to poor, rural persons or inner-city Hispanic populations? It would be a mistake to assume that older adults are either a homogeneous or a unique population, that all of them are frail, or that all measurement applications will always require intensive training in special methods. When selecting a measure, it is imperative to know the spectrum of individuals who will be measured and to plan for any special problems. A carefully planned pilot application of a potential measure is always wise and worth the investment of time and resources. Fortunately, some commonly used instruments have a substantial literature on their applicability in special groups (e.g., the MMSE reviewed in Chapter 4).

Understanding the various statistical or psychometric properties of measurement tools can be daunting to the uninitiated. A number of authors give general overviews of methods for health status measurement (Fitzpatrick et al., 1992; Fletcher, Gore, et al., 1992; Kane & Kane, 1981; Kirshner & Guyatt, 1985; Lawton & Lawrence, 1994; McDowell & Newell, 1987; Patrick & Erickson, 1993; Streiner & Norman, 1989; Teresi & Holmes, 1994; Ware, 1987) or explain the rationale for specific measures (Brook et al., 1979; Fillenbaum & Smyer, 1981; Stewart & Ware, 1992). The authors of the present book provide some details of the statistical evidence for the strengths and weaknesses of the selected measures. Each chapter is accompanied by a text interpretation comparing the relevant evidence. Generally, the most important psychometric properties to examine are reliability and validity. *Reliability* refers to tests of a measure's ability to give the same answer in a consistent fashion (internal consistency) or a repeated fashion (test-retest or interobserver). *Validity* refers to tests of an instrument's ability to measure what it intends to measure, either theoretically or biologically. Practically, validity testing often relies on comparing a new method with standard, well-known measures. In selecting a measure, older tools will generally have more extensive psychometric testing results in the published literature than newer ones. However, their disadvantages include the possibility that theoretical constructs have evolved since their development and that newer measures may capture important new ideas or needs (with regard to measurement and evaluation) for use in our changing society. Furthermore, statistical techniques and their interpretation may have evolved. For example, retest reliability of instruments that provide scores on a continuous measurement scale should be tested using the intraclass correlation coefficient. However, virtually all studies prior to the mid-1990s provide evidence based on other correlational statistics (e.g., Pearson's or Spearman's). Such evidence should not be discarded, but the issues raised underscore the benefit of assessing an instrument during a pilot for a study or as a formal substudy. Interpretation of the results of any particular study should include a thorough understanding of the strengths and weaknesses of its measurement tools.

THE FUTURE OF HEALTH STATUS ASSESSMENT: QUALITY IMPROVEMENT AND CLINICAL PRACTICE

Many of the health measurement techniques described in this book have strong track records in research applications but have not been broadly applied in medical care settings. This is especially true of the general multidimensional measures described in Chapter 2. There are emerging arguments for using health status assessment in regular clinical or hospital settings (Applegate, 1987; Fitzpatrick, Fletcher, et al., 1992; Fletcher, Dickinson, & Philp, 1992; Lohr, 1992; Thier, 1992). This idea is intriguing but not yet widely accepted. Acceptance may come more quickly for the use of multidimensional health status measures in institutional quality improvement efforts, as discussed below. Regarding clinical use, there is skepticism that these general measures can be translated usefully in the same way as familiar clinical diagnostic tools. Patient-oriented health status assessment is best described as an appealing possibility, tempered with a healthy dose of reality about obstacles to its development and dissemination.

Assessing the functional health of older patients was cautiously endorsed by a task force of the Society of General Internal Medicine (Rubenstein et al., 1989; the participants had met on April 29, 1987, in San Diego, California). The task force included physical, social, mental, and sexual function in its recommendations and also urged changes in medical training to incorporate the newer assessments that are not based on diagnosis of disease. In a 1992 supplement to the journal *Medical Care* guest-edited by K. N. Lohr, an excellent series of articles discusses the potential strengths and limitations of using health status tools for clinical assessment. In this series as well as in other publications, authors voice enthusiasm but also raise concerns (Blim, 1992; Deyo & Carter, 1992; Deyo & Patrick, 1989; Feinstein, 1992; Golden, 1992; Greenfield & Nelson, 1992; Mac-Keigne & Pathak, 1992; Nelson & Berwick, 1989; Patrick, 1992; Thier, 1992; Ware, 1992). Among the supporters, a nephrologist (Thier, 1992) reminisced on the historical definition of patient outcomes as ''tangible'' clinical measures. He portrayed the emerging interest in assessment of health status and quality of life as indicating that a curative approach to medicine is giving way to one of slowing or stopping the loss of function. A laboratory value is easier to understand than a health status assessment, but it does not supply information about function or well-being. As Thier points out, however, few clinicians are prepared to use and understand the newer assessment tools.

Even among the knowledgeable researchers who are proponents of these health status measures, Deyo and Carter (1992) acknowledge that certain practical issues—of cost, the training of physicians and clinicians, and doubts as to the ''hardness'' of the measures—may hamper their clinical use. Golden (1992) approaches the problem of acceptance as a matter of assessing technology and disseminating information; he notes a general failure of continuing medical education strategies to effect change in physicians' behaviors. Cogent discussions from a skeptical viewpoint raise a doubt that clinicians will be able to translate the new measures into useful treatment strategies; a concern that these new techniques may not be sensitive enough to serve as measures of individual-level indicators of health or changes in health; and concerns about practical issues, such as cost and increased time demanded of clinicians (Blim, 1992; Feinstein, 1992; Rubenstein et al., 1989; Thier, 1992; Tuteur, 1992). However, nurses or clinical support personnel, and not physicians, could be the health care providers who implement the clinical use of the measures (Golden, 1992). Certainly the usefulness of general health status measures would be best proved by formal tests of their utility and effectiveness in real clinical settings. A few of these studies have concluded that such assessment may be useful (Nelson, Landgraf, Hays, Wasson, & Kirk, 1990; Parkerson, Broadhead, & Tse, 1992; Street, Gold, & McDowell, 1994; Wasson et al., 1992), although the research has not yet shown the pragmatic benefits of such assessment.

A very cogent demonstration of the utility of expanded clinical diagnostic tools was suggested by a study by Calkins and colleagues (1991). A 12-item questionnaire about physical and social function was completed by patients and their physicians; the latter underestimated or missed 66% of the disabilities reported by patients. Perhaps the brevity of the tool or difficulty in interpretation explains the apparent failure of medical care providers to anticipate patients' reports of their functioning. Pinholt and colleagues (1987) also reported that physicians made an inadequate assessment of moderate impairment among older adults using traditional clinical methods. The concept of multidimensional and multidisciplinary assessment of geriatric medicine is obviously not new (Deyo, Applegate, Kramer, & Meehan, 1991; Epstein et al., 1990; National Institute of Health, 1987; Pinholt et al., 1987; Stuck, 1993; U.S. General Accounting Office, 1994; Williams, Williams, Zimmer, Hall, & Podgorski, 1987), despite the rather novel feel of the specific instruments reviewed in Chapter 2.

Employers and third-party payers could provide a considerable impetus for using health status measures in clinical or hospital settings. There is already some interest in incorporating measures of general health status into assessment of quality of care (Gouveia, Bungay, Massaro, & Ware, 1991; Winslow, 1992). Some authors speculate that insurers are the ones most likely to pay for patient assessments (Deyo & Carter, 1992; Golden, 1992). One such model of an imposed assessment is the Minimum Data Set (MDS) used for nursing home placement and Medicare/Medicaid reimbursement (Hawes et al., 1995; Morris et al., 1990; Morris, Hawes, Murphy, & Nonemaker, 1992), which is also being extended to home care settings via MDS-HC (V. Mor, personal communication, July 1, 1996). Another example is provided in a recent report by the Health Maintenance Organization Work Group on Care Management (1994), which recommends a brief health screening tool for older adults as a strategy for risk management.

Another aspect of applying the tools to patient care is their use in fostering communication with patients themselves. Nelson and Berwick (1989) suggest that in addition to its medical and clinical relevance, health status assessment may actually enhance patient-physician communication and provide some reassurance for patients. Street and colleagues (1994) have demonstrated that patients seeking prenatal care prefer that their physician inquire into the general and physical aspects of their health as measured by the SF-36, but they vary considerably in their feelings about questions regarding their psychosocial health. These results cannot be generalized to older adults, but it is important to note also that clinicians themselves did not appear to use the SF-36 information at all in their encounters with patients. If general health status instruments are to be used in clinical settings with older adults, more research is needed. The real or perceived benefits of such assessment—including its utility for the patient—should be formally evaluated. If clinicians raise concerns about how to use the information gathered from these instruments, it is germane to ask how patients would use the same assessment information. How do older adults use the information that they score above or below other people of their age on a specific scale? If their scores deteriorate over time, is there a reasonable explanation? Is there an appropriate intervention? So far, the evidence in favor of using general health status instruments comes from studies of groups, not individuals. The psychometric properties of these instruments are demonstrated with aggregate data and have not been evaluated thoroughly at the individual level. In fact, two studies suggest that the SF-36 has too much individual variability to provide sufficiently precise scores for patient-level assessment and monitoring (McHorney & Tarlov, 1995; Weinberger, Oddone, Samsa, & Landsman, 1996). McHorney and Tarlov (1995) tested four other health-status instruments, and found they all lacked sufficient reliability for clinical applications. They recommend further work on existing instruments or the development of new tools.

The future use of general health status assessment in clinical or institutional settings is unclear. To foster their use among institutions, clinicians, and patients, benchmarks and normal standards must be provided and must be easy to interpret. There is a need for more pragmatic research projects in clinical settings. There is also a need to demonstrate that the considerable effort required to collect the data provides enough additional information to enhance quality of care and improve clinical care.

REFERENCES

Applegate WB. (1987). Use of assessment instruments in clinical settings. *J Am Geriatr Soc*, *35*, 45–50.

*Bergner M, Bobbitt RA, Carter WB, & Gilson BS. (1981). The Sickness Impact Profile: Development and final revision of a health status measure. *Med Care*, *19*, 787–805.

Blim RD. (1992). Strategies for improving and expanding the application of health status measures in clinical settings: Discussion. *Med Care*, *30*, MS196–MS197.

Boult C, Kane RL, Louis TA, Boult L, & McCaffrey D. (1994). Chronic conditions that lead to functional limitation in the elderly. *J Gerontol*, *49*, M28–M36.

Brook RH, Ware J, Davies-Avery A, Stewart AL, Donald WH, Williams KN, & Johnston SA. (1979). Overview of adult health status measures fielded in Rand's health insurance study. *Med Care*, *17* (Suppl. 7), 1–131.

*Butland RJA, Pang J, Gross ER, Woodcock AA, & Geddes DM. (1982). Two-, six-, and twelve-minute walking tests in respiratory disease. *Br Med J*, *284*, 1607–1608.

Calkins DR, Rubenstein LV, Cleary PD, Davies AR, Jette AM, Fink A, Kosekoff J, Young R, Brook RH, & Delbanco TL. (1991). Failure of physicians to recognize functional disability in ambulatory patients. *Ann Intern Med*, *114*, 451–454.

Camacho TC, Strawbridge WJ, Cohen RD, & Kaplan GA. (1993). Functional ability in the oldest old. *J Aging Health*, *5*, 439–454.

Deniston OL, & Jette A. (1980). A functional status assessment instrument: Validation in an elderly population. *Health Serv Res*, *15*, 21–34.

Deyo R, Applegate WB, Kramer A, & Meehan S. (Eds.). (1991). The future of geriatric assessment. *J Am Geriatr Soc*, *39* (Suppl.), 1S.

Deyo RA, & Carter WB. (1992). Strategies for improving and expanding the application of health status measures in clinical settings: A researcher-developer viewpoint. *Med Care*, *30* (Suppl. 5), MS176–M186.

Deyo RA, & Patrick DL. (1989). Barriers to the use of health status measures in clinical investigation, patient care, and policy research. *Med Care*, *27* (Suppl. 3), S254–S268.

Epstein AM, Hall JA, Fretwell M, Feldstein M, DeCiantis ML, Tognetti J, Cutler C, Constantine M, Besdine R, Rowe J, & McNeil BJ. (1990). Consultative geriatric assessment for ambulatory patients: A randomized trial in a health maintenance organization. *JAMA, 263*, 538–544.

Feinstein AR. (1992). Benefits and obstacles for development of health status assessment measures in clinical settings. *Med Care, 30*, MS50–MS56.

Fillenbaum GG, & Smyer MA. (1981). The development, validity and reliability of the OARS multidimensional functional assessment questionnaire. *J Gerontol, 34*, 428–434.

Fitzpatrick R, Fletcher A, Gore S, Jones D, Spiegelhalter D, & Cox D. (1992). Quality of life in health care: I. Applications and issues in assessment. *BMJ, 305*, 1074–1077.

Fletcher A, Gore S, Jones D, Fitzpatrick R, Spiegelhalter D, & Cox D. (1992). Quality of life measures in health care: II. Design, analysis, and interpretation. *BMJ, 305*, 1145–1148.

Fletcher AE, Dickinson EJ, & Philp I. (1992). Review: Audit measures. Quality of life instruments for everyday use with elderly patients. *Age Aging, 21*, 142–150.

Foley DJ, Branch LG, Madans JH, Brock DB, Guralnik JM, & Williams TF. (1990). Physical function. In J. C. Coroni-Huntley, R. R. Huntley, J. J. Fledman (Eds.), *Health status and well-being of the elderly* (pp. 221–236). New York: Oxford University Press.

Fredman L, Droge JA, & Rabin DL. (1992). Functional limitations among home health care users in the National Health Interview Survey Supplement on Aging. *Gerontologist, 32*, 641–646.

George LK. (1994). Multidimensional assessment instruments: Present status and future prospects. In MP Lawton & JA Teresi (Eds.), *Annual review of gerontology and geriatrics: Vol. 13. Focus on assessment techniques* (pp. 353–375). New York: Springer.

Golden WE. (1992). Health status measurement: Implementation strategies. *Med Care, 30* (Suppl. 5), MS187–MS195.

Gouveia WA, Bungay KM, Massaro FJ, & Ware JE. (1991). Paradigm for the management of patient outcomes. *Am J Hosp Pharm, 48*, 1912–1916.

Grauer H, & Birnbom F. (1975). A geriatric functional rating scale to determine the need for institutional care. *J Am Geriatr Soc, 23*, 472–476.

Greenfield S, & Nelson EC. (1992). Recent developments and future issues in the use of health status assessment measures in clinical settings. *Med Care, 30* (Suppl. 5), MS23–MS41.

*Guyatt GH, Sullivan MJ, & Thompson PJ. (1985). The 6-minute walk: A new measure of exercise capacity in patients with chronic heart failure. *Can Med Assoc J, 132*, 919–923.

Hawes C, Morris JN, Phillips CD, Mor V, Fries BE, & Nonemaker S. (1995). Reliability estimates for the minimum data set for nursing home facility resident assessment and care screening (MDS). *Gerontologist, 35*, 172–178.

HMO Workgroup on Care Management. (1996). *Identifying high-risk Medicaid HMO members: A report from the HMO Workgroup on Care Management.* Princeton, NJ: Robert Wood Johnson Foundation.

Kane RA, & Kane RL. (1981). *Assessing the elderly: A practical guide to measurement.* Lexington, MA: Lexington.

Katz S, Downs TD, Cash HR, & Grotz RC. (1970). Progress in the development of the index of ADL. *Gerontologist, 10,* 20–30.

Kirshner B, & Guyatt G. (1985). A methodological framework for assessing health indices. *J Chron Dis, 38,* 27–36.

Kovar MG, & Lawton MP. (1994). Functional disability: activities and instrumental activities of daily living. In MP Lawton & JA Teresi (Eds.), *Annual review of gerontology and geriatrics: Vol. 13. Focus on assessment techniques* (pp. 57–75). New York: Springer.

Kuriansky J, & Gurland B. (1976). The performance test of activities of daily living. *Int J Aging Hum Dev, 7,* 343–352.

Lawton MP, & Brody EM. (1969). Assessment of older people: Self-maintaining and Instrumental Activities of Daily Living. *Gerontologist, 9,* 179–186.

Lawton MP, & Herzog AR. (1989). Special research methods for gerontology. In JA Hendricks (Ed.), *Society and Aging Series.* Amityville, NY: Baywood.

Lawton MP, & Lawrence RH. (1994). Assessing health. In MP Lawton & JA Teresi (Eds.), *Annual review of gerontology and geriatrics: Vol. 13. Focus on assessment techniques* (pp. 23–56). New York: Springer.

Lawton MP, & Teresi JA. (Eds.). (1994). *Annual review of gerontology and geriatrics: (Vol. 14). Focus on assessment techniques.* New York: Springer.

Lohr KN. (1992). Applications of health status assessment measures in clinical practice: Overview of the Third Conference on Advances in Health Status Assessment. *Med Care, 30,* MS1–MS14.

MacKeigan LD, & Pathak DS. (1992). Overview of health related quality-of-life measures. *Am J Hosp Pharm, 49,* 2236–2245.

Maddox J. (1981). Medical care and the arthritis sufferer: A survey in outer Melbourne. *Aust Fam Physician, 10,* 876–882.

McDowell I, & Newell C. (1987). *Measuring health: A guide to rating scales and questionnaires.* New York: Oxford University Press.

McHorney CA, & Tarlov AR. (1995). Individual-patient monitoring in clinical practice: Are available health status surveys adequate? *Qual Life Res, 4,* 294–307.

National Institutes of Health Consensus Development Conference Statement. (1988). Geriatric assessment methods for clinical decision making. *J Am Geriatr Soc, 36,* 342–347.

*Mathias S, Nayak USL, & Isaacs B. (1986). Balance in elderly patients: The "Get-Up and Go" test. *Arch Phys Med Rehabil, 67,* 387–389.

Morris JN, Hawes C, Fries BE, Phillips CD, Mor V, Katz S, Murphy K, Drugovich ML, & Friedlob AS. (1990). Designing the national resident assessment instrument for nursing home facilities. *Gerontologist, 30,* 293–307.

Morris JN, Hawes C, Murphy K, & Nonemaker S. (1992). *Multistate nursing home case mix and quality demonstration training manual.* Natick, MA: Eliot.

Nelson EC, & Berwick DM. (1989). The measurement of health status in clinical practice. *Med Care, 27* (Suppl. 3), S77–S90.

Nelson EC, Landgraf JM, Hays RD, Wasson JH, & Kirk JW. (1990). The functional status of patients: How can it be measured in physicians' offices? *Med Care, 28,* 1111–1126.

Parkerson GR, Broadhead WE, & Tse CJ. (1992). Quality of life and functional health of primary care patients. *J Clin Epidemiol, 45,* 1303–1313.

Patrick DL. (1992). Strategies for improving and expanding the application of health status measures in clinical settings: Discussion. *Med Care, 30,* MS198–MS201.

Patrick DL, & Erickson P. (1993). *Health status and health policy: Allocating resources to health care.* New York: Oxford University Press.

Pinholt EM, Kroenke K, Hanley JF, Kussman MJ, Twyman PL, & Carpenter JL. (1987). Functional assessment of the elderly: A comparison of standards with clinical judgment. *Arch Intern Med, 147,* 484–488.

Plutchik R, Conte H, Lieberman M, Bakur M, Grossman J, & Lehrman N. (1970). Reliability and validity of a scale for assessing the functioning of geriatric patients. *J Am Geriatr Soc, 18,* 491–500.

*Podsiadlo D, & Richardson S. (1991). The Timed "Up & Go": A test of basic functional mobility for frail elderly persons. *J Am Geriatr Soc, 39,* 142–148.

Rubenstein LV, Calkins DR, Greenfield S, Jette AM, Meenan RF, Nevins MA, Rubenstein LZ, Wasson JH, & Williams ME. (1989). Health status assessment for elderly patients: Report of the Society of General Internal Medicine Task Force on Health Assessment. *J Am Geriatr Soc, 37,* 562–569.

Stewart AL, & Ware JE. (Eds.). (1992). *Measuring functioning and well-being. The Medical Outcomes Study approach.* Durham, NC: Duke University Press.

Street RL, Gold WR, & McDowell T. (1994). Using health status surveys in medical consultations. *Med Care, 32,* 732–744.

Streiner DL, & Norman GR. (1989). *Health measurement scales: A practical guide to their development and use.* New York: Oxford University Press.

Stuck AE, Siu AL, Wieland GD, Adams J, & Rubenstein LZ. (1993). Comprehensive geriatric assessment: A meta-analysis of controlled trials. *Lancet, 342,* 1032–1036.

Teresi JA, & Holmes D. (1994). Overview of methodological issues in gerontological and geriatric measurement. In MP Lawton & JA Teresi (Eds.), *Annual review of gerontology and geriatrics. Vol. 13: Focus on assessment techniques* (pp. 1–22). New York: Springer.

Thier SO. (1992). Forces motivating the use of health status assessment measures in clinical settings and related clinical research. *Med Care, 30,* MS15–MS22.

Tuteur PG. (1992). Strategies for improving and expanding the application of health status measures in clinical settings: Discussion. *Med Care, 30,* MS202–MS204.

U.S. General Accounting Office. (1994). *Long-term care: The need for geriatric assessment in publicly funded home and community-based programs.* (Publication No. GAO/T-PEMD-94-20). Washington, DC: U.S. Government Printing Office.

Van Nostrand JF. (1993). Selected issues in long-term care: Profile of cognitive disability of nursing home residents and the use of informal and formal care by the elderly in the community. In JF Nostrand, SE Furner, & R Suzman (Eds.), *Vital and health statistics: Health data on older Americans: United States 1992* (DHHS Publication No. PHS 93-1411, pp. 143–159). Hyattsville, MD: U.S. Department of Health and Human Services.

Wallace RB, & Woolson RF. (Eds.). (1992). *The epidemiologic study of the elderly.* New York: Oxford University Press.

Ware JE. (1987). Standards for validating health measures: Definition and content. *J Chron Dis*, *40*, 473–480.

Ware JE. (1992). Comments on the use of health status assessment in clinical settings. *Med Care*, *30*, MS205–MS209.

Wasson J, Keller A, Rubenstein L, Hays R, Nelson E, & Johnson D. (1992). Benefits and obstacles of health status assessment in ambulatory settings: The clinician's point of view. Dartmouth Primary Care COOP Project. *Med Care*, *30*, MS42–MS49.

Weinberger M, Oddone EZ, Samsa GP, & Landsman PB. (1996). Are health-related quality of life measures affected by mode of administration? *J Clin Epidemiol*, *49*, 135–140.

*Williams ME, & Hadler NM. (1981). Musculoskeletal components of decrepitude. *Sem Arthritis Rheum*, *11*, 284–287.

*Williams ME, Hadler NM, & Earp JA. (1982). Manual ability as a marker of dependency in geriatric women. *J Chron Dis*, *35*, 115–122.

Williams ME, Williams TF, Zimmer JG, Hall WJ, & Podgorski CA. (1987). How does the team approach to outpatient evaluation compare with traditional care: A report of a randomized controlled trial. *J Am Geriatr Soc*, *35*, 1071–1078.

Winslow R. (1992, July 7). Questionnaire probes patients' quality of life. *Wall Street Journal*, p. B1.

Functional Assessment

James G. Zimmer, Barbara M. Rothenberg,
Elena M. Andresen

OVERVIEW

There is wide agreement that physical functioning is a highly important outcome
of treatment of illness and disability as well as a predictor of future health
problems and utilization of health care. Its importance is acknowledged from
both clinical and research perspectives. It is hardly the only outcome of importance; death, pain, and discomfort of various kinds have been recognized probably
since the origin of our species as undesirable outcomes. However, apart from
mortality and specific morbidities and symptoms, physical functioning is one of
the first components of health status to be measured and studied systematically
in modern times. Unlike some of the broader measures of general health status,
the measurement of rather basic physical functions pertains mainly to older adults
who are "frail," or at least less robust, and often chronically ill, or to younger
people with disabilities. We concentrate here on measures of function for
older adults.

A regular, systematic assessment of the function of older adults was recommended by the American College of Physicians (1988), although no specific
measures were endorsed. They considered a broad range of self-reported general
health status tools to have potential (e.g., the Sickness Impact Profile, Short-
Form 36, Dartmouth COOP). Because of their concern for brief screening in
clinical settings and because of potential reimbursement issues, the recommendations lean toward traditional measures of activities of daily living (ADLs) and

instrumental activities of daily living (IADLs), described below. They suggest more focused assessment tools for follow-up on some patients. ADLs and IADLs provide information for clinicians and researchers about the self-care ability of high risk patients, that is, those who are relatively frail or those likely to deteriorate to a state of questionable independent function or frank dependence.

The National Institutes of Health (NIH) also included functional status as one of the elements of geriatric assessment important to clinical decision making in their 1988 Consensus Statement (Consensus Development Panel, 1988). Like the American College of Physicians, they limited their recommendations to the use of ADLs and IADLs. However, they also pointed to the need for tools to assess the function of those with mild and moderate impairment whose capabilities are not well measured by either ADLs or IADLs. Self-reported health status, as in the measures reported in Chapter 2, may already meet the assessment needs of relatively robust older adults. But physical function remains a cornerstone of assessment of, and research about, those older adults who are at the ''frail'' end of the health spectrum.

In spite of efforts spanning at least the past half century, a true, widely accepted ''gold standard'' for measurement of physical function does not yet exist. Many general approaches to this measurement have been used, described, and advocated, and each has used and promoted a number—in some cases myriads—of different constructs, wordings, scalings, weightings, and scoring systems. The general approaches include measures that are self-administered, administered by a proxy or surrogate, administered by a caregiver or provider, administered by an interviewer, abstracted from medical records, taken from direct observation of activities, and, more recently, based on performance tests. Finally, the use of combinations of these measures has been advocated, on the presumption that this will provide multiple perspectives and thus will come closer to true validity. This chapter will give an overview of these various approaches. We will refer to some of the more highly regarded methods and measures and outline some of the main problems associated with their use. Finally, we will focus in more detail on some of the more recent performance-based measures. One measure of upper body function, the Timed Manual Performance Test, and two measures of lower body function (broadly defined), the Get Up and Go test and the 6-minute walk test, have been selected for more detailed assessment.

Excellent reviews of the earlier history of assessment of physical function are provided by Stewart, Ware, Brook, and Davies-Avery (1978); Kane and Kane (1981, especially chapter 2); Katz (1983, especially on the numerous measures developed in the 1950s); and Feinstein, Josephy, and Wells (1986), who cite 43 of the earlier ADL indexes. More recent reviews and discussions of problems are presented by Applegate, Blass, and Williams (1990); Foley and colleagues (1990); Guralnik, Branch, Cummings, and Curb (1989); Law (1993), who writes largely from the perspective of occupational therapy; Reuben, Valle, Hays, and

Siu (1995); Kovar and Lawton (1994); and the book on the Medical Outcomes Study edited by Stewart and Ware (1992, especially chapter 6).

ADLs AND IADLs

Activities of Daily Living

As a matter of historical interest, the earliest physical function measure cited in the thorough review by Feinstein et al. (1986) had been developed by Sheldon (1935) for use with "crippled" children. However, the cornerstone instrument, probably the most familiar to researchers and clinicians, is the ADL Index that was developed by Katz, Ford, Moskowitz, Jackson, and Jaffe, at the Benjamin Rose Hospital (1963), with further developments and uses described later (Katz, 1983; Katz, Downs, Cash, & Grotz, 1970). This caregiver-administered instrument evaluates functional ability in what are now the "classic" six self-care domains of activities of daily living: bathing, dressing, using the toilet, transferring (e.g., in and out of bed or chairs), continence, and feeding.

A number of other instruments were developed around the time of and subsequent to the Katz ADL measure, and they contain the same or similar elements. Some of those more widely used are the Barthel Index, which has 10 items (Mahoney & Barthel, 1965); the Rapid Disability Rating Scale (RDRS), which has 16 items rated by medically oriented staff members (Linn, 1967); the Older Adults Rehabilitation Services (OARS) instrument, which makes a relatively comprehensive assessment of health in general and includes essentially the same ADL items as the Katz measure but uses self-reports rather than caregivers' reports (Pfeiffer, 1975); and the PULSES Profile (standing for Physical, Upper limbs, Lower limbs, Sensory, and Social factors), which measures wider dimensions of function but also includes ADLs (Moskowitz & McCann, 1957; modified in Sherwood, Morris, Mor, & Gutkin, 1977). One of the most recent widely used instruments, which includes ADL assessment, is the Minimum Data Set (MDS, now evolved into the MDS+) for use primarily with nursing home residents, which is based on direct observations by clinical professionals as well as on review of clinical records (Morris et al., 1990; Morris, Hawes, & Murphy, 1991). It includes a comprehensive assessment of a rather broad array of residents' functional, medical, psychosocial, and cognitive status, and of their needs for care; its use is required of all Medicare- and Medicaid-certified nursing homes under the Omnibus Reconciliation Act of 1987 (Omnibus Reconciliation Act, OBRA, 1987). Two benefits of the required Minimum Data Set (MDS) version of ADL are that it can be collected relatively easily from administrative records for all nursing home subjects (Morris et al., 1990, 1991) and that it provides for a descriptive analysis of the functional status of research subjects. However, data routinely collected for purposes other than those of the researchers (in this case, administration and reimbursement) may not meet all of the needs of a specific study, especially as regards the quality of the information and its applicability to a particular research question.

Instrumental Activities of Daily Living

The other major measures of physical functioning look at more complex and less basic self-care functions and are called instrumental activities of daily living (IADL) scales. The term *instrumental* refers to the fact that most of the tested items require external objects or entities in order to be performed. Clearly, performance of complex activities, as measured by the many instruments which include IADL questions and also by the performance-based measures, is highly dependent on mental ability at a considerably higher level than required by the basic ADLs. Thus, it must be recognized that these functions are by no means purely physical. This is also the case for the ADLs, though at a much more basic level.

One of the first instruments to measure IADLs, the Functional Health Status Test of Rosow and Breslau (1966), was designed for use in the general population and is not very useful for severely compromised populations. The most widely adopted IADL scale currently in use is probably that developed by Lawton and others, which includes nine items for housekeeping, "handyman" work, telephone use, shopping, food preparation, laundering, use of transportation, use of medicine, and financial behavior (Lawton, 1988; Lawton & Brody, 1969; Lawton et al., 1982). The reliability and validity of this IADL instrument is well established, and it has been widely recognized as a suitable standard in geriatric and gerontological research for more than two decades (Gallo, Reichel, & Andersen, 1995; Kane & Kane, 1981). The psychometric measurement properties of this version have been studied in a variety of national studies, including the Longitudinal Study on Aging (Johnson & Wolinsky, 1993, 1994; Wolinsky & Johnson, 1991), the National Long-Term Care Survey (Clark, Stump, & Wolinsky, 1997), and the Survey on Assets and Health Dynamics among the Oldest Old (Stump, Clark, Johnson, & Wolinsky, 1997), and in a survey of hospitalized veterans (Fitzgerald, Smith, Martin, Freedman, & Wolinsky, 1993).

Other early IADL measures are included in more comprehensive assessment tools, such as the OARS (Pfeiffer, 1975), mentioned above, and the PACE II (U.S. Department of Health, Education, and Welfare, DHEW, 1978). The Functioning for Independent Living Scale (FIL) includes 11 items on highly detailed ordinal scales with weights, and it reflects considerable specificity of activities, such as hand movement assessed in common household tasks (Gross-Andrew & Zimmer, 1978). The Performance Activities of Daily Living (PADL) is a provider-observed set of 16 relatively simple tasks, usually considered in the category of IADLs (Kane & Kane, 1981) but including some that are ADLs. It was designed to overcome the problem of lack of opportunity to perform some of the usual IADLs (i.e., the issue of capacity versus actual performance), particularly in institutional settings (Kuriansky & Gurland, 1976). This issue is discussed further below, in the section on performance-based measures. The Pilot Geriatric Arthritis Project (PGAP) functional status measure is an example of an ADL and IADL instrument designed specifically to assess people with a particular condition; it adds two additional dimensions, the rating of pain and difficulty in performance (Deniston & Jette, 1980; Jette & Deniston, 1978).

More recently, a brief 5-item screen for IADL function was developed from the OARS questionnaire (Fillenbaum, 1985); it is useful for targeting individuals potentially in need of further assessment and service. A self-administered 50-item questionnaire was developed by Myers (1992) for use through the mail; it showed good reproducibility over a 2-week period. Spector, Katz, Murphy, and Fulton (1987) reported that both ADLs and IADLs demonstrate a negative association with a number of variables, including age, risk of decline in ADLs, death, and hospitalization (i.e., *lower* ADL status is correlated with *higher* risk).

Methods of Assessment and Problems with ADLs and IADLs

The various methods or modes of administration of ADL and IADL measures have been compared by a number of researchers. Rubenstein, Schairer, Wieland, and Kane (1984) studied the effects of different data sources on functional status assessment. Using the Lawton Personal Self-Maintenance and IADL scales, they compared patients' self-reports with reports by their nurses and their significant others and found that the results were not interchangeable. Weinberger et al. (1992) compared the patient's self-report with the proxy's reports of both ADLs and IADLs. Concordance was significantly greater for ADLs than for IADLs. When there was disagreement, patients rated themselves as more independent than did the proxies, especially for IADLs. While there is little agreement among studies as to the details of agreement and bias in reporting by proxies compared with subjects, it is a relatively well-accepted generalization that family proxies tend to report more functional disability than subjects themselves (Magaziner, 1992; Rubenstein et al., 1984). In spite of the problems and the need for further research in this area, the use of proxies will continue, especially with the "oldest old" (Herzog & Rogers, 1992; Magaziner, 1992). A major difficulty of research comparing proxies' responses with subjects' responses is that the only comparable pairs are those in which the subject is able to respond. This eliminates the possibility of comparison when subjects are very disabled and have cognitive dysfunction; thus it leads to bias in interpretation and generalization (Herzog & Rodgers, 1992). Furthermore, when there is disagreement, it is difficult to ascertain who is "overreporting" and who is "underreporting" disability (Kovar &

Lawton, 1994). Magaziner (1992) provides a thorough review of the issues in the use of proxy respondents and a discussion of ways to approach the problems in research, especially in epidemiological studies of older adults.

Burns et al. (1992) compared self-report versus medical record abstraction for ascertainment of ADL ability on a sample of 2,504 patients in 52 hospitals. The total number of areas on dependency was greater from self-reports than from the medical records (average of 3.2 versus 2.3). In a pilot for this study, these researchers found that nurses' notes documented functional status better than physicians' notes. Further evidence of problems with reliability regarding ADLs was presented by Sager and colleagues (1992), who found that among hospitalized older adults agreement (as measured by the κ coefficient) between self-reported ADLs and performance as assessed by occupational therapists ranged from a poor 0.27, for dressing, to a maximum of 0.63, for eating. The κ (kappa) coefficent is a measure of agreement beyond agreement expected by chance alone; κ is considered poor at 0.30 or lower and excellent at 0.75 or higher (Fleiss, 1981).

Of relatively recent interest has been the comparison of self-reported functional status with performance-based testing. The usual assumption has been that the latter is more statistically valid, although this is yet to be completely verified, and there are pitfalls in both approaches, which will be discussed below. *Falconer et al. (1991) compared the ability of several tests of hand function (to be discussed later in this chapter) with discriminate degree of dependency in older adults as measured by self-reported multidimensional functional status measures. They found that hand function does correlate with self-reported functional dependency. Kelly-Hayes, Jette, Wolf, D'Agostino, and Odell (1992) compared differences as measured by self-report of disability and observation by a trained nurse during a physical examination of six ADL tasks in older adults in the Framingham study. When differences were observed, subjects ranked disability higher than observers 89% of the time. The authors concluded that observed functional limitation and self-perception of disability may be two distinct concepts and that choice of method should be determined by the purposes of the assessment. Comparison of self-administered, interviewer-administered, and performance-based measures of physical function revealed inconsistent and weak relationships in a study of 83 subjects by Reuben et al. (1995). Again, the results suggest that the different methods are not measuring the same construct and that perhaps a composite measure—including self-reported ADLs and IADLs, caregiver-reported ADLs and IADLs, or both as well as performance-based measures—might be the best approach.

In recent years, a number of attempts have been made to evaluate the many functional measurement instruments and to articulate the various limitations in their administration and interpretation. In a very thorough review of earlier indexes of functional disability, Feinstein et al. (1986) identified the six most prominent "generic" problems with the 43 ADL measures they analyzed. Briefly summarized, these include the following: First, omission of attention to the collaborative effort of the patient in performance of the activities in the areas of personal effort and support by a caregiver. Second, neglect of the role of personal preferences in respect to what is important in function and activities. Third, inadequacy in measurement of change in functional abilities due to coarseness of rating scales and the obscuring of specific abilities within aggregate scores. Fourth, difficulty in interpretation of indexes that are constructed as profiles of separate attributes or are aggregated into combined-score ratings. Fifth, lack of justification and rationale for development of new instruments. Sixth, unsatisfactory selection and inappropriate use of instruments for the specific goals of the application or study.

Many of the issues raised by Feinstein and colleagues, or variations on them, are echoed in later analyses of conceptual and methodological issues in measuring physical functioning. Stewart and Kamberg (1992) identify several unresolved issues, some of which are interrelated, that were problems during the development of the Medical Outcomes study. These include identification of appropriate content, coarseness of scaling (i.e., too few scale levels in many measures), too narrow a range of activities measured, and the patient's *potential* for performance of an activity as opposed to *actual* degree of difficulty in performing it or *actual* need for help. There were also problems in aggregating different categories of function. There was a lack of consideration of personal values regarding levels of function and satisfaction with the current level of function. Finally, there were difficulties in methods of scoring, which often use overly complicated algorithms. Problems in eliciting valid and accurate reports of functional status from older disabled subjects by direct interview are reported by Keller, Kovar, Jobe, and Branch (1993) and relate to difficulties in understanding questions and to differences in interpretation between what is intended by the questioner and what is understood by the respondent. Reuben et al. (1995) reflect on the reasons for the discrepancies in the three methods of administration of their instruments: self-administered, interviewer-administered, and performance-based. These include the probability that the instruments evaluate different levels of function and that response items diverge in reflecting respondents' perceptions, such as their perception of "difficulty" versus "amount of limitation."

Problems with IADL instruments and their interpretation are similar to those with ADLs but are intensified by the much greater complexity of what they attempt to measure. There is obviously a far wider spectrum of abilities that relate to the IADL functions, including not only physical but mental and social variables, and a much greater diversity of interpretations and perspectives on the relative importance of different functions, levels of ability, and other aspects of measurement.

The validity of IADL measures was examined by Myers (1992), who acknowledged the problem of the many definitions of validity used by different researchers (e.g., face, discriminant, and construct) and the fact that solid evidence for validation is limited, especially in light of the multiplicity of scales in use. She used a 50-item self-administered IADL questionnaire and found good reproducibility over a 2-week period, internal consistency, reasonably predictable correlations with other measures of health status, and an ability to distinguish users of formal home health care services from nonusers. However, her other findings demonstrate a need for caution in choosing rating formats and scoring methods and in interpreting subjects' responses. The ratings of difficulty in performing an activity, nonperformance, and the need for assistance should not be considered interchangeable or reflective of basic physical ability, which perhaps is better measured by performance. Her scalogram analysis (i.e., Guttman scaling) showed that the common assumption of hierarchical ordering is not justified. Also, there are many other potentially confusing factors in administration and interpretation, including problems in understanding questions, the fact that some subjects may find some questions insulting or disturbing, and the variable degree of motivation and cooperation among subjects. In addition, there are likely to be differing perceptions of the effects of the social and physical environment, effects based on whether activity occurs indoors or outdoors, whether assistive devices are or are not used, and multiple possible interpretations of answers. Moreover, there is no general agreement on the universe of content that constitutes IADL status. Finally, even though directly observed performance-based measures are appealing and are considered by some to be the preferred technique when feasible, they are not the single or ultimate solution. This is addressed further below.

The perspective of occupational therapy is of interest, particularly from a clinical viewpoint, since problems with ADLs and IADLs are often assessed and treated by occupational therapists, particularly in rehabilitation-oriented settings. This perspective is presented by Law (1993), who raises many of the issues discussed above and offers some suggestions as to what needs to be done in the future.

PERFORMANCE-BASED MEASURES

Performance-based measures of physical function have been available for many years. A very complex and thorough protocol for manual function was described by Carroll (1965) and modified by Jefferys, Millard, Hyman, and Warren (1969) to include lower-body tests and the use of a portable props kit for testing in the homes of clients and research subjects. Another early tool, proposed by Jebson, Taylor, Trieshmann, Trotter, and Howard (1969), was designed to measure fine motor skills of the hands. The test was envisioned as a fairly brief and easy assessment of tasks that could distinguish among older adults with different functional levels. A number of the tasks first described by Jebson have been adopted in later performance tests (e.g., Reuben & Siu, 1990; *Williams & Hadler, 1981). These directly observed, standardized tests of functional ability continue to be part of the tool kit for the research and clinical assessment of older adults, especially those at the "frail" end of the health spectrum and those with actual or suspected limitations in their ability to perform self-care activities.

Performance-based measures serve two goals of testing, as the tasks combine physical and mental ability. However, as such, they may be limited to older adults with some minimum level of cognitive ability (e.g., Weiner, Duncan, Chandler, & Studenski, 1991). Performance-based measures summarize across these two constructs, and their use might be augmented with measures of cognition (see Chapter 4) if it is necessary to disentangle purely physical function from the combination of cognitive and physical performance. However, the use of performance-based measures is sometimes recommended precisely for individuals who are cognitively impaired, to avoid the potential biases that can be introduced by the use of proxy respondents (Zimmerman & Magaziner, 1994).

There are advantages and drawbacks to the use of performance-based measures. They are generally considered more *objective* measures of function than traditional self-reported or caretaker-reported measures like the ADL and IADL scales. They have excellent face validity for the tasks being performed (Zimmerman & Magaziner, 1994), which often are tasks required in daily life, especially compared with corresponding laboratory measures such as postural sway or maximum oxygen consumption on a bicycle ergometer.

Differences in subjects' motivation or their ability to perform tasks may create difficulties, however (*Applegate et al., 1987; Cress et al., 1995; Myers, Holliday, Harvey, & Hutchinson, 1993; Reuben & Siu, 1990). In a study by *Guyatt, Sullivan, and Thompson (1985) of the 6-Minute-Walk test, 14 of the original sample of 57 (25%) dropped out of the study. Among the reasons given (p. 921) were feeling ill after the test, "The walks did not seem beneficial," and "A doctor wasn't present." In *Berg, Maki, Williams, Holliday, and Wood-Dauphinee's (1992) assessment of the several performance-based measures of balance, 5 of 36 (14%) subjects were unable to complete the laboratory tests because of "fatigue, hot laboratory conditions, or inability to stand independently for the minimum required time" (p. 1076). When subjects do not complete some of the tasks, it is unclear whether this is due in part to insufficient motivation, inability to perform the task, or both. The completion of tasks on a test may be related to their difficulty; Reuben and Siu (1990) found that among individual tasks in their Physical Performance Test (PPT), completion ranged from 91% of the subjects (for climbing stairs) to 100% (for simulated eating). However, Myers and colleagues (1993) found no obvious pattern in refusal or inability to perform tasks similar to IADLs. Even if the reason why subjects do not complete tasks is simply that they are unable to do so, this creates difficulties in scoring the test, since poorer performance should be associated with longer test times. *Ostwald,

Snowdon, Rysavy, Keenan, and Kane (1989) dealt with the problem of missing data in the Williams Timed Manual Performance Test by assigning the maximum time of subjects who completed the test to those who were unable to complete it. However, there are no straightforward and accepted scoring guides for replacing missing values in performance tests due to refusals to participate and subjects' dropping out.

The benefits and disadvantages of using performance-based measures of function are also reviewed by Guralnik and colleagues (1989; see also Zimmerman & Magaziner, 1994, for a general review as well as a discussion of the use of these measures in the cognitively impaired). These authors advocate using performance-based measures to supplement more commonly used self-reported and proxy-reported measures. However, they also caution that continued formal studies of the tests' psychometric and practical properties are needed. In addition, they note that most performance-based methods are not necessarily direct measures of actual functional ability. One exception is the Performance of Activities of Daily Living (PADL) test developed by Kuriansky and Gurland (1976), which literally requires subjects to use specific props to demonstrate their ability with clothing, a clock, a cup, etc. Another pragmatic test of hand function is demonstrated in a study of medication packaging by Keram and Williams (1988); they found that a sizable proportion of older adults could not open childproof and other difficult-to-open packages (even nitroglycerin patches). Myers and colleagues (1993) concluded that performance-based measures provide different information from self-reported physical function, but that the former are not necessarily superior in terms of their psychometric properties, as was proposed, in theoretical terms, by Guralnik and colleagues (1989). Some performance measures may require specially trained observers or testers or special props (e.g., *Williams, Hadler, & Earp, 1982); this makes their application impractical in some settings. Finally, the issue of the subjects' safety and the appropriateness of testing some persons has been raised (Duncan & Studenski, 1994).

Other studies have combined performance and self-reported or observer-assessed function, with varying results. In a multivariate analysis, both the PPT and the ADL measures independently predicted death and nursing home placement in a cohort study, which suggests that they each contribute different information about frailty and might be used in tandem (Reuben, Siu, & Kimpau, 1992). A study of various measures of health, including an early version of the Short Form 36 (SF-20), the Quality of Well-Being (QWB) Scale, ADLs, and performance-based measures used factor analysis to test for similarities among measures and found that manual performance and the other measures "loaded" on different factors (Siu et al., 1993). In another study, Reuben and colleagues (1995) found weak relationships among similar measurement constructs from ADL measures, the PPT, and the SF-36. This finding also suggests that self-reported and performance-based measures may tap different health domains. This study found higher, but still somewhat modest, correlations between IADL scales and performance-based measures. It may be best to combine measurement strategies when it is relatively easy to administer ADL measures, IADL measures, or both at the same time as performance-based measures.

Performance Tests of Upper-Body and Hand Function

Overview

Performance-based methods for the upper body include the Timed Manual Performance Test (TMP) (*Williams & Hadler, 1981; *Williams et al., 1982) and a short version of the TMP (*Gerrity, Gaylord, & Williams, 1993), functional reach (Weiner, Duncan, Chandler, & Studenski, 1991), and measures that evaluate other categories of hand function, including fine motor skills such as timed signature and simulated eating (Jebson et al., 1969) and grip strength (Buchner et al., 1993; Lee, Baxter, Dick, & Webb, 1974). Technically, the functional reach measure (Weiner et al., 1991) is a measure of balance more than upper-body function; it measures subjects' "maximal safe forward reach" and is strongly related to physical frailty.

There are also measures that combine performance of the upper and lower extremities, for example, simulated household and self-care activities (Myers et al., 1993), which are formalized in the Physical Performance Test (Reuben & Siu, 1990; Reuben et al., 1992, 1995) and the Physical Disability Index (PDI; Gerety et al., 1993). The PDI is a 54-task assessment conducted by physical therapists that includes a broad range of upper- and lower-extremity functions. It is clear that lower-body function is strongly related to falling. However, interestingly, timed signature testing was independently related to both "fall-related efficacy" and fear of falling in a large cohort study conducted as part of the New Haven Project Safety Cohort, even when other measures of function were added to statistical models as covariates (Tinetti, Mendes de Leon, Doucette, & Baker, 1994).

Observing older adults' ability to reach while standing has been used in conjunction with measures of balance for research on mobility (Duncan, Chandler, Studenski, Hughes, & Prescott, 1993). However, the Functional Reach (FR) test was found to have very strong correlations both with more complex performance measures of function and with self-reported limitations (Weiner et al., 1991). It might serve as a single independent measure in some studies of frailty.

Grip strength is often used in tandem with other performance measures in research (e.g., Buchner et al., 1993; *Falconer et al., 1991; *Ostwald et al., 1989; Williams & Hornberger, 1984). All sites of the Frailty and Injuries: Cooperative Studies of Intervention Techniques (FICSIT) use grip strength as one measure of physiologic status; this is in combination with lower-body measures of gait and balance (Buchner et al., 1993). Buchner and colleagues report that grip strength has a low correlation, while lower-body performance measures have moderate correlations, with several scales of the Sickness Impact Profile (SIP; Cress et al., 1995). Measures of grip strength have a particular relevance to clinical evaluation and research with arthritis patients (e.g., Lee et al., 1974).

Timed Manual Performance (TMP) Test

Background and Use. The Timed Manual Performance Test (TMP; *Williams & Hadler, 1981; *Williams et al., 1982) is a composite test of manual ability. There are 27 items, and these include hand tasks derived from Jebson and colleagues (1969) such as writing, simulated eating, and picking up small objects. A unique component is the "Williams board," a 2- by 3-ft board with nine fastened doors; subjects are timed on their ability to open the fasteners after a demonstration. The functioning of both the dominant hand and the nondominant hand is tested. Performance is timed, and the total score is computed by summing the time (in seconds) that it takes to complete all of the tasks. The test protocol is reported to take about 15 to 20 minutes, on average, to complete (Williams, 1987; *Williams & Hadler, 1981). The TMP is administered by a trained interviewer (e.g., *Applegate et al., 1987; *Falconer et al., 1991; Ostwald et al., 1989). Some studies use an occupational therapist to administer the test (e.g., Scholer, Potter, & Burke, 1990), while others use a nurse (e.g., Williams, 1987) or a physician (*Williams et al., 1982). As with other performance measures, some older adults may have difficulty completing the tasks, owing to poor vision or other physical impairments (*Applegate et al., 1987; Ostwald et al., 1989). Analysis of the reliability of the TMP has been restricted to measuring internal consistency, which is moderate (*Williams, Gaylord, & Gerrity, 1994); test-retest and interrater reliability have, to our knowledge, not been assessed.

The TMP was found to be the most responsive measure of improved visual acuity in a study of cataract surgery compared with ADLs and other measures (*Applegate et al., 1987). Fifty-one percent of the subjects were scaled as "completely independent" using ADLs, so no improvement was possible on this scale. The TMP test has also been found to be a strong predictor of long-term care (Williams, 1987) and of dependent living (*Falconer et al., 1991; Ostwald et al., 1989; *Williams et al., 1982). In the study conducted by Falconer and colleagues, the prevalence of poor manual performance was 16.1% among community-dwelling older adults in North Carolina; even when writing tasks were omitted from the TMP (because of the subjects' low level of formal education), the prevalence was 8.3%. Poor manual performance in this cohort was linked to older age, poor health, lower socioeconomic status, and race and ethnicity (African American; *Williams et al., 1990). This cohort study found that the TMP was a good predictor of mortality, but not of hospitalization, among older adults (*Williams et al., 1994).

Scaling Variations. *Gerrity and colleagues (1993) propose shortening the TMP and have identified two groups of tasks that do not overlap and can be used independently. One (Doors) requires five of the Williams board tasks, and the second (Table) consists of six "table" tasks. These short forms were apparently easier to complete and had fewer missing responses, and the resulting scores may have been less biased by subjects' educational status and race or ethnicity. A subsequent analysis of a large cohort of older adults also supports the use of these shorter versions, especially the TMP-Table version (*Williams et al., 1994). Ostwald and colleagues had previously reported the TMP-Doors test to be strongly correlated to dependent living among Catholic nuns (1989). However, the timed performances yielded a very broad distribution, skewed toward shorter times but with outliers with very long times. The median time for those tasks was 56 seconds, and the range was 29 to 197 seconds. An automated TMP has also been developed and is described below.

Some studies (Falconer et al., 1992; Scholer et al., 1990; Williams, 1987; *Williams, Gaylord, & McGaghie, 1990) have used the TMP test as a dichotomous variable dividing subjects into two categories using a cutoff of 350 seconds. Falconer and colleagues (1992) found an elevated, but not statistically significant, relationship between performance on the TMP and subsequent dependency in a cohort of older adults using this scoring method, while Williams and colleagues (1987, *1990) found that the ability to complete the test items was as predictive of subsequent dependency as the dichotomous timed performance. Scholer, Potter, and Burke (1990) found this dichotomous scoring method insensitive as a prediction of future formal long-term care and use of other services. This study is also instructive in that an analysis of subjects' actual TMP completion time showed some relationship to the outcome when group means were compared, but the variability of times within groups was substantial and may account for the lack of statistical significance. *Williams and colleagues (1994) also report on the long version and two short versions of the TMP using timed scores in quartiles; this categorization worked relatively well in predicting death, but not hospitalization, in their large cohort study. Williams and colleagues have also used the TMP to produce a "manual skill index" based on the items with the three best manual skill times (*Williams et al., 1982), plus another unusual computed scaling variation that does not appear to have been repeated (Williams & Hornberger, 1984).

If the TMP does provide some discriminant ability with a two-category score or with some subset of items, this suggests that it may be overly complex in its full form. Possibly, however, performance time should not be collapsed into a single binomial classification but should be tested as a "continuous" (rather than "categorical") measure or at least broken into discrete, ranked time categories. Analyses clearly have been hampered by some combination of the timed score variance, and perhaps by the skewed distribution of scores. Analyses that examine other, more complex relationships with the timed test (e.g., log transformation of scores, polynomial functions) might be instructive. For example, researchers found that the correlation between the timed Get Up and Go test (discussed below) and several measures of balance and function (Berg Balance scale, gait speed, and Barthel Index of ADL) improved substantially after the latter three were log-transformed (*Podsiadlo & Richardson, 1991). If the TMP is the primary measure for a research trial, investigators might also consider other methods of reducing individual variability—for example, by summarizing across multiple tests (Armstrong, White, & Saracci, 1992). At the present, researchers appear to have a choice of scoring methods available to them and may need to pilot the TMP to determine the method best suited to their needs. Of potential interest is the recent development of a three-door electronic computer-based device marketed under the name *Cognatemp* by Quantum Research Services (5410 Apex Highway, Suite W, Durham, NC 27713-9434). This automated TMP is not yet well described in gerontological scientific journals.

Performance Tests of Lower-Extremity Function

Overview

A variety of tests have been developed to assess older adults' mobility and balance. Many of these are aimed at identifying individuals at risk of falling (e.g., Duncan et al., 1992; Tinetti, Williams, & Mayewski, 1986); they have also been used to assess individuals' capacity to maintain their independence (*Podsiadlo & Richardson, 1991). There are laboratory-based measures, such as measures of postural sway (used, for example, in *Berg et al., 1992), and performance-based clinical measures, such as Tinetti's Performance-Oriented Mobility Assessment (Tinetti, 1986), the Balance Scale (Berg, Wood-Dauphinee, Williams, & Gayton, 1989; *Berg et al., 1992), the Get Up and Go Test (*Mathias, Nayak, & Isaacs, 1986; *Podsiadlo & Richardson, 1991), and Functional Reach (e.g., Duncan et al., 1992; Weiner et al., 1991). The performance-based measures do not require specialized equipment, are easier to administer, and may be more directly relevant to the functions that older adults need to perform. In many cases they are also easier or more acceptable to subjects. For example, the 6-minute walk test was developed in part to test chronically ill individuals who found it difficult to perform the exercise tests that had been traditionally used to assess individuals with chronic lung disease.

The development of some performance-based measures, e.g., of balance, has been complicated, however, by the lack of a definitive laboratory test that can serve as the "gold standard" in assessing the clinical measures (*Berg et al., 1992). Nevertheless, there are a number of studies that compare performance-based measures both to each other and to a variety of laboratory measures of balance (e.g., *Berg et al., 1992; *Duncan, Chandler, Studenski, Hughes, & Prescott, 1993; *Mathias et al., 1986), as well as to the risk of actually falling or having fallen (*Anacker & Di Fabio, 1992; *Salgado, Lord, Packer, & Ehrlich, 1994).

Two measures of mobility and balance are reviewed in greater detail in this chapter. The first is the Get Up and Go Test, which is one of the simplest and quickest measures to administer. The second is the 6-minute walk test (*Butland, Pang, Gross, Woodcock, & Geddes, 1982; *Guyatt et al., 1985). The 6-minute walk test has been used extensively to measure exercise capacity among individuals with chronic lung disease or congestive heart failure, but it has also been used as a more general measure of mobility (*Duncan et al., 1993). Both measures are also simple to administer and have been used quite extensively among frail, older adults.

Get Up and Go Test

One of the simplest performance-based measures of mobility and balance is the Get Up and Go Test, which was developed by *Mathias and colleagues in the mid-1980s (1986). The original test consists of getting up from a straight-backed chair with armrests, walking 3 meters, turning around, returning to the chair, and sitting down. The test has sometimes been modified by changing the distance walked (e.g., to 5 meters) or by using a chair without arms. The subject's performance is then assessed by a trained observer and scored on a 5-point scale where 1 equals "normal" (i.e., showing no evidence of being at risk of falling) and 5 equals "severely abnormal" (i.e., the subject appeared at risk of falling during the test). In the original study, subjects practiced the required moves once to familiarize themselves with the test before they were graded.

Because of a concern about interrater reliability, especially in assigning the intermediate scores (whose meaning is less clear), *Podsiadlo and Richardson (1991) modified the scoring of the test. They replaced the 5-point scale with simply recording the time it took to complete the test. They found that both the intrarater and the interrater reliability of this scoring system were excellent (intraclass correlation coefficient = 0.99 in both cases). They also found that the scores differentiated subjects in terms of their ability to go outside alone safely and to perform ADLs, i.e., to be independently mobile.

Both the original Get Up and Go Test and the timed version have been tested in older adult populations, although the samples have been relatively small. The performance of these tests has been compared both with laboratory measures of balance (e.g., *Mathias et al., 1986) and with other clinical measures (e.g., *Berg et al., 1992). Their use as part of a screening mechanism to identify potential fallers has also been examined (*Anacker & Di Fabio, 1992; *Salgado et al., 1994), although additional studies are needed to explore more fully their sensitivity and their specificity in diverse populations. The simplicity of Get Up and Go and its obvious relevance in assessing older adults' ability to perform tasks essential for maintaining independence make it an attractive candidate for an instrument to use in evaluating older adults. However, additional studies on its reliability and predictive power in a variety of populations are clearly needed.

Six-Minute-Walk Test

Walking tests were first proposed for evaluating the impact of treatments in patients with chronic lung disease (*McGavin, Gupta, & Harvey, 1976); they were modified from the 12-minute running test originally proposed to measure physical fitness in healthy young men (Cooper, 1968). They provide an alternative to conventional exercise testing, measures of functional status, and hemodynamic studies, which can be less than ideal for patients with chronic lung disease (*Guyatt et al., 1985). In McGavin's original test, patients were asked to walk as far as they could during 12 minutes. Alternative time periods were subsequently tested, and 6 minutes was found to perform equally well (*Butland et al., 1982; but see Bernstein et al., 1994, for an alternative view). The 6-minute test has been used quite extensively; there are more than 50 citations in the online database Medline (1995), and many of them focus on older adults. Most of them report on its use in patients with chronic lung or heart disease (e.g., *Bittner et al., 1993; *Goldstein, Gort, Stubbing, Avendano, & Guyatt, 1994; *Guyatt et al., 1985; Guyatt, Townsend, Keller, Singer, & Nogradi, 1989; *Kennedy, Desjardins, Kassam, Ricketts, & Chan-Yeung, 1994; Mak, Bugler, Roberts, & Sprio, 1993). The test has been used in other patient groups as well, for example, those who have undergone hip replacement (*Laupacis et al., 1993) or are on hemodialysis (Laupacis et al., 1991).

The 6-minute-walk test is simple to administer and requires no specialized equipment. However, several recommendations about its administration should be taken into account (Guyatt et al., 1984, *1985):

1. The persons administering the test should be blinded to the patients' treatment assignment, so they will not inadvertently encourage one group more than another.
2. There is no clear evidence on whether or not it is advisable to encourage patients, but whichever strategy is chosen should be used consistently.
3. Two trial tests should be undertaken before the baseline measurement is taken, to take into account an initial learning effect.
4. In studies of treatment effects, the age distribution in the groups should be taken into account, since there is evidence that younger persons improve more on the test over time.

The 6-minute-walk test has been found reliable (after allowing for two practice walks). It also correlates reasonably well with a maximal exercise test (e.g., $r = 0.58$ with cycle ergometer scores; *Guyatt et al., 1985), and it appears to compare well with the more demanding 12-minute-walk test ($r = 0.955$; *Butland et al., 1982). In one study, it correlated weakly with one measure of health-related quality of life, the Sickness Impact Profile ($r = -0.02$ to -0.26 for the various scales of the SIP; *Kennedy et al., 1994). As with the 12-minute-walk test, the correlations with measures of lung function were weak to modest (e.g., *Kennedy et al., 1994).

Although the 6-minute-walk test was developed to provide an alternative to more demanding exercise tests among chronically ill populations, dropouts may pose a problem. In one large study (*Bittner et al., 1993), for example, 65 of 898 subjects did not perform the walk test, for reasons such as inability or unwillingness to walk, and their physicians' judgment. Another 49 patients began the test but were unable to complete it. As with all tests, it is difficult to know what effect the omission of these individuals has on the reported performance of the test.

RECOMMENDATIONS

Self-reports or proxy reports and performance-based measures provide alternative methods of assessing individuals' functional ability. While there is some overlap between the two types of measures, it appears that they capture different aspects of functioning. It is therefore worthwhile to consider combining them in some way, especially if a broad definition of functioning is required and if there are no practical constraints.

The selection of specific performance-based measures depends on the purposes of the research or on the clinical use. For example, the TMP is more likely to be useful in assessing arthritis patients, while the 6-minute-walk test would be more appropriate in evaluating individuals with COPD. In all cases, the training requirements of the testers, the special equipment needed, and the length of the test should be reviewed as practical considerations before selecting a measure.

ANNOTATED BIBLIOGRAPHY

Williams Timed Manual Performance (TMP) Test

Development and Methods

Williams ME, & Hadler NM. (1981). Musculoskeletal components of decrepitude. *Sem Arthritis Rheum, 11,* 284–287.

Design.   The authors compared two groups in terms of their manual function; the groups were expected to be different, on the basis of the degree of independence of their living situations. Both the Williams board test and the Jebson hand function test were used.

Sample.   Two groups of older women were surveyed. One group consisted entirely of all ambulatory "self-care" patients aged 60 and older in an intermediate care nursing home ($n = 17$), and the others were ambulatory members of an independent retirement living community ($n = 11$). Not surprisingly, with this small sample, there were no significant differences in the groups' mean ages; no additional information on the groups' demographics is given.

Summary.   The evaluation is reported to take about 20 minutes. Mean times for each task are given for both groups; seven of nine board tasks required significantly longer times ($p < 0.01$) for the nursing home group. Six of seven Jebson tasks also took significantly longer ($p < 0.001$) for the nursing home group, with the largest differences occurring in tasks performed with the nondominant hand.

Discussion.   This article provides the first description of the "Williams board," but Williams, Hadler, and Earp (1982) is usually considered the definitive developmental article for the Timed Manual Performance Test (TMP). The authors point to the group differences as evidence of the face validity of the TMP.

Williams ME, Hadler NM, & Earp JA. (1982). Manual ability as a marker of dependency in geriatric women. *J Chron Dis*, 35, 115–122.

Design.   This was a cross-sectional study of correlates of dependent status among older women. The Timed Manual Performance Test was administered along with the Philadelphia Geriatric Center Scale of Morale, the Lawton-Brody Instrumental Activities of Daily Living instrument, a measure of social support, and Jacob's Mental Status Evaluation. Subjects also underwent a limited exam for rheumatologic and neurologic disorders. Regression analysis was used to examine the relationship of various indicators (physical performance, cognition, etc.) to dependency status (dependent variable); the latter was classified according to the subjects' living situation.

Sample.   White women over the age of 65 were selected from three settings representing a range of dependency. Two nursing homes yielded 61 eligible women, of whom 2 refused and 20 were selected randomly for the study (mean age = 78.1 years). All 16 eligible women from a group with intermediate dependency were enrolled. They were clients of a hot meal program (mean age = 75.6). The last dependent group were subscribers to a newsletter for senior citizens; 240 women met the criteria for eligibility, of whom 20 were randomly selected and agreed to participate in the study (mean age = 74.5).

Summary.   A variety of indicators showed differences related to dependency status. For example, more dependent women were older, had more medical problems, took more medications, and had lower mental status scores. Each component of the Williams board test and Jebson's hand function test is shown with its average time per group. In general, the most dependent group took twice as long to perform the tasks as the intermediate group, which averaged twice as long as the independent group. No overall mean times are provided. The authors computed a "manual skills index" based on the items with the three best manual times and used this as an independent variable in subsequent multivariate analyses; used in this manner, it represented the largest explained variance in dependency status ($R^2 = 0.86$) of any measured variable. The authors report that any combination of the 27 measured hand tests produced larger R^2 values than other measured covariates.

Discussion. The sample was chosen to be racially homogeneous; however, the variability of function produced an interesting range of subjects for comparison. From the analyses, it is difficult to extrapolate about how to score the TMP test for other research. Apparently all of the tasks have strong relationships with dependency, and it is not clear whether one should select their quoted ''best three'' (closing one of the panel doors with the doorknob, writing with the nondominant hand, and simulated eating with the dominant hand), some other subset of tasks, or all 27 tasks. In addition, this is a correlational study of TMP with dependency, and it is not clear whether low TMP produces the dependency status or is, in part, a result of it.

Gerrity MS, Gaylord S, & Williams ME. (1993). Short versions of the Timed Manual Performance Test: Development, reliability, and validity. *Med Care, 31*, 617–628.

Design. The authors considered the 27 items of the Timed Manual Performance Test (TMP) too lengthy for many assessment uses and tested components of the long version for their potential to provide meaningful brief measures. Item reduction was followed by psychometric tests of internal consistency and validity compared with other measures of function (e.g., IADLs), health status (self-reported health status and the Quality of Well-Being or QWB scale), and depression (the CES-D).

Sample. The sample was drawn from a 2,535-member study of the effects of preventive services among older adults in North Carolina. The sample was drawn beginning about midway through study enrollment and included 1,286 individuals. The mean age of subjects was 75.2 (range, 66–98); 61% were women and 32% African American. See also *Williams et al. (1990) for results of this cohort study.

Summary. Principal components analyses yielded two factor structures for the Williams tests. Five items of the board series were retained (Door), as well as six additional tasks (Table). Although only 77% of subjects performed all 27 TMP tasks, the two derived task sets had 28% higher completion. The long version of the TMP took an average of 200 seconds, but the TMP Doors took only 7.5 seconds on average and the TMP Table took 38 seconds on average. The shorter versions were correlated with each other and with the longer version at about $r = 0.50$. The TMP short versions were moderately correlated with IADLs at about $r = 0.40$, which was higher than for the 27-item TMP. The correlations were higher between the short versions of the TMP and the QWB ($r = -0.26, -0.27$) than between the longer version and the QWB ($r = -0.16$). Importantly, there was a moderate negative correlation between the long TMP and education; this correlation decreased for each of the shorter versions. African Americans took longer to complete all versions of the TMP, even after controlling for education. Other multivariate relationships are not presented.

Discussion. Remarkably, the shorter versions of the TMP seem to perform better than the longer one when compared with other measures. Subsequent tests should consider whether they also predict utilization of health care and functional decline similarly to the original TMP. Given the difficulties for many individuals in completing the long version, the brief version shows promise.

Applications

Applegate WB, Miller ST, Elam JT, Freeman JM, Wood TO, & Gettlefinger TC. (1987). Impact of cataract surgery with lens implementation on vision and physical function in elderly patients. *JAMA*, *257*, 1064–1066.

Design. The study prospectively studied a cohort of older adults from shortly before to 12 months after cataract surgery for changes in visual acuity and subjective and objective function. Interviews were conducted before surgery and 4 and 12 months after the surgery. Assessments included the Functional Assessment Inventory (FAI), the Short Portable Mental Status Questionnaire (SPMSQ) for cognitive function, and the Timed Manual Performance (TMP) Test.

Sample. Patients age 70 or older who were scheduled for cataract surgery during a 15-month period in two physicians' practices were eligible. The total eligible sample is not given, but the authors report that 70% were enrolled and 30% either were not interviewed or refused to participate, leaving 293 subjects with baseline information; however, only 222 (76%) could complete the TMP at baseline. Four-month data were available for 280 (96%) patients, of whom 160 could complete the TMP; 12-month data were collected for 246 individuals (84%), and 126 (51%) had TMP results. Patients' ages ranged from 70 to 95 years (mean = 77). They were 77% women and 97% white; 36% had formal education beyond high school.

Summary. At baseline, patients were fairly independent, and fully 51% needed no assistance on ADLs. The authors report that visual acuity improved for patients in tandem with the results of their Timed Manual Performance Test, but that other measures of function did not change as dramatically. Specifically, ADL items improved significantly at 4 months but then deteriorated to nearer baseline levels at 1 year. TMP tasks all improved significantly at the 4-month assessment and were maintained with slight improvements after 1 year, with the exception of the simulated eating tasks, which reverted to near baseline levels at 1 year. After classifying patients by level of general vision improvement, the authors found a corresponding "dose-response" improvement in the sentence-writing task but no regular pattern in ADL functions.

Discussion. The study began with a good-size sample but was hampered in the analyses by the relatively poor completion of the TMP test. However, the study suggests that the test is very responsive to changes in these patients. Perhaps the TMP is best used in a somewhat selected subset of patients who demonstrate basic competence in visual and physical skills.

Falconer J, Hughes SL, Naughton BJ, Singer R, Chang RW, & Sinacore JM. (1991). Self report and performance-based hand function tests as correlates of dependency in the elderly. *J Am Geriatr Soc*, *39*, 695–699.

Design. These analyses were part of a larger study of dependency; the present analyses were conducted to determine the best measures to use in such research. Self-reported or proxy-reported function was measured using the Dexterity Scale of the Geriatrics-Arthritis Impact Measurement Scale (GERI-AIMS), and the performance-based items used were the Jebson Test of Hand Function plus the Williams Test of Hand Function (basically the Williams Timed Manual Performance test), the Williams board items only, and grip strength. The dependent variable was "dependency" based on living status categorized by three levels.

Sample. Adults aged 60 and older (*n* = 764) were selected from three populations in the Chicago area on the basis of their living situation (community-dwelling, retirement community, etc.). No data on selection methods or refusals are given. There were incomplete data on 62 enrolled subjects, and analyses were performed on 702 (92%). These subjects were 75% women and 86% white, with a mean age of 76.8 years (*SD* = 8.8).

Summary. The mean age rose significantly for increased dependency classifications, and these groups varied by other demographic variables also. Nearly all performance-based and self-reported measures were predictably different among the groups. Of the hand performance measures, the Williams board discriminated best among the three levels of dependency, explaining 12.5% of the variance; however, the GERI-AIMS added another 16.9% of explained variance, even with demographic variables in the model.

Discussion. This is an impressive effort to select, with strong formal analyses, the best instrument or instruments for research on dependency. The "outcome" or dependent variable may have caused some analytic problems, in that the variability of function within each of the three levels is likely to have been quite high and might obscure an understanding of the difference among dependency categories.

Ostwald SK, Snowdon DA, Rysavy DM, Keenan NL, & Kane RL. (1989). Manual dexterity as a correlate of dependency in the elderly. *J Am Geriatr Soc*, 37, 963–969.

Design. The Williams Timed Manual Performance Test (Doors only) was tested for its ability to predict dependence among Catholic nuns. Tests also included grip strength, timed 6-foot walk, vision, and the Short Portable Mental Status Questionnaire (SPMSQ). If a subject was not able to perform a task, she was assigned the maximum time of any subject who completed the task (for the TMP-Doors, this was 198.6 seconds). Because of skewed time distribution and extreme scores, the authors analyzed the scores as ranked performance (1–128). Three levels of dependence were used to classify subjects on the basis of their living situation (independent, retirement center, nursing home). Median scores for groups were used for analyses.

Sample. The sample was chosen to provide for maximum homogeneity. The subjects were Catholic sisters (i.e., nuns) aged 75–94 years. These were selected from 366 listed sisters, of whom 20 had left the order, 191 had died, and 155 had survived; of the latter, 128 (83%) completed the study assessments. They were living independently in the community (*n* = 21), in a retirement community (*n* = 64), or in a nursing home (*n* = 43).

Summary. Correlations were moderate to strong between the TMP-Doors and grip strength (*r* = −0.55) and 6-foot walk (*r* = 0.63). The TMP-Doors was strongly correlated with mental status (*r* = 0.67) and with near vision (*r* = 0.63, corrected vision). Completion time for the TMP-Doors test was shortest among the community-living sisters, followed by those in the retirement center, and it was longest among those living in the nursing home; this relationship was statistically significant. The discriminant analysis equation using manual dexterity predicted living site correctly for 63% of the sisters in the nursing home, with a specificity of 99%, a positive predictive value of 96%, and a negative predictive value of 84%. The addition of age and mental status to the equation improved the prediction only slightly.

Discussion. The analyses are unusual and suggest that timed tests cause difficulties because of their skewed distribution. Using age in the statistical models as a dichotomous variable (cutoff at age 85) also seems unusual. However, the TMP-Doors clearly delineates between levels of dependency among these sisters.

Williams ME, Gaylord SA, & McGaghie WC. (1990). Timed manual performance in a community elderly population. *J Am Geriatr Soc*, **38**, 1120–1126.

Design. The TMP was added to a large study of the effectiveness of preventive services for older adults in North Carolina. Other measures included function (e.g., the IADL), health status (self-reported health status and quality of well-being, or QWB; the QWB is reviewed in Chapter 2), and depression (the Center for Epidemiologic Studies Depression Scale, or CES-D, which is reviewed in Chapter 5). "Good" versus "poor" performance on the TMP was based on (1) subjects' completing the protocol in under or over 350 seconds or (2) subjects' inability to complete one or more items. Because of the potential for those who were functionally illiterate to bias the results, inability to complete the writing task was omitted for the latter classification.

Sample. The study sample was drawn beginning about midway through study enrollment and included 1,286 individuals. The mean age of subjects was 75.2 years (range, 66–98); 61% were women and 32% African American. See also *Gerrity et al. (1993) for a subsequent analysis of this cohort using an abbreviated TMP.

Summary. A total of 8.3% of the subjects were classified as having performed "poorly" on the basis of one of the two study criteria. A substantial number of individuals did not complete the protocol, because of unexplained equipment problems or refusals. The ADL mean (items requiring assistance) was 1.8 for those who were able to complete the TMP versus 5.7 for noncompleters. The ADL means for the two "time" groups were 2.1 and 9.0, respectively. Other univariate associations were found. Age was significantly greater for those whose performance was "poor," as was level of depression and poorer self-perceived health, and QWB scores were lower (indicating worse health).

Discussion. These results suggest some response limitations to the TMP owing to refusals, technical problems, or inability to complete the tasks. Despite this, the dichotomized classification suggests that about 8% of community-dwelling older adults in this population may have substantial problems with manual dexterity and that poor performance on the TMP is related to a number of indicators of function and health.

Williams ME, Gaylord SA, & Gerrity MS. (1994). The Timed Manual Performance test as a predictor of hospitalization and death in a community-based elderly population. *J Am Geriatr Soc*, **42**, 21–27.

Design. The results of this prospective cohort study follow the results of the cross-sectional research described by *Gerrity et al. (1993) and *Williams et al. (1990). The TMP had been added about midway through recruitment and was included in a substantial assessment protocol described previously by Gerrity. Both the full 27-item version of the TMP and two of its components (Doors, 5 tasks; Table, 6 tasks) are analyzed. Two years later, mortality and hospitalization data were obtained from the Medicare database and were classified for the analyses as (1) any hospitalization, (2) the number of hospitalizations, (3) the average length of stay per hospitalization, and (4) total hospital charges.

Sample. As described by Gerrity, there were 1,286 persons for this cohort analysis. The mean age was 75.2 years, 61% were women, and 32% were African American.

Summary. The three tests gave the following mean times and standard deviations: Long TMP, 200.8±102.1 seconds; TMP-Doors, 7.5±2.9 seconds; TMP-Table, 38.0±14.7 seconds. There were substantial ranges for all versions, with median scores lower than these means. Cronbach's α (internal consistency), was only moderate for the full TMP (0.58; a standardized α was higher at 0.91) but relatively higher for the TMP-Doors and TMP-Table versions (0.74 and 0.82, respectively).

There were 127 deaths (10%), and 200 subjects were hospitalized at least once (16%). The adjusted relative risk (RR) of dying strongly increased for each quartile of TMP time in all three versions. Hospitalizations were significantly associated only with the TMP-Table test; no other hospital-based outcomes were associated with any of the TMP versions. Correlations among IADLs and the two short TMP versions were modest: $r = 0.42$ for the TMP-Doors and $r = 0.40$ for the TMP-Table. The correlation between IADLS and the long TMP was weak ($r = 0.25$) until the two writing tasks were eliminated; it then rose to $r = 0.52$. The IADLs were also a significant predictor of death and of hospitalization after 2 years. When both IADLs and the TMP were included in a single model, only the long TMP was independently associated with mortality.

Discussion. Scores on both short TMP versions were associated with mortality. They were more weakly related to hospitalization, which was associated more strongly with traditional IADLs. The number of models used in these analyses gives rise to some caution in interpretation; replication with other populations would reinforce the findings that the TMP-Table performed somewhat better than the long or TMP-Doors versions.

Get Up and Go Test

Development and Testing

Mathias S, Nayak USL, & Isaacs B. (1986). Balance in elderly patients: The 'Get-Up and Go' Test. *Arch Phys Med Rehabil, 67*, 387–389.

Design. This article describes the initial development of the Get Up and Go Test. Its purpose was to devise a simple test of balance that could serve as an alternative to laboratory tests (e.g., measurement of postural sway and gait speed) and could be used by clinicians in routine care of their older patients. The results were examined for interrater reliability and were compared with the measurement of sway, which is a standard laboratory test of balance. Subjects also performed a gait test. All of the tests were videotaped and reviewed by different types of health care professionals, including doctors, medical students, physiotherapists, occupational therapists, and laboratory technicians. The performances of the professional groups were compared by examining the means and standard deviation of the summed scores for each group.

Sample. The sample consisted of 40 inpatients or outpatients with some degree of balance disturbance from a hospital in England. The mean age was 73.8 years (range, 52–94); 50% were women. Eight patients did not complete the gait test.

Summary. The Pearson correlation coefficient between the Get Up and Go score and the measure of sway was 0.50 ($p < 0.001$). Get Up and Go was more likely to detect problems when there were none (e.g., with stroke patients whose gait appeared abnormal but whose balance actually was good) than vice versa. The article also reports on the correlation between test scores and other measures of gait. The article contains some suggestions on pitfalls to avoid in rating the test (e.g., confusing gait and balance).

As for interrater reliability, the authors report that the Kendall coefficient of concordance test shows that the agreement within each group was higher than would be expected by chance ($p < 0.001$ for both physiotherapists and senior doctors). However, there was a significant difference in scores between the two groups; doctors scored subjects half a point higher than therapists did.

Discussion.   This article presents a simple test for measuring balance among older adults and shows that it performs quite well compared with more sophisticated, laboratory-based measures of balance and gait. It would have been useful to see how the test performed in healthy control subjects as well. The results on interrater reliability emphasize the need to train those scoring the test and to look for systematic biases in the way scoring is done before the test is used in practice.

Podsiadlo D, & Richardson S. (1991). The Timed "Up & Go": A test of basic functional mobility for frail elderly persons. *J Am Geriatr Soc*, *39*, 142–148.

Design.   The purpose of this study was to develop and test the reliability of a modified version of the Get Up and Go test. The authors replaced the original scoring system, which they argue is imprecise, especially in the middle ranges, with a timed version of the test. Instead of rating subjects' performance on a scale from 1 to 5, the time that it took them to complete the test was measured. Both intra- and interrater reliability were assessed using intraclass correlation coefficients, and the relationship to other measures of balance, gait speed, and functional ability was examined using Pearson correlation co-efficients.

Sample.   The sample consisted of 60 community-dwelling older adults referred to a geriatric day hospital (mean age = 79.5 years, range = 60–90; 37 were women) and 10 healthy control subjects (mean age = 75 years; range = 70–84; 4 were women). The reliability studies were performed on 22 patients.

Summary.   All of the healthy control subjects performed the test in 10 seconds or less (mean = 8.5; range, 7–10 seconds). The scores for the patients ranged from 10 to 240 seconds; 3 were unable to complete the test. The Timed Up and Go Test had a correlation of −0.72 with the Berg Balance Scale, −0.55 with gait speed, and −0.51 with the Barthel Index of ADL. The correlations are stronger when the latter three measures are log-transformed. Dividing the subjects into three groups on the basis of their time scores shows that the test provides some indication of the patient's functional skills. Most patients in the fastest group (less than 20 seconds) were able to go outside alone safely, while none in the slowest group (30 or more seconds) were able to do so; the middle group fell in between in terms of their functional abilities.

The Timed Up and Go Test was shown to be very reliable. The intraclass correlation coefficient was 0.99 both between raters and for the same rater on two consecutive visits. The variation in time between the two tests was 5 seconds or less for all but two subjects. The authors also suggest that this test can be used to measure clinical change, but they report only anecdotal information as supportive evidence.

Discussion.   The scoring change recommended in this article appears to strengthen the Get Up and Go Test considerably and to simplify its administration (by reducing the need for training those who administer it, for example). It would be interesting to compare the two versions of the test directly, but that was not done here. The authors also point out that they tested this measure in individuals with a middle range of functional abilities; it would be useful to examine its performance in other populations as well. However, the results on inter- and intrarater reliability are impressive. The effort to correlate this test with other standard measures of balance, gait, and functional ability is also informative. The one source of ambiguity is what this test is intended to measure. In the original development article (*Mathias et al., 1986) the focus was on balance and preventing falls, whereas here it is on physical mobility and maintaining independence. The performance of the test for purposes of research may vary with the end point of interest.

Applications

Anacker SL, & Di Fabio RP. (1992). Influence of sensory inputs on standing balance in community-dwelling elders with a recent history of falling. *Phys Ther, 72, 575–584.*
Design. The purpose of this study was to determine how conflicting visual or ankle somatosensory inputs affect standing balance in older adults with and without a history of falling. A secondary objective was to examine the correlation between scores on a sensory organization test (SOT) and scores on a test of general mobility (in this case, the Get Up and Go Test). This abstract will focus on the latter results. A 5-point scale was used to score the test.
Sample. The sample consisted of 47 relatively healthy community-dwelling older adults (39 women; mean age = 80.5 years; SD = 9.0, range, 65–96). Sixteen of the 47 were in the ''fall'' group, that is, they had fallen two or more times during the previous 6 months. The mean age of this group was 85 years (SD = 7.73, range, 67–96); the median number of falls was 3.5 (mean = 5; range, 2–24).
Summary. The adjusted mean score on the Get Up and Go Test was significantly different for ''fallers'' (2.65; SD = 1.48) than ''nonfallers'' (1.47; SD = 0.77; $p < 0.01$). The Spearman correlation coefficient between the Get Up and Go scores and the total SOT scores was −0.67 for ''fallers'' versus −0.44 for ''nonfallers.'' Test-retest reliability was assessed in 10 subjects who repeated the test within 7 days ($r = 0.96, p < 0.05$; $\kappa = 0.52$).
Discussion. The primary focus of this article is on the performance of the SOT and on furthering our understanding of the mechanisms responsible for maintaining balance. It also does provide some useful information on the performance of the Get Up and Go Test. However, it would be useful to follow this up with a prospective study that measures the sensitivity and specificity of the SOT and Get Up and Go Test in predicting falls.

Berg KO, Maki BE, Williams JI, Holliday PJ, & Wood-Dauphinee SL. (1992). Clinical and laboratory measures of postural balance in an elderly population. *Arch Phys Med Rehabil, 73, 1073–1080.*
Design. The purpose of this study is to assess the performance of the Balance Scale in comparison with laboratory measures of postural sway and clinical measures of mobility and balance, including the Timed Up and Go Test. They also compared the test results with the use of a walking aid, which was used as an indicator of balance (given the lack of a ''gold standard'' measure of balance). Only the results relating to the Timed Up and Go Test are reported in this abstract.

Sample.   Thirty-six subjects were recruited from residential care facilities and acute and extended care wards at a health science center in Canada; five did not complete the laboratory tests and were excluded from the analysis. The mean age of the remaining 31 subjects was 83.0 years (SD = 6.9); 71% were female. The subjects were selected so that approximately one third used no walking aid, one third used a cane, and one third used a walker. The mean Barthel Index score of 93 (SD = 9.8) indicates that most were functionally independent in the basic ADLs.

Summary.   The mean score on the Timed Up and Go was 26.9 seconds (SD = 18.0; range, 10–70). The correlation between the Timed Up and Go and the other tests was as follows: Balance Scale, −0.76 ($p < 0.001$); Tinetti balance subscale, −0.74 ($p < 0.001$); mobility section of the Barthel index, −0.48 ($p < 0.01$); use of mobility aids, 0.70 ($p < 0.001$); total diagnoses, 0.38; and numbers of total medications, 0.43. The mean Timed Up and Go score was 14.0 seconds for those using no walking aid (n = 10; 95% confidence interval, CI, 11.9–16.1); 19.9 for those using a cane (n = 9; 95% CI, 13.7–20.3), and 40.9 for those using a walker (n = 11; 95% CI, 28.1–53.7). The Balance Test was best able to distinguish among subjects according to their use of walking aids, but the Timed Up and Go test was the next best measure. However, the Timed Up and Go could distinguish only between those who used walkers and those who used canes or nothing; it did not distinguish between those who used nothing and those who used canes.

Discussion.   This article provides useful data comparing the performance of the Timed Up and Go Test with other measures of functional balance. The Timed Up and Go appeared to perform well compared with these other measures. Although it did not distinguish among walking aids quite as well as the Balance Scale, the use of aids is also an imprecise measure of balance.

Salgado R, Lord SR, Packer J, & Ehrlich F. (1994). Factors associated with falling in elderly hospital patients. *Gerontology, 40,* 325–331.

Design.   This is a case control study to examine the factors associated with falls in an acute care hospital. Subjects underwent a variety of tests of balance, gait, and posture, including the Get Up and Go Test as well as a number of clinical tests.

Sample.   The sample consisted of 44 individuals who fell while in the hospital in Australia and 44 hospitalized control subjects matched for age, sex, type (medical or surgical), and primary diagnosis. The mean age of the "fallers" was 80.7 years (SD = 8.2), and that of the "nonfallers" was 80.0 years (SD = 6.8). There were 23 men and 21 women in each group. "Fallers" were examined within 48 hours of falling; "nonfallers" were examined sometime during their hospital stay.

Summary.   Impaired performance on the Get Up and Go Test (inability to undertake two or more of the following tasks: stand up, walk 5 meters, turn around) was one of 7 factors significantly associated with falling. In a multivariate analysis that included impaired orientation, use of psychoactive drugs, evidence of stroke, and impaired performance on the Get Up and Go Test, the adjusted odds ratio for the Get Up and Go Test was 4.63 (95% CI, 1.39–15.36). The equation correctly classified 80% of the patients as "fallers" or "nonfallers."

Discussion.   This study provides evidence of the utility of the Get Up and Go Test in identifying individuals at risk of falling. However, individuals were categorized according to their ability to do all components of the test; it is not clear why this scoring method was used. It would be interesting to see whether the test scores themselves—with either the original 5-point scale or the timed version—would have yielded similar results. The authors also point out the potential weaknesses of this retrospective design, in which "fallers" and "nonfallers" were tested at different times during their hospitalization. They acknowledged the possibility that the test performance of "fallers" might have been affected by the fall itself, although none of them suffered serious injuries as a result of falling. Nevertheless, the study does suggest the utility of four easily measured variables for identifying individuals at risk of falling.

Six-Minute-Walk Test

Development and Testing

McGavin CR, Gupta SP, & McHardy GJR. (1976). Twelve-minute walking test for assessing disability in chronic bronchitis. *Br Med J, 1,* 822–823.

Design. This article evaluates the use of the 12-minute-walk test for assessing tolerance for exercise among patients with chronic bronchitis. A 12-minute running test was initially developed by Cooper (1968) as a guide to physical fitness. It was later modified by other researchers to become the 6-minute-walk test. Performance on this test was compared with the results of test of lung function and bicycle ergometer testing. Test-retest reliability was assessed in 12 subjects who performed the test on 3 different days and in 29 patients on 2 days.

Sample. The sample consisted of 35 men aged 40 to 70 with chronic bronchitis.

Summary. Among those who repeated the test three times, the mean distance walked was 891 (SD = 286) meters for the first test, 955 (SD = 313) meters for the second test, and 996 (SD = 336) meters for the third test. The overall range was 238 to 1,463 meters. The difference between the first and second days, after allowance for a change in the forced expiratory volume in 1 second (FEV_1) was significant ($p < 0.05$). In the group of 29 subjects with two tests, the difference in the distance walked between the first and second tests was also significant. Using data from all 35 patients, the correlation between the distance walked and FEV_1 was weak and not significant ($r = 0.283$; $p>0.05$), while the correlation with the forced vital capacity (FVC) was modest and significant ($r = 0.406$; $p < 0.05$). Using data from the progressive exercise test, the correlation between the distance walked in 12 minutes and oxygen uptake was $r = 0.52$ ($p < 0.01$) and with ventilation was $r = 0.53$ ($p < 0.01$).

The authors suggest that the advantages of this test are that (1) the results are reproducible (if the test is repeated twice), (2) it requires no apparatus, (3) it is applicable to patients with diseases of varying severity, (4) it involves a skill familiar to everyone, and (5) patients can set their own pace. They assert that the lack of correlation between the 12-minute test and FEV_1 demonstrates the "range of performance found in patients with established airways obstruction" (p. 823).

Discussion. This article provides data on the precursor to the 6-minute-walk tests and emphasizes the importance of providing practice runs of this test before measurements are taken.

Butland RJA, Pang J, Gross ER, Woodcock AA, & Geddes DM. (1982). Two-, six-, and 12-minute walking tests in respiratory disease. *Br Med J, 284,* 1607–1608.

Design.   This study compares the performance of the 2-, 6-, and 12-minute-walk tests in assessing patients with respiratory disease. The objective was to find a test that would be less time-consuming for investigators and less exhausting for patients than the 12-minute-walk test. The results include three substudies. (1) The first compared pacing during 2-minute intervals of the 12-minute test. Participants performed the test 5 times at 4-week intervals. (2) The second substudy compared the 2-, 6-, and 12-minute-walk tests. Subjects performed each of the tests once. (3) The third substudy assessed the reproducibility of the 2-minute test. Subjects repeated the 2-minute test four times, with at least an hour between walks.

Sample.   There were three samples, corresponding to the three substudies: (1) The first sample consisted of 10 patients with stable chronic airflow obstruction. The mean age was 61 years ($SD = 11$). (2) The second sample consisted of 30 patients with stable chronic respiratory disability. The mean age was 61 years ($SD = 12$). (3) The third sample consisted of 13 patients with a range of respiratory disease and exercise tolerance (54–215 meters on the 2-minute-walk test). Their mean age was 51 ($SD = 14$) years.

Summary.   (1) In the first substudy, the distance walked in 12 minutes ranged from 400 to 1,100 meters. Patients usually covered more during the first 2 minutes than during subsequent 2-minute intervals, but after the first 2 minutes the distances covered in subsequent 2-minute intervals were quite similar (mean correlation coefficient = 1.000; range, 0.996–1.000; $n = 50$). (2) For the second group, the mean distance walked in 6 minutes was 413 ($SD = 107$) meters. The correlation between the 6- and 12-minute tests was 0.955; while between the 6- and 2-minute tests, it was 0.892. The variance was 23.4 for the 2-minute test, 26.0 for the 6-minute test, and 29.6 for the 12-minute test. (3) For the third substudy, the mean distances walked were 137 ($SD = 46$) meters for the first 2-minute walk and 141 ($SD = 43$), 146 ($SD = 41$), and 147 ($SD = 40$) meters for the subsequent walks. The authors conclude that ''the time chosen to assess exercise tolerance is not critical. Shorter times are easier for both patient and investigator and are as reproducible, but they discriminate slightly less well and have less of a training role. The six-minute walk may represent a sensible compromise'' (p. 1608). The authors also note the need for two practice walks to account for the initial training effect.

Discussion.   This study provides solid evidence on the use of the 6-minute-walk test as an acceptable alternative to the 12-minute-walk test. It reinforces the need for practice walks before the first measurement is taken. An alternative view is provided by Bernstein and his colleagues (1994), who favor the 12-minute walk over the 6-minute walk because they found that changes in maximal oxygen intake were more closely correlated with changes in the 12-minute walk ($r = 0.72$) than with the 6-minute walk ($r = 0.64$); however, they do not indicate whether this difference is significant. It also would be useful to know the subjects' gender in Bernstein's study.

Guyatt GH, Sullivan MJ, & Thompson PJ. (1985). The 6-minute walk: A new measure of exercise capacity in patients with chronic heart failure. *Can Med Assoc J, 132,* 919–923.

Design.   The purpose of this study is to assess the use of the 6-minute-walk test in patients with chronic heart failure and to compare its utility for this group with its use for patients with chronic lung disease, for whom walking tests have been assessed previously. The impact of encouraging patients during the test was also assessed. Patients completed the 6-minute-walk tests 6 times at 2-week intervals. They were stratified by disease and then randomized to receive encouragement every 30 seconds during the walk or to receive no encouragement. Their performance on the walk test was compared with the results of a maximal exercise test using a bicycle ergometer and functional status as measured by the Specific Activity Scale for all subjects and the New York Heart Association criteria for patients with heart failure. The article also briefly reviews the use of walking tests, primarily a 12-minute-walk test, among patients with chronic lung disease.

Sample.   The sample consisted of individuals who experienced dyspnea or fatigue while performing activities of daily living. More specific clinical criteria are discussed in the article. Of 57 individuals enrolled in the study, 43 completed all 6 tests. There were 34 men and 9 women; 25 were respiratory patients and 18 were cardiac patients (8 apparently met the criteria for both groups, but the authors do not explain how the assignments were made for these 8). The mean age was 64.7 ($SD = 8.3$) years.

Summary.   The patients' scores increased during the first two walks and then leveled off (the difference in the distance walked between the first two walks and the last four was significant, $p < 0.001$). Encouragement increased the distance walked in both groups ($p < 0.02$). The patients with chronic lung disease improved more over time than the cardiac patients, independent of the effect of encouragement. The within-person standard deviation was less than 6% of the mean score; according to the authors, this compares favorably with most clinical and laboratory tests. The correlation between the scores on the 6-minute test and the cycle ergometer scores was 0.58; with the Specific Activity Scale, the correlation was −0.47. They report that in other studies the walking test scores have correlated well with other measures of functional status. The authors conclude that the 6-minute-walk test provides a promising, simple measure of functional exercise capacity. The results after the first two walks were sufficiently consistent, they assert, that the test can be used to detect small treatment effects with samples of reasonable sizes.

In another article reporting the results of the same study, Guyatt et al. (1984) compare the results of the 2- and 6-minute-walk tests and also compare the magnitude of the encouragement effect with the size of the treatment effect reported in a number of studies using a walking test. They conclude the following: (1) It does not appear to matter whether or not encouragement is given as long as the same approach is applied consistently. (2) The individual administering the test should be blinded to the treatment assignment, since in some studies the treatment and encouragement effects are quite similar in magnitude. In other words, the results could be biased if the test supervisor inadvertently provided greater encouragement to treatment subjects than to control subjects. (3) Subjects should be randomized by age as well, since younger subjects tend to improve more over time than older ones. (4) Two practice tests should be performed before baseline measurements are made. (5) The 6-minute-walk test is more appropriate than the 2-minute-walk test for measuring treatment effects.

Discussion.   These articles provide valuable information both on the performance of the 6-minute-walk test and on the optimal mode of administration. They suggest that the test is useful for evaluating potential treatments in patients with chronic lung disease and heart failure. However, the samples were quite small and were limited to two diagnoses. It would be useful to assess the test in a more diverse population that included healthy individuals and heterogeneous samples with a broad range of chronic diseases common among older adults.

Applications

Bittner V, Weiner DH, Yusuf S, Rogers WJ, McIntyre KM, Bangdiwala SI, Kronenberg MW, Kostis JB, Guillotte M, Greenberg B, Woods PA, Bourassa MG, for the SOLVD Investigators. (1993). Prediction of mortality and morbidity with a 6-minute-walk test in patients with left ventricular dysfunction. *JAMA, 270*, 1702–1707.

Design.   This study examines the usefulness of the 6-minute-walk test in predicting morbidity and mortality in patients with left ventricular dysfunction. Subjects underwent a clinical evaluation that included the walk test and then were followed for an average of 242 (*SD* = 82) days. Their performance on the walk test was compared with (1) all-cause mortality, (2) all hospitalizations, (3) hospitalizations for congestive heart failure (CHF), and (4) a combination of (1) and (3). Performance on the walk test was divided into four categories, with cutoff points of 300, 375, and 450 meters.

Sample.   The subjects consisted of a subsample of the individuals who participated in the Studies of Left Ventricular Dysfunction (SOLVD), designed as a randomized controlled trial of enalapril maleate. (The results of that trial are not reported here.) The patients were from 20 hospitals in the United States, Canada, and Belgium. A random sample of 898 patients was selected out of 6,273 patients with an ejection fraction of 0.45 or less or radiological evidence of CHF (see the article for more details on the sampling strategy). These patients were compared with 40 age- and sex-matched controls with no history of left ventricular dysfunction. Three of the 898 patients were lost to follow-up; 65 did not participate in the 6-minute walk. The article compares subjects in the larger registry with those in the substudy; it also compares those in the substudy who participated in the walking test with those who did not. The controls had a significantly lower body mass index and were less likely to have ever smoked. The mean age of the 833 patients who participated in the walking test was 60 (*SD* = 12) years; 78% were men; and 86% were white. Of the 833 test takers, 49 did not complete the test and 43 stopped or rested during the test. All of the control subjects completed the test. Thirty-four percent of the patients reported symptoms during the walk, including angina, dyspnea, fatigue, and dizziness; all symptoms resolved quickly after the walk.

Summary.   The mean distance walked was 374.3 (*SD* = 117.1) meters among patients and 555.2 (*SD* = 114.5) meters among controls ($p < 0.0001$). The distance walked was inversely related to age and was less for women and African Americans. Those with no symptoms (New York Heart Association, NYHA, class I) tended to walk longer distances, and those with severe symptoms (NYHA classes III/IV) tended to walk shorter distances. However, those in between (NYHA class II) showed a wide range of performance. The correlation between the distance walked and the ejection fraction was weak (*r* not reported).

Fifty-two of the participants died during the follow-up period, 252 were hospitalized, and 78 of those were hospitalized for CHF. The distance walked was inversely related to mortality ($p < 0.02$) and to both hospitalizations of any kind and hospitalizations for CHF ($p < 0.001$ for both), but not to hospitalizations for noncardiovascular reasons. In a stepwise logistic regression that initially included distance walked, ejection fraction, age, sex, cause of left ventricular dysfunction, and NYHA class (nonsignificant variables other than cause were subsequently dropped), distance walked was a significant predictor of mortality (odds ratio (OR) = 1.5 for each 120 meter decrement; 95% CI, 1.1–2.0) and of the combined mortality and hospitalization for CHF outcome (OR = 1.8; 95% CI,

1.4–2.3). The odds ratios are based on the reduced model. Only walking distance and ejection fraction were significant independent predictors of mortality. The test is particularly useful in patients with mild to moderate CHF or asymptomatic left ventricular dysfunction.

The authors reported that the test was easy to administer, was well accepted by patients, and more closely mimics patients' day-to-day activities than maximal exercise testing.

Discussion. The study is valuable in documenting the utility of the 6-minute-walk test in predicting outcomes as opposed to measuring treatment effects. The sample size was large, and the locations were diverse. However, it included only a single category of patients, so its applicability to more diverse populations, whether healthy or sick, is unknown. It is interesting that Lipkin, Scriven, Crake, and Poole-Wilson (1986) reported a much longer distance walked among normal subjects: 683 meters (with a mean age in the study population of 58 years), compared with the 552 meters reported among controls in this study. The reason for the difference is not clear. As the authors also point out, patients performed the test only once, and that did allow for the training effect reported in other studies (e.g., *Guyatt et al., 1985). However, they note that the performances on the first and second walks were highly correlated. It would also have been interesting to know how reproducible the results were, especially given the variety of settings in which the test was used.

Duncan PW, Chandler J, Studenski S, Hughes M, & Prescott B. (1993). How do physiological components of balance affect mobility in elderly men? *Arch Phys Med Rehabil, 74,* **1343–1349.**

Design. This study assesses the relationship between physiological components of balance and mobility. More specifically, the hypothesis was that function is affected more by an accumulation of modest impairments than by a single impairment. Older men from Veterans Affairs outpatient clinics were divided into three categories of mobility on the basis of their ability to climb stairs step over step without using a handrail and to tandem-walk. The authors believed that the ability to do these two tasks demonstrates "excellent balance and a high degree of physical function and low risk for falls" (p. 1343). Sensory, central processing, and effector functions were tested as physiological components of balance. Functional performance was evaluated using the 6-minute-walk test, the Duke Mobility Skills Test, 10-ft walking speed, and functional reach.

Sample. The subjects were participants in an ongoing cohort study of risk factors for falls among older male veterans aged 70 to 104. Thirty-nine of the original cohort of 310 were selected as a convenience sample. The subjects did not have "significant disease" (see the article for further details). The mean age in the three mobility groups ranged from 73.8 to 76.2 years ($p = 0.61$).

Summary. The mean distance walked in 6 minutes was 1,010.7 ($SD = 198$) feet in the low-mobility group, 1,190 ($SD = 260$) feet in the intermediate-mobility group, and 1,354 ($SD = 214$) feet in the high-mobility group ($p = 0.0008$). The differences between both the high and low groups and the intermediate and low groups were statistically significant. The differences in single physiological components of balance across the three groups were seldom significant. However, in accordance with the authors' hypothesis, there was a statistically significant difference in the number of impaired components. In a linear regression model, after controlling for age, neurodiagnosis, and orthodiagnosis, the number of impaired domains was a significant predictor of performance on the 6-minute-walk test ($R^2 = 0.25$).

Discussion. This study provides some useful information on the performance of the 6-minute-walk test compared with physiological measures of balance and with an alternative classification of mobility. It would be interesting to know the relationship between the 6-minute-walk test and each of the individual physiological components of balance, but the 6-minute-walk test is not the primary focus of this article. It should also be noted that subjects performed it only once, contrary to the recommendation (e.g., *Guyatt et al., 1985) that subjects should be given several trial runs before the baseline measurement is taken. In addition, the generalizability of these results is limited by the fact that the subjects were male veterans; further studies would be needed to determine whether these results hold up in other populations.

Goldstein RS, Gort EH, Stubbing D, Avendano MA, & Guyatt GH. (1994). Randomised controlled trial of respiratory rehabilitation. *Lancet*, *344*, 1394–1397.

Design. This article reports on the results of a randomized controlled trial of the use of respiratory rehabilitation programs among patients with severe but stable chronic obstructive pulmonary disease (COPD). Patients were assigned at random to either 8 weeks of inpatient rehabilitation followed by 16 weeks of outpatient follow-up or to conventional care from their own physicians. Measures of tolerance for exercise and quality of life were administered three times before randomization (the third measurement was used as the baseline) and 12, 18, and 24 weeks after randomization. The outcome measures included measurements of pulmonary function, the 6-minute-walk test, use of a cycle ergometer, and health-related quality of life using the interviewer-administered Chronic Respiratory Disease Questionnaire.

Sample. The sample consisted of 89 nonsmoking patients who had severe but stable COPD; 78 completed the study. They were selected from 244 subjects who were screened (see the article for more details on selection and randomization). The mean age was 66 years ($SD = 7$); 44 were men and 45 were women. Subjects were stratified by their performance on the 6-minute-walk test, using 350 meters as the cutoff point.

Summary. The mean distance walked at baseline among all participants was 366 ($SD = 99$) meters. Twenty-four weeks after randomization, the treatment group walked 37.9 meters farther than the control group (95% CI, 10.8–65.0). The authors reported that in their experience, the coefficient of variation of the 6-minute-walk test is 4%–10% and that a difference of 30 meters is clinically significant. The treatment group also showed significant improvements compared with the control group in submaximal cycle time; in the baseline dyspnea index; and in responses to the Chronic Respiratory Disease Questionnaire regarding dyspnea, fatigue, emotional functional, and mastery. The magnitude of the reported changes in dyspnea and mastery were considered to be clinically significant. There was no change in the pulmonary function tests.

Discussion. This study provides an example of the use of the 6-minute-walk test to assess the efficacy of a treatment (in this case, a rehabilitation program) among patients with COPD. It also demonstrates the ability of the 6-minute-walk test to measure change among individuals whose condition had changed according to other measures of exercise and quality of life. In terms of assessing the rehabilitation program itself, it would have been useful to have a longer follow-up period to determine whether the treatment effect was sustained after the end of the rehabilitation program (although the intensity of the rehabilitation program did diminish over the time covered by the study).

Kennedy SM, Desjardins A, Kassam A, Ricketts M, & Chan-Yeung M. (1994). Assessment of respiratory limitation in activities of daily life among retired workers. *Am J Respir Crit Care Med*, 149, 575–583.

Design. This article describes the development and testing of an instrument, the Q-ADL, to measure the impact of respiratory dysfunction on the ability to perform activities of daily living. The instrument was tested among retired workers and was compared with performance on the 6-minute-walk test, lung function tests, the Medical Research Council dyspnea scale, and the Sickness Impact Profile (SIP, reviewed in Chapter 5). Performance on the 6-minute-walk was measured not only by the traditional measure of the distance walked but also by asking the subject immediately after the walk about the magnitude of the breathing effort, using a modified Borg Scale. Only the results relating to the 6-minute-walk test are summarized here.

Sample. Out of 171 eligible subjects, 120 participated in part of the study. Complete spirometry and questionnaire results were obtained on 112 subjects; 75 were retired grain elevator workers and 37 were civic retirees. The mean age was 68.5 ($SD = 4.7$) years, and all were white men. Fourteen subjects did not perform the 6-minute-walk test.

Summary. The mean distance walked in 6 minutes was 554.9 ($SD = 78.4$) meters. The distance walked in 6 minutes was correlated only weakly with most of the other parameters reported. The Pearson correlation coefficients are as follows: with Q-ADL score, -0.13; with lung function, -0.07 to 0.44; with the SIP, -0.02 to -0.26. The only significant correlations were with FEV_1 ($r = 0.28$; $p < 0.01$), FVC ($r = 0.44$; $p < 0.001$), the SIP physical scale ($r = -0.22$; $p < 0.05$), and the SIP ambulation scale ($r = -0.26$; $p < 0.01$). The Borg Scale measuring the effort required by the test was significantly but only weakly to modestly correlated with the Q-ADL score ($r = 0.32$; $p < 0.01$) and FEV_1 ($r = 0.24$; $p < 0.05$). The score on the 6-minute-walk test was more closely correlated with FEV_1 and FVC than with the Q-ADL score but was less closely correlated than the Q-ADL with the Borg Scale and most of the SIP scales.

Discussion. This study provides additional data on the performance of the 6-minute-walk test in comparison with other measures of both lung function and more general health status (the SIP). The generally low correlations suggest that the 6-minute-walk test may be measuring a different construct, but more formal tests would be needed to verify this. Two other notes are in order: First, it is not clear from the description whether test runs of the 6-minute-walk test were taken before the distance was measured. Second, the generalizability of these results is limited by the fact that all of the subjects were white men from two professions.

Laupacis A, Bourne R, Rorabeck C, Feeny D, Wong C, Tugwell P, Leslie K, & Bullas R. (1993). The effect of elective total hip replacement on health-related quality of life. *J Bone Joint Surg*, 75-A, 1619–1626.

Design. This study assesses the impact of total hip replacement on health-related quality of life in patients with osteoarthritis. Patients completed a variety of measures, including the Harris Hip Score, Sickness Impact Profile (SIP), Western Ontario and McMaster

University Osteoarthritis Index, a time trade-off measure of quality of life, and the 6-minute-walk test. They were evaluated at 3, 6, 12, and 24 months.

Sample.   This article reports on subjects in a randomized controlled trial assessing a femoral head prosthesis inserted with and without cement. For the purposes of this article, the groups are combined and a single set of results is reported. Of 251 eligible patients, 188 agreed to participate. The mean age was 64 years (range, 40–75); and 53% were men. Three patients died, three refused to return for the quality-of-life assessments, and another 17 did not take the 6-minute-walk test (because of pain, chronic pulmonary disease, a motor vehicle accident, or refusal). The patients had been followed for varying lengths of time, ranging from a minimum of 3 months to 2 years.

Summary.   There was a significant improvement ($p < 0.01$) in all of the measures following the hip replacement surgery (except the work section of the SIP). Much of the improvement occurred within the first 3 months. The distance walked increased from 231 ($SD = 90.0$) meters preoperatively to 327 meters 3 months later ($n = 188$) and from 247 meters preoperatively for a subsample with longer follow-up ($n = 90$) to 408 meters 2 years later. No further details on the test's performance are reported.

Discussion.   Although the primary focus of this article is not the 6-minute-walk test, it does provide a useful example of use of the test in a different patient population (i.e., among individuals undergoing hip replacement). Not surprisingly, the distance walked does increase substantially following the operation. The study also shows that unlike some of the other measures of health-related quality of life, scores on the 6-minute-test continue to improve throughout at least 2 years of follow-up.

REFERENCES

American College of Physicians, Health and Public Policy Committee. (1988). Comprehensive functional assessment for elderly patients. *Ann Intern Med, 109*, 70–72.

*Anacker SL, & Di Fabio RP. (1992). Influence of sensory inputs on standing balance in community-dwelling elders with a recent history of falling. *Phys Ther, 72*, 575–584.

Applegate WB, Blass JP, & Williams TF. (1990). Instruments for the functional assessment of older patients. *N Engl J Med, 322*, 1207–1214.

*Applegate WB, Miller ST, Elam JT, Freeman JM, Wood TO, & Gettlefinger TC. (1987). Impact of cataract surgery with lens implementation on vision and physical function in elderly patients. *JAMA, 257*, 1064–1066.

Armstrong BK, White E, & Saracci R. (1992). Reducing measurement error and its effects. In *Monographs in epidemiology and biostatistics: Vol 21. Principles of exposure measurement in epidemiology* (pp. 115–124). New York: Oxford University Press.

Benjamin Rose Hospital, Staff of. (1959). Multidisciplinary studies of illness in aged persons: II. A new classification of functional status in activities of daily living. *J Chronic Dis, 9*, 55–62.

*Berg KO, Maki BE, Williams JI, Holliday PJ, & Wood-Dauphinee SL. (1992). Clinical and laboratory measures of postural balance in an elderly population. *Arch Phys Med Rehabil, 73*, 1073–1080.

Berg K, Wood-Dauphinee S, Williams JI, & Gayton D. (1989). Measuring balance in the elderly: Preliminary development of an instrument. *Physiother Can, 41*, 304–311.

Bernstein ML, Despars JA, Singh NP, Avalos K, Stansbury DW, & Light RW. (1994). Reanalysis of the 12-minute walk in patients with chronic obstructive pulmonary disease. *Chest*, *105*, 163–167.

*Bittner V, Weiner DH, Yusuf S, Rogers WJ, McIntyre KM, Bangdiwala SI, Kronenberg MW, Kostis JB, Guillotte M, Greenberg B, Woods PA, & Bourassa MG, for the SOLVD Investigators. (1993). Prediction of mortality and morbidity with a 6-minute walk test in patients with left ventricular dysfunction. *JAMA*, *270*, 1702–1707.

Buchner DM, Hornbrook MC, Kutner NG, Tinetti ME, Ory MG, Mulrow CD, Schechtman KB, Gerety MB, Fiatarone MA, Wolf SL, Rossiter J, Arfken C, Kanten K, Lipsitz LA, Sattin RW, & DeNino LA [FICSIT Group]. (1993). Development of the common data base for the FICSIT trials. *J Am Geriatr Soc*, *41*, 297–308.

Burns RB, Moskowitz MA, Ash A, Kane RL, Finch MD, & Bak SM. (1992). Self-report versus medical record functional status. *Med Care*, *30*, MS85–MS95.

*Butland RJA, Pang J, Gross ER, Woodcock AA, & Geddes DM. (1982). Two-, six-, and twelve-minute walking tests in respiratory disease. *Br Med J*, *284*, 1607–1608.

Carroll D. (1965). A quantitative test of upper extremity function. *J Chron Dis*, *18*, 479–491.

Clark DO, Stump TE, & Wolinsky FD. (in press). A race-and gender-specific replication of five dimensions of functional limitation and disability. *J Aging Health*.

Consensus Development Panel. (1988). National Institutes of Health Consensus Development Conference Statement: Geriatric assessment methods for clinical decision-making. *J Am Geriatr Soc*, *36*, 342–347.

Cooper KH. (1968). A means of assessing maximal oxygen intake: Correlation between field and treadmill testing. *JAMA*, *203*, 201–204.

Cress ME, Schectman KB, Mulrow CD, Fiatarone MA, Gerety MB, & Buchner DM. (1995). Relationship between physical performance and self-perceived physical function. *J Am Geriatr Soc*, *43*, 93–101.

Deniston OL, & Jette A. (1980). A functional status assessment instrument: Validation in an elderly population. *Health Serv Res*, *15*, 21–34.

*Duncan PW, Chandler J, Studenski S, Hughes M, & Prescott B. (1993). How do physiological components of balance affect mobility in elderly men? *Arch Phys Med Rehabil*, *74*, 1343–1349.

Duncan PW, & Studenski S. (1994). Balance and gait measures. In MP Lawton & JA Teresi (Eds.), *Annual review of gerontology and geriatrics: Vol. 13. Focus on assessment techniques* (pp. 76–92). New York: Springer.

Duncan PW, Studenski S, Chandler J, & Prescott B. (1992). Functional reach: Predictive validity in a sample of elderly male veterans. *J Gerontol*, *47*, M93–M98.

*Falconer J, Hughes SL, Naughton BJ, Singer R, Chang RW, & Sinacore JM. (1991). Self report and performance-based hand function tests as correlates of dependency in the elderly. *J Am Geriatr Soc*, *39*, 695–699.

Falconer J, Naughton BL, Hughes SL, Chang RW, Singer RH, & Sinacore JM. (1992). Self-reported functional status predicts change in level of care in independent living residents of a continuing care retirement community. *J Am Geriatr Soc*, *40*, 255–258.

Feinstein AR, Josephy BR, & Wells CK. (1986). Scientific and clinical problems in indexes of functional disability. *Ann Intern Med*, *105*, 413–420.

Fillenbaum GG. (1985). Screening the elderly: A brief instrumental activities of daily living measure. *J Am Geriatr Soc, 33*, 698–706.

Fitzgerald JF, Smith DM, Martin D, Freedman JM, & Wolinsky FD. (1993). Replication of the multidimensionality of activities of daily living. *J Gerontol, 48*, S28–S31.

Fleiss, JL (1982). *Statistical methods for rates and proportions* (2nd ed.). New York: Wiley.

Foley DJ, Branch LG, Madams JH, Brock DB, Guralnik JM, & Williams TF. (1990). Physical function. In JC Cornoni-Huntley, RR Huntley, & JJ Feldman (Eds.), *Health Status and well-being of the elderly: National Health and Nutrition Examination Survey I—Epidemiologic Follow-Up Study* (pp. 221–236). New York: Oxford University Press.

Gallo JJ, Reichel W, & Andersen LM. (1995). *Handbook of geriatric assessment* (2d ed.). Gaithersburg, MD: Aspen.

Gerety MB, Mulrow CD, Tuley MR, Hazuda HP, Lichtenstein MJ, Bohannon R, Kanten DN, O'Neil MB, & Gorton A. (1993). Development and validation of a physical performance instrument for the functionally impaired elderly: The Physical Disability Index (PDI). *J Gerontol, 48*, M33–M38.

*Gerrity MS, Gaylord S, & Williams ME. (1993). Short versions of the Timed Manual Performance Test: Development, reliability, and validity. *Med Care, 31*, 617–628.

*Goldstein RS, Gort EH, Stubbing D, Avendano MA, & Guyatt GH. (1994). Randomised controlled trial of respiratory rehabilitation. *Lancet, 344*, 1394–1397.

Gross-Andrew S, & Zimmer A. (1978). Incentives to families caring for disabled elderly: Research and demonstration project to strengthen the natural support system. *J Gerontol Soc Work, 1*, 119–135.

Guralnik JM, Branch LG, Cummings SR, & Curb JD. (1989). Physical performance measures in aging research. *J Gerontol, 44*, M141–M146.

Guyatt GH, Pugsley SO, Sullivan MJ, Thompson PJ, Berman LB, Jones NL, Fallen EL, & Taylor DW. (1984). Effect of encouragement on walking performance. *Thorax, 39*, 818–822.

*Guyatt GH, Sullivan MJ, & Thompson PJ. (1985). The 6-minute walk: A new measure of exercise capacity in patients with chronic heart failure. *Can Med Assoc J, 132*, 919–923.

Guyatt GH, Townsend M, Keller J, Singer J, & Nogradi S. (1989). Measuring functional status in chronic lung disease: Conclusions from a randomized controlled trial. *Respir Med, 83*, 293–297.

Herzog AR, & Rodgers WL. (1992). The use of survey methods in research on older Americans. In RB Wallace & RF Woolson (Eds.), *The epidemiologic study of the elderly* (pp. 60–90). New York: Oxford University Press.

Jebson RH, Taylor N, Trieschmann RB, Trotter MJ, & Howard LA. (1969). An objective and standardized test of hand function. *Arch Phys Med Rehabil, 50*, 311–319.

Jefferys M, Millard JB, Hyman M, & Warren MD. (1969). A set of tests for measuring motor impairment in prevalence studies. *J Chron Dis, 22*, 303–319.

Jette AM, & Deniston OL. (1978). Inter-observer reliability of a functional status assessment instrument. *J Chronic Dis, 31*, 573–580.

Johnson RJ, & Wolinsky FD. (1993). The structure of health status among older adults: A model of disease, disability, limitations, and perceived health. *J Health Soc Behav, 34*, 105–121.

Johnson RJ, & Wolinsky FD. (1994). Gender, race, and health: The structure of health status among older adults. *Gerontologist, 34,* 24–35.

Kane RA, & Kane RL. (1981). Measures of physical functioning in long-term care. In *Assessing the elderly: A practical guide to measurement* (pp. 25–67). Lexington, MA: Lexington Books.

Katz S. (1983). Assessing self-maintenance: Activities of daily living, mobility, and instrumental activities of daily living. *J Am Geriatr Soc, 31,* 721–727.

Katz S, Downs TD, Cash HR, & Grotz RC. (1970). Progress in the development of the index of ADL. *Gerontologist, 10,* 20–30.

Katz S, Ford AB, Moskowitz RW, Jackson BA, & Jaffe MW. (1963). Studies of illness in the aged: The Index of ADL: A standardized measure of biological and psychosocial function. *JAMA, 185,* 914–919.

Keller DM, Kovar MG, Jobe JB, & Branch LG. (1993). Problems eliciting elder's reports of functional status. *J Aging Health, 5,* 306–318.

Kelly-Hayes M, Jette AM, Wolf PA, D'Agostino RB, & Odell PM. (1992). Functional limitations and disability among elders in the Framingham Study. *Am J Public Health, 82,* 841–845.

*Kennedy SM, Desjardins A, Kassam A, Ricketts M, & Chan-Yeung M. (1994). Assessment of respiratory limitation in activities of daily life among retired workers. *Am J Respir Crit Care Med, 149,* 575–583.

Keram S, & Williams ME. (1988). Quantifying the ease or difficulty older persons experience in opening medication containers. *J Am Geriatr Soc, 36,* 198–201.

Kovar MG, & Lawton MP. (1994). Functional disability: Activities and instrumental activities of daily living. In MP Lawton & JA Teresi (Eds.), *Annual review of gerontology and geriatrics: Vol. 14. Focus on assessment techniques* (pp. 57–75). New York: Springer.

Kuriansky J, & Gurland B. (1976). The performance test of activities of daily living. *Int J Aging Hum Dev, 7,* 343–352.

*Laupacis A, Bourne R, Rorabeck C, Feeny D, Wong C, Tugwell P, Leslie K, & Bullas R. (1993). The effect of elective total hip replacement on health-related quality of life. *J Bone Joint Surg, 75-A,* 1619–1626.

Laupacis A, Wong C, Churchill D, and the Canadian Erythropoietin Study Group. (1991). The use of generic and specific quality-of-life measures in hemodialysis patients treated with erythropoietin. *Controlled Clin Trials, 12,* 168S–179S.

Law M. (1993). Evaluating activities of daily living: Directions for the future. *Am J Occup Ther, 47,* 233–237.

Lawton MP. (1988). Scales to measure competence in everyday activities. *Psychopharm Bull, 24,* 609–614.

Lawton MP, & Brody EM. (1969). Assessment of older people: Self-maintaining and instrumental activities of daily living. *Gerontologist, 9,* 179–186.

Lawton MP, Moss M, Fulcomer M, & Kleban, MH. (1982). A research and service-oriented Multilevel Assessment Instrument. *J Gerontol, 27,* 91–99.

Lee P, Baxter A, Dick WC, & Webb J. (1974). An assessment of grip strength measurement in rheumatoid arthritis. *Scand J Rheumatol, 3,* 17–23.

Linn MW. (1967). A rapid disability rating scale. *J Am Geriatr Soc, 15,* 211–214.

Lipkin DP, Scriven AJ, Crake T, & Poole-Wilson PA. (1986). Six-minute walking test for assessing exercise capacity in chronic heart failure. *Br Med J*, *292*, 653–655.

Magaziner J. (1992). The use of proxy respondents in health studies of the aged. In RB Wallace & RF Woolson (Eds.), *The epidemiologic study of the elderly* (pp. 120–129). New York: Oxford University Press.

Mahoney FI, & Barthel DW. (1965). Functional evaluation: The Barthel Index. *Md State Med J*, *14*, 61–65.

Mak VHF, Bugler JR, Roberts CM, & Sprio SG. (1993). Effect of arterial oxygen desaturation on six-minute-walk distance, perceived effort, and perceived breathlessness in patients with airflow limitation. *Thorax*, *48*, 33–38.

*Mathias S, Nayak USL, & Isaacs B. (1986). Balance in elderly patients: The 'Get-up and Go' test. *Arch Phys Med Rehabil*, *67*, 387–389.

*McGavin CR, Gupta SP, & McHardy GJR. (1976). Twelve-minute walking test for assessing disability in chronic bronchitis. *Br Med J*, *1*, 822–823.

Medline. (1995). (CD-ROM). Bethesda, MD: National Library of Medicine (Producer). Available from OVID Technologies, Inc.

Morris JN, Hawes C, Fries BE, Phillips CD, Mor V, Katz S, Murphy K, Drugovich ML, & Friedlob AS. (1990). Designing the national resident assessment instrument for nursing facilities. *Gerontologist*, *30*, 293–307.

Morris JN, Hawes C, & Murphy K. (1991). *Resident assessment instrument training manual and resource guide*. Natick, MA: Eliot.

Moskowitz E, & McCann CB. (1957). Classification of disability in the chronically ill and aging. *J Chronic Dis*, *5*, 342–346.

Myers AM. (1992). The clinical Swiss army knife: Empirical evidence on the validity of IADL functional status measures. *Med Care*, *30*, MS96–MS111.

Myers AM, Holliday PJ, Harvey KA, & Hutchinson KS. (1993). Functional performance measures: Are they superior to self-assessments? *J Gerontol*, *48*, M196–M206.

Omnibus Budget Reconciliation Act of 1987 (OBRA).

*Ostwald SK, Snowdon DA, Rysavy DM, Keenan NL, & Kane RL. (1989). Manual dexterity as a correlate of dependency in the elderly. *J Am Geriatr Soc*, *37*, 963–969.

Pfeiffer E. (Ed.). (1975). *Multi-dimensional functional assessment: The OARS methodology. A manual*. Durham, NC: Duke University.

*Podsiadlo D, & Richardson S. (1991). The Timed "Up & Go": A test of basic functional mobility for frail elderly persons. *J Am Geriatr Soc*, *39*, 142–148.

Reuben DB, & Siu AL. (1990). An objective measure of physical function of elderly outpatients: The Physical Performance Test. *J Am Geriatr Soc*, *38*, 1105–1112.

Reuben DB, Siu AL, & Kimpau S. (1992). The predictive validity of self-report and performance-based measures of function and health. *J Gerontol*, *47*, M106–M110.

Reuben DB, Valle LA, Hays RD, & Siu AL. (1995). Measuring physical function in community-dwelling older persons: A comparison of self-administered, interviewer-administered, and performance-based measures. *J Am Geriatr Soc*, *43*, 17–23.

Rosow I, & Breslau N. (1966). A Guttman health scale for the aged. *J Gerontol*, *21*, 556–559.

Rubenstein LZ, Schairer C, Wieland GD, & Kane R. (1984). Systematic biases in functional status assessment of elderly adults: Effects of different data sources. *J Gerontol*, *39*, 686–691.

Sager MA, Dunham NC, Schwantes A, Mecum L, Halverson K, & Harlowe D. (1992). Measurement of activities of daily living in hospitalized elderly: A comparison of self-report and performance-based methods. *J Am Geriatr Soc, 40,* 457–462.

*Salgado R, Lord SR, Packer J, & Ehrlich F. (1994). Factors associated with falling in elderly hospital patients. *Gerontology, 40,* 325–331.

Scholer SG, Potter JE, & Burke WJ. (1990). Does the Williams Manual Test predict service use among subjects undergoing geriatric assessment? *J Am Geriatr Soc, 38,* 767–772.

Sheldon MP. (1935). A physical achievement record for use with crippled children. *J Health Phys Ed, 6,* 30–31, 60.

Sherwood SJ, Morris J, Mor V, & Gutkin C. (1977). *Compendium of measures for describing and assessing long term care populations.* Boston: Hebrew Rehabilitation Center for Aged.

Siu AL, Hays RD, Ouslander JG, Osterwell D, Valdez RB, Krynski M, & Gross A. (1993). Measuring functioning and health in the very old. *J Gerontol, 48,* M10–M14.

Spector WD, Katz S, Murphy JB, & Fulton JP. (1987). The hierarchical relationship between activities of daily living and instrumental activities of daily living. *J Chron Dis, 40,* 481–489.

Stewart AL, & Kamberg CV. (1992). Physical functioning measures. In AL Stewart & JE Ware (Eds.), *Measuring functioning and well-being: The Medical Outcomes Study approach* (pp. 86–101). Durham, NC: Duke University.

Stewart, AL, & Ware, JE (Eds.). (1992). *Measuring functioning and well-being: The medical outcomes approach.* Durham, NC: Duke University Press.

Stewart AL, Ware JE, Brook RH, & Davies-Avery A. (1978). *Conceptualization and measurement of health for adults in the health insurance study: Vol II. Physical health in terms of functioning.* Santa Monica, CA: Rand Corporation.

Stump TE, Clark DO, Johnson RJ, & Wolinsky FD. (in press). The structure of health status among Hispanic, African-American, and White older adults. *Gerontol.*

Tinetti ME. (1986). Performance-oriented assessment of mobility problems in elderly patients. *J Am Geriatr Soc, 34,* 119–126.

Tinetti ME, Mendes de Leon CF, Doucette JT, & Baker DI. (1994). Fear of falling and fall-related efficacy in relationship to functioning among community-living elders. *J Gerontol, 49,* M140–M147.

Tinetti ME, Williams TF, & Mayewski R. (1986). Fall risk index for elderly patients based on number of chronic disabilities. *Am J Med, 80,* 429–434.

U.S. Department of Health, Education, and Welfare (DHEW). (1978). *Working document on patient care management.* Washington, DC: U.S. Government Printing Office.

Weinberger M, Samsa GP, Schmader K, Greenberg SM, Carr DB, & Wildman DS. (1992). Comparing proxy and patients' perception of patients' functional status: Results from an outpatient geriatric clinic. *J Am Geriatr Soc, 40,* 585–588.

Weiner DK, Duncan PW, Chandler J, & Studenski SA. (1991). Functional reach: A marker of physical frailty. *J Am Geriatr Soc, 40,* 203–207.

Williams ME. (1987). Identifying the older person likely to require long-term care services. *J Am Geriatr Soc, 35,* 761–766.

*Williams ME, Gaylord SA, & Gerrity MS. (1994). The Timed Manual Performance test as a predictor of hospitalization and death in a community-based elderly population. *J Am Geriatr Soc, 42,* 21–27.

*Williams ME, Gaylord SA, & McGaghie WC. (1990). Timed manual performance in a community elderly population. *J Am Geriatr Soc*, *38*, 1120–1126.
*Williams ME, & Hadler NM. (1981). Musculoskeletal components of decrepitude. *Sem Arthritis Rheum*, *11*, 284–287.
*Williams ME, Hadler NM, & Earp JA. (1982). Manual ability as a marker of dependency in geriatric women. *J Chron Dis*, *35*, 115–122.
Williams ME, & Hornberger JC. (1984). A quantitative method of identifying older persons at risk for increasing long term care services. *J Chron Dis*, *37*, 705–711.
Wolinsky FD, & Johnson RJ. (1991). The use of health services by older adults. *J Gerontol*, *46*, S345–S357.
Zimmerman SI, & Magaziner J. (1994). Methodological issues in measuring the functional status of cognitively impaired nursing home residents: The use of proxies and performance-based measures. *Alzheimer Dis Assoc Disord*, *8*(Suppl. 1), S281–S290.

2

Measures of General Health Status

Elena M. Andresen

OVERVIEW

All of the other chapters in this book describe questionnaires and methods that measure rather narrowly defined aspects of health status. The present chapter, however, takes on the challenge of defining general health status and reviews three key measures. Researchers, and more recently clinicians, may wish to describe the health of individuals, groups, or populations in a generic and multidimensional fashion. Historically, these broader measures followed functional assessment methods, as described in Chapter 1. Today, in addition to measures of physical function, health status measurement includes social and mental health and even role functions. This chapter will (1) describe the evolution of terminology and definitions of health status, (2) briefly describe some of the broad array of choices, and (3) describe three candidate measures in detail.

The three measures chosen for the present chapter are the Sickness Impact Profile, or SIP (*Bergner, Bobbitt, Carter, & Gilson, 1981); the Short-Form 36, or SF-36 (Hayes, Sherbourn, & Mazel, 1993; *Ware & Sherbourne, 1992); and the Quality of Well-Being Scale, or QWB (*Patrick, Bush, & Chen, 1973, Kaplan, Anderson, & Ganiats, 1993). They have been chosen because all three are respected and have impressive developmental and testing histories and also because they represent three very different types of measurement.

What the three have in common, though, is their use across the age spectrum. As the name implies, the SIP is primarily useful for measuring the impact of illness in persons who are not completely well. It has been used extensively for studies of patients with chronic diseases and with frail older adults. The newest, the SF-36, is able to measure health at the more "positive" or healthy end of the spectrum. It may be a poor choice for measuring the health of frail persons. But it is brief, and it now has a respectable number of publications on older adults to use as normative or comparison data. The QWB, the most complex and difficult measure to use, is based on a very sound theoretical foundation in which health is measured on a scale that ranges from normal, good health to death. In addition to these principles of measurement, it is a preference-weighted measure, and this makes the QWB a good choice for health services research applications where there is a need to calculate quality-adjusted life years (QALYs) as an outcome (e.g., Ganiats, Miller, & Kaplan, 1995). It also comes closer to the pure quality-of-life measures, for example, the time trade-off and the standard gamble methods (Gafni, 1994; for a review of these methods, see Patrick & Erickson, 1993, pp. 164–174).

At this point, few researchers would find these three measures interchangeable in the same settings or for similar populations. Underscoring their differences, the Medical Outcomes Trust (MOT, Boston, MA) has recently announced that it will distribute the SIP and QWB in addition to its own measure, the SF-36. The three tools represent a broad range of strategies for measuring general health status. This chapter is highly selective, for the sake of brevity, but it will provide the reader with an understanding of the issues that should be considered in using other health status measurement options as well. The order in which the instruments are presented below and in the annotated bibliography section is (1) the SIP, (2) the SF-36, (3) the QWB, and (4) a final section on studies that use combinations of these and other instruments.

There are other, briefer methods of measuring health status among older adults. The National Center for Health Statistics has used a variety of restricted and limited activity day measures in the National Health Interview Surveys (NHIS) to monitor the health status of Americans. These measures, well-described by Patrick & Erickson (1993, pp. 87–89, 120–121), rely on self-reports of days lost from usual activities (work, school, etc.) and also on "bed days" and days with restricted (usual) activities. The Behavioral Risk Factor Surveillance System (BRFSS) conducted by the Centers for Disease Control and Prevention (CDC) also uses questions about "poor health" days as part of its survey tool (CDC, 1994, 1995). The BRFSS offers a core four-question and an optional 10-question module for the state-based surveys. Adaptations of the NCHS measures were found to be somewhat successful in a study of health promotion among fairly healthy older adults (Kosorok, Omenn, Diehr, Koepsell, & Patrick, 1992), but they seem to suffer from "ceiling" effects. In a recent study, over 70% of community-dwelling older adults reported that they had no days with restricted activity or "bed days" in a year (Andresen, Rothenberg, Panzer, Katz, & McDermott, 1997).

Another very brief option is represented by asking a single question for self-rating health as excellent, very good, good, fair, or poor (E, VG, G, F, P; this is also a response choice to a question on the SF-36). This question, plus restricted activity days, is used by the Centers for Disease Control and Prevention (CDC, 1994, 1995; Hennessy, Moriarty, Zack, Scherr, & Brackbill, 1994) and was used for a large, randomized health promotion intervention among seniors (Wagner, LaCroix, Grothaus, & Hecht, 1993). A similar combination adding questions about activities of daily living (ADLs) was used in the 1984 national sample of the Survey of Income and Program Participation (Mutchler & Burr, 1991). A question about general health was asked even more briefly (E, G, F, P) in the MacArthur Field Study of Successful Aging (Schoenfeld, Malmrose, Blazer, Gold, & Seeman, 1994). Epstein and colleagues (1990) asked clinicians to rate geriatric patients on the basis of six categories of health (adding "very poor" to the usual five categories) as a screening device for potential consultive services, and a similar five-category question was used in the New Haven site of the Epidemiologic Study of the Elderly (Idler, 1993). Another short option, the SHORT-CARE (Gurland, Golden, Teresi, & Challop, 1984), measures health status among older patients who may require supervised or institutional care and includes the dimensions of function, self-care, cognitive function, and mental health. There are also longer and quite comprehensive instruments, for example, the OARS Multidimensional Assessment Questionnaire of Older Americans (Fillenbaum & Smyer, 1981) and the Nottingham Health Profile (e.g., Wikland & Karlberg, 1991); the latter has a strong tradition in British research. Finally, there is also a multinational instrument, WHOQOL, developed by the World Health Organization (anonymous, 1993, 1995), which is intended to cross age, cultural, and language barriers. This instrument is an impressive effort at a simultaneous development of a measure, rather than the usual translation and cultural adaptation of other instruments (Mathias, Fifer, & Patrick, 1994).

One of the drawbacks to measuring general health status is that it requires the personal report of individuals about their perceptions, and perhaps their symptoms and even their role functions. Among people whose health is relatively poor, including some older adults, there may be a need to rely on proxy or surrogate respondents for this complex information. Proxy methods are relatively straightforward for measures of physical function (see Chapter 1). The validity of using proxy respondents is less clear and poorly documented in the literature on general health status measures, except for the SIP, and (to a limited degree) the SF-36 (Epstein, Hall, Tognetti, Son, & Conant, 1989; *Longstreth, Nelson, Linde, & Munoz, 1992; McCusker & Stoddard, 1984; Pierre, Korner-Bitensky, Hanley, & Wood-Dauphinee, 1995; Reimer, Thurston, & Russell, 1995). This evidence is presented in more detail in the following discussions of each questionnaire.

Generally, it would be wise to reconsider the use of one of the complex multidimensional health status questionnaires if it is necessary to rely heavily on surrogate responders, or at least it would be wise to test formally the ability of the instrument to measure health by proxy. Methods for research using proxy respondents are thoroughly reviewed by Nelson, Longstreth, Koepsell, and van Belle (1990). The potential for measurement error may outweigh the theoretical allure of using some questionnaires when relying on proxies. In some cases, a simple, accurate functional assessment, such as those reviewed in Chapter 1, may still be the best measure.

Not only have health status measures changed; the terminology used to describe them has also changed (Liang, Cullen, & Larson, 1982). The early measures of health status, which were restricted to physical function and self-care (for example, the ADL-type scales), were often called just that: measures of function. With the advent of multidimensional measures, like the Sickness Impact Profile, the term *health status* was more appropriate. Some measures, even the SIP, are now called measures of *quality of life* or *health-related quality of life* (HRQoL or HRQL, e.g., Pocock, 1991; CDC, 1994, 1995). Each of these changes in terminology has expanded the meaning and importance of this area of measurement. The increasing interest in promotion of health, rather than prevention and diagnosis of disease, may have provided some of the impetus for expanded definitions of health status (Breslow, 1989). "Health promotion" strategies presuppose that interventions will improve both the health and the well-being of patients. These concepts are often very difficult to measure; not all benefits are measurable, and not all measurable outcomes are important (Liang, Cullen, & Larson, 1982). One of the slipperiest areas of measurement is well-being, yet we all understand, perhaps intuitively, that this is an important construct in the definition of health. Some criticism is aimed at the variety of applications of the term *quality of life* (e.g., Gill & Feinstein, 1994). For the purposes of this book, the term *health status* is used because it represents the broadest array of measures. This use conforms to the terminology of the Task Force of the Society of General Internal Medicine (Rubenstein et al., 1988). For a thorough discussion of the definitions and taxonomy of measures of health status, quality of life, and health-related quality of life, the reader is directed to the book by Patrick and Erickson (1993). There is also a journal, *Quality of Life Research*, devoted to these issues.

There is no single source for a health status or quality-of-life compendium for older adults. This deficiency, and the lack of a set of instruments that cut across care settings and a broad spectrum of health states for older adults, are among recommended research areas in a report issued by the Institute of Medicine (Feasley, 1996). The report notes, "Health-related quality of life is perhaps the most important dimension of health outcomes for older individuals" (p. 16). However, the report does not make specific recommendations about current assessment tools and recommends further testing and development of a "toolbox"

(p. 23). A bibliography of health status instruments and published papers, without comment, is given in *Medical Care* (Spilker, Molinek, Johnston, Simpson, & Tilson, 1990), organized by author, instrument, and diseases and therapies. A book by McDowell and Newell (1987) reviews health measures for a broad age range. Both may serve as useful references for a spectrum of questionnaires and tests. Another review of health status instruments, including disease-specific options and their use in special groups such as older adults, is provided by Patrick and Erickson (1993, pp. 113–142). A general report on issues involved in measuring health or quality of life in older adults is provided by Fletcher, Dickinson, and Philp (1992). A review of health status measurement, research, and human considerations specific to clinical cancer research is provided by Aaronson (1988). Additional discussions of health status measures are provided by Jette (1980), Kirshner and Guyatt (1985), Patrick and Deyo (1989), Pocock (1991), and Ware (1987). A formal study of randomized trials published in three leading medical journals concluded that such measures are underutilized, despite their usefulness (Van Zanten, 1991); possibly the interpretation of these "softer" outcomes limits their popularity. Some studies use multiple health status measures as a "battery" approach to measurement. For example, in a study of employment among liver transplant patients, researchers used the SF-36 and SIP (Adams, Ghent, Grant, & Wall, 1995); and the ongoing Beaver Dam Health Outcomes Study (*Fryback et al., 1993) uses both the SF-36 and the QWB. Other researchers have combined generic tools with disease-specific measures, for example, Callahan and colleagues (1994) combine the SIP and a measure of depression, and Kantz, Harris, Levitsky, Ware, and Ross Davies (1992) used the SF-36 and the Knee Society's Clinical Rating System. The Patient Outcome Research Teams (PORTs) have also carefully considered the potential of a variety of health status instruments as their outcome measures (including the SIP and SF-36). As in the Institute of Medicine report (Feasley, 1996), the PORTs have concluded that there is no currently available universal tool for such research; the selection of an instrument depends on the needs of specific studies. They also assert that there is still a need for specific, comparative research on health status assessment (Fowler, Cleary, Magaziner, Patrick, & Benjamin, 1994).

THE SICKNESS IMPACT PROFILE

Background and Development

The Sickness Impact Profile (SIP) was developed in the 1970s as a generic measure of health status that incorporates multiple dimensions (Bergner, Bobbitt, Kressel, et al., 1976; Bergner, Bobbitt, Pollard, Martin, & Gilson, 1976; *Bergner et al., 1981; Carter, Bobbitt, Bergner, & Gilson, 1976; Gilson et al., 1975; Pollard,

Bobbitt, Bergner, Martin, & Gilson, 1976). It is a measure that provides a health status profile from its multiple subscales. The SIP is copyrighted by the Health Services Research and Development Center (HSR&D) at the Johns Hopkins School of Hygiene and Public Health. Potential users should obtain permission to use it by writing to the center (HSR&D Center, Department of Health Policy and Management, Johns Hopkins, 624 N. Broadway, Baltimore, MD 21205) or to the Medical Outcomes Trust (20 Park Plaza, Suite 1014, Boston, MA 02116-4313).

The SIP contains 136 statements that a subject affirms only if the statement is true at the time of the SIP administration and is related to his or her health. Statements are arranged into 12 scales: Sleep and Rest, Eating, Work, Home Management, Recreation and Pastimes, Ambulation, Mobility, Body Care and Movement, Social Interaction, Alertness Behavior, Emotional Behavior, and Communication. The SIP provides a global score as well as scores for two dimensions (Physical and Psychosocial). The statements represent adverse impacts on health in a wide range of areas, including emotional, social, role, and physical function. Sample statements are "I do not maintain balance," from the Body Care and Movement scale; and "I walk more slowly," from the Ambulation scale.

A score of zero on any component (scale, dimension, or total score) of the SIP indicates that a person has no dysfunction due to his or her health; increasing scores indicate increasing disability or decreasing health status. Scores are computed by adding "weights" assigned to each statement (statements with greater dysfunction have greater weights) and are expressed as a percentage of the total dysfunction possible (100%). The SIP can be administered by an interviewer, either in person or over the telephone, or it can be self-administered. A computer-administered SIP form was developed and used successfully among rehabilitation clients by Maitland and Mandel (1994), and at least one study has piloted both card-read and optically scanned versions of SIP subscales and the SF-36 among nursing home patients, with mixed results (D. Ossip-Klein, personal communication, September 1995). The SIP takes between 15 and 45 minutes to complete, depending on the health status, age, and communication skills of the respondent. The SIP has been studied and found to be useful when completed by proxy or surrogate responders for deceased subjects or patients who are too impaired to answer for themselves (Epstein et al., 1989; Krenz, Larson, Buchner, & Canfield, 1988; *Longstreth et al., 1992; McCusker & Stoddard, 1984). In addition, the SIP is unique in having a published study of research subjects' favorable acceptance. Despite worries on the part of professionals about the content of questions that are personal and perhaps stressful, Carter and Deyo (1981) found that older arthritic patients rated the SIP very favorably from among a battery of questionnaires.

The SIP has been studied extensively for its validity in disease-specific populations by comparing it with biomedical and clinical rating scales. It has been found to be especially useful for arthritis research (Bendtsen & Hörnquist, 1993; Deyo, Inui, Leininger, & Overman, 1982, 1983; Katz, Larson, Phillips, Fossel, & Liang, 1992; *Sullivan, Ahlmen, Archenholtz, & Svensson, 1986; *Weinberger, Samsa, Tierney, Belyea, & Hiner, 1992) and back-pain (Deyo, 1984, 1986; Deyo & Centor, 1986; Follick, Smith, & Ahern, 1985; Roland & Morris, 1983; Stucki, Liang, Lipson, Fossel, & Katz, 1994). The SIP was judged insensitive to health improvements in a highly selected group of post–myocardial infarction patients undergoing rehabilitation (Ott et al., 1983). It was also found to be limited in assessing changes in hospitalized persons (MacKenzie, Charlson, DiGioia, & Kelley, 1986), although a more recent study found the SIP useful in predicting function among hospitalized persons (Wu et al., 1995). The SIP has been used effectively for other research on heart disease (Bergner, Bergner, Hallstrom, Eisenberg, & Cobb, 1984, 1985; Clark et al., 1992; O'Brien, Buxton, & Patterson, 1993; *Visser, Fletcher, Parr, Simpson, & Bulpitt, 1994) and lung diseases (Anthonisen, Wright, & Hodgkin, 1986; Bergner et al., 1988; Hasley, Brancati, Rogers, Hanusa, & Kapoor, 1993; the Intermittent Positive Pressure Breathing Trial Group, 1983; Jones, Baveystock, & Littlejohns, 1989; Juniper, Guyatt, Ferrie, & Griffith, 1993; McSweeny, Grant, Heaton, Adams, & Timms, 1982; the Nocturnal Oxygen Therapy Trial Group, 1980; Schrier, Dekker, Kaptein, & Dijkman, 1990). Other examples of studies using the SIP for diseases common among older adults include a study of depression (*Callahan et al., 1994), dementia (Krenz et al., 1988), hearing loss (Lichtenstein, Bess, Logan, & Burger, 1990), cataracts (Steinberg et al., 1994), stroke (de Haan, Horn, Limburg, & Van Der Mueien, 1993; Granger, Cotter, Hamilton, & Fiedler, 1993; Nydevik & Hulter-Asberg, 1991, 1992; Schuling, Greidanus, & Meyboom-de Jonghe, 1993), Parkinson's disease (*Longstreth et al., 1992), and incontinence (Hunskaar & Vinsnes, 1991; *Kutner, Schechtman, Ory, & Baker, 1994). The Physical Dimension of the SIP is used as one of multiple measures of function in the Frailties and Injuries (FICSIT) multicenter study (Cress et al., 1995). The SIP was used as an outcome measure in an assessment of adult day health care (Rothman, Diehr, Hedrick, Erdly, & Nickinovich, 1993), and it has been used in nursing home research (*Mulrow, Gerety, Cornell, Lawrence, & Katen, 1994; Rothman, Hedrick, & Inui, 1989). Four SIP physical function scales were used in studies of geriatric assessment and satisfaction among patients over age 70 (Epstein et al., 1990; Hall, Milburn, & Epstein, 1993). A variety of other health problems have been studied using the SIP, although many studies do not include an adequate number of older adults to allow comment on its usefulness. The health problems examined include end-stage renal disease (*Hart & Evans, 1987; Revicki, 1992), major depressive episodes resulting in hospitalization (Goethe & Fischer, 1995), chronic fatigue syndrome (Swanink et al., 1995), multiple sclerosis (Zeldow &

Pavlou, 1988), and head injury (Temkin, Dikman, Machamer, & McLean, 1989). Mean SIP scores for a wide variety of studies on patient groups are summarized by Patrick and Deyo (1989).

The SIP has also been evaluated for its cross-cultural use in British studies (Patrick, Sittampalam, Somerville, Carter, & Bergner, 1985) and among Mexican Americans in a Spanish language form (Deyo, 1984; Hendricson et al., 1989). The SIP has been translated and used in a broad variety of other languages (e.g., DeBruin, Buys, DeWitte, & Diederiks, 1994; Feio, Batel Marques, Borges Alexandrino, & Salek, 1995; GIVIO, 1994; Hunskaar & Vinsnes, 1991; Schrier et al., 1990; Schuling et al., 1993; Sullivan et al., 1986).

Scaling Variations of the SIP

The SIP is usually used in its full form, but its length has prompted some investigators to shorten it for specific populations. A 24-item version was developed specifically for studies of back pain (Roland & Morris, 1983); this has not gained wide acceptance, although it was independently tested and judged to be acceptable (Deyo, 1986). Hasley and colleagues (1993) felt that the SIP categories of Home Maintenance, Work, and Mobility contained statements that would offend persons hospitalized for acute pneumonia and removed them. Since the SIP asks about changes in activity because of health, the rationale here seems puzzling. However, the Work subscale can be especially problematic and confusing for people of retirement age and is occasionally omitted (e.g., McCusker & Stoddard, 1984; S. Hedrick, personal communication, September 15, 1995). There is also a short (68-item) Dutch version (DeBruin, Buys, et al., 1994; DeBruin, Diederiks, DeWitte, & Stevens, 1994) that has not been tested among older Americans. Some researchers have used a response format with a forced choice ("yes," "no") rather than making the usual assumption that every blank response is a "no" (Karlsson, Sjostrom, & Sullivan, 1995; Sullivan et al., 1993; Andresen, Rothenberg, et al., 1996), although this format may bias responses toward higher scores.

Gerety proposes a more salient version of the SIP for nursing homes, the SIP-NH (*Gerety et al., 1994). This 66-item version, although not yet used in many settings, is very thoroughly justified and yields a score that can be compared with other populations using the full SIP. Items that have been dropped are those (e.g., home maintenance, work) that simply do not apply to people in long-term care facilities and those found to have little predictive value for the total score.

SHORT-FORM 36

Background and Use

The Short-Form 36 Health Survey, or SF-36, is increasingly being used to assess health status in survey and clinical research and to monitor medical care outcomes

(Tarlov et al., 1989). It is a profile health status measure and its subscales do not provide a single unified index score. The development of the SF-36 followed the impressive work of the Medical Outcomes Study (MOS). An early version with 20 items and other measures from the MOS are well described by Stewart and colleagues in a book (Stewart & Ware, 1992) and other scientific publications (Stewart, Hays, & Ware, 1988; Stewart et al., 1989). An early publication described a potential "floor" phenomenon with the 20-item version (Bindman, Keane, & Lurie, 1990), and that is given as one reason for promoting the longer 36-item version (*Ware & Sherbourne, 1992).

The SF-36, as the name implies, has 36 questions about health that provide eight distinct scales as well as one item used to score "transition" in health during the previous year. Two of the eight scales (Social Functioning, Bodily Pain) are as brief as 2 items; the longest (Physical Functioning) has 10. Other scales include two role scales (Role-Physical, 4 items; and Role-Emotional, 3 items) and scales measuring Mental Health (5 items), Vitality (4 items), and General Health (5 items). Responses to each question are scored from 0 (negative health) to 100 (positive health). The subscale scores of the SF-36 increase as a person's health status improves. The SF-36 can be self-administered or interviewer-administered. Formal tests of data quality with different administration modes suggest that self-administration, especially for older adults, may yield problems such as missing data (*Andresen, Bowley, Rothenberg, Panzer, & Katz, 1996; *McHorney, Ware, Lu, & Sherbourne, 1994) and biased scale results (Weinberger, Oddone, Samson, & Landsman, 1996) but a higher overall response (Lyons, Perry, & Littlepage, 1994; *McHorney, Kosinski, & Ware, 1994). Special, large-print versions have been used (Kurtin, Davies, Meyer, DeGiacomo, & Kantz, 1992; Meyer et al., 1994), and card-read or optically scanned forms have been used or recommended for some applications (Anderson et al., 1995; Kurtin et al., 1992; Lansky, Butler, & Waller, 1992; D. Ossip-Klein, personal communication, September 1995). A computer-assisted telephone interview has also been used (*McHorney, Kosinski et al., 1994). A recent summary of methods among older adults suggests that no one administrative mode is favored, because of conflicting problems of literacy, hearing, and vision among older adults (McHorney, 1996). The review also suggests pretesting among a small group representative of the target population for which the SF-36 is intended. The SF-36 has been translated into a number of languages (e.g., Alonso, Prieto, & Antó, 1995; Bullinger, 1995; Dela Cruz, 1995; Perenger, Leplège, Etter, & Rougemont, 1995; Persson, Karlson, Bengtsson, Steen, & Sullivan, 1995; Sullivan et al., 1995; Ware, Keller, et al., 1995) and adapted to other English-speaking countries (Brazier et al., 1992; McCallum, 1995). For a current list of language options, contact the Medical Outcomes Trust or RAND (see "Scaling Variations," below).

Evidence continues to be published about the relative merits and potential problems of using the SF-36 for older adult populations. Internal reliability and validity are considered excellent from reports of the development and testing phases of the questionnaire (McHorney, Ware, & Raczek, 1993; *McHorney, Kosinski, & Ware, 1994; *McHorney, Ware, et al., 1994; Stewart, Hays, & Ware, 1988; Stewart et al., 1989; *Ware & Sherbourne, 1992), and in subsequent tests among patient populations (Bousquet, Bullinger, et al., 1994; Bullinger & Heidrich, 1995; Bousquet, Knani, et al., 1994; Jacobson, Samson, & DeGroot, 1994; *Weinberger et al., 1994) and other older adult groups (*Andresen, Bowley et al., 1996; Lyons et al., 1994; *Reuben, Valle, Hays, & Siu, 1995; Weinberger et al., 1996). Some investigators report that the SF-36 results in problems with inaccuracy or nonresponse problems for older adults (*Andresen, Bowley, et al., 1996; *Johnson et al., 1995; *McHorney, Kosinski, & Ware, 1994; *McHorney, Ware, et al., 1994; *Reuben et al., 1995; Sherbourne & Meredith, 1992; Tennant, Fear, Hillman, & Chamberlain, 1995), although one report found that both telephone and face-to-face interviews were acceptable to older veterans with multiple chronic conditions (*Weinberger et al., 1994). In a study of French- and English-speaking proxy respondents of older adults by Pierre and colleagues (1995), agreement with patients was judged "substantial" only on the Physical Functioning scale of the SF-36 and relatively poor or moderate on all other scales. In a study of a cohort of Swedish 92-year-olds, only about half were judged capable of completing an SF-36 with the assistance of a nurse, but among these respondents, a substantial "floor effect" was found only for the Role and Physical Functioning scales (Sullivan, Karlsson, & Persson, & Steen, 1995). Additional evidence on potential response and scaling problems with the SF-36 among older adults will be helpful in suggesting whether there are specific groups for which the scales are not useful.

There is conflicting evidence about the test-retest reliability of the SF-36. Andresen, Bowley, and colleagues (1996) reported good correlation estimates for the eight scales (from 0.65 to 0.87) for a mailed version of the SF-36 repeated after 1 month among community-living adults above age 65. Aydelotte, Andresen, and Podgorski (1997) also report adequate scale retest correlations for SF-36 among nursing home residents selected for relatively intact cognition; intraclass correlation coefficient ranged from 0.52 to 0.82. Another study of the reliability of the SF-36 conducted among older veterans reported considerable individual variation in SF-36 scale scores, including lower retest correlations for scales in the range of 0.26 to 0.37 (Weinberger et al., 1996).

For community-living older adults, there may be a "ceiling" phenomenon for scales measuring physical function (*Andresen, Patrick, Carter, & Malmgren, 1995), and some evidence of both ceiling and floor effects is reported by others (Reuben et al., 1995; Weinberger, Oddone et al., 1996). The ability to summarize across scales may ameliorate this scaling limitation (see "Scaling Variations," below; Andresen et al., 1997; Aydelotte et al., 1997). The use of the SF-36 among patients with debilitating chronic illness or acute events, frail older adults, and nursing home residents, where one might encounter "floor" effects, is not yet well documented (Aydelotte et al., 1996; Weinberger et al., 1996). Bousquet and colleagues reported encouraging results for the French version of the SF-36 among two patient groups (with chronic asthma and rhinitis); however, these patients were, on average, under 40 years old and could self-administer the survey (Bousquet, Bullinger, et al., 1994; Bousquet, Knani, et al., 1994). It is not clear that the additional items and scales contained in the SF-36 will completely remove the "floor" phenomenon found in the SF-20. Reports on further experience with the SF-36 need to be published to clarify its strengths and limitations for measuring the health of older adults. Testing of the SF-36 among older adults with cognitive deficits is especially needed (McHorney, 1996).

Use of the SF-36 (Brazier et al., 1992; Garratt, Ruta, Abdalla, Buckingham, & Russell, 1993; Lyons et al., 1994) in Britain has resulted in a number of tests of its utility in the general population and among older adults. It is unclear whether these experiences can be translated directly to American applications, but the careful documentation of these methods is instructive to any research audience. For example, the SF-36 was administered successfully by mail with an 80% response after up to three repeat mailings (Brazier et al., 1992).

The SF-36 was developed specifically for use in general populations, and it has been used in a variety of research and some clinical settings. The applications of the SF-36 are numerous, and a thorough bibliographic aid is available through a publication of the Health Institute (Shiely, Bayliss, Keller, Tsai, & Ware, 1996). It has been nominated as a potential tool for assessing functional status after total knee replacement (*Kantz et al., 1992) and has been used in research with patients undergoing total hip replacement (Katz et al., 1992); it has also been discussed as an outcome measure in hospital settings (Lansky et al., 1992) and as a predictor of the costs associated with health care in general medical patients (Litaker, Bronson, & Solomon, 1995). Researchers have used the SF-36 to investigate a variety of chronic and acute diseases including low back pain (Ruta, Garratt, Leng, Russell, & MacDonald, 1994), arthritis (Tennant et al., 1995), lupus (Fortrin, Neville, & Abrahamowicz, 1995), soft-tissue injuries (Beaton, Erdeljan, Hogg-Johnson, & Bombardier, 1995; Beaton & Richards, 1995), duodenal ulcer (Martin, Marquis, & Bonfils, 1994), Hodgkin's disease (van Tulder, Aaronson, & Bruning, 1994), renal disease (Kurtin et al., 1992; *Meyer et al., 1994), elective surgery (*Mangione et al., 1993), cancer (Muller et al., 1995), heart disease (Jette & Downing, 1994; *Johnson et al., 1995; Kromholz, McHorney, Clark, Levesque, Baim, & Goldman, 1996; Shaw, Miller, Romeis, Kargl, Younis, & Chaitman, 1994), peripheral artery disease (Bullinger & Heidrich, 1995; Schneider, McHorney, Malenka, McDaniel, Walsh, & Cronenwett, 1993), asthma (Bousquet, Knani, et al., 1994; Noonan et al., 1985; Okamoto, Noonan, DeBoisblanc, & Kellerman, 1996), allergy (Bousquet, Bullinger, et al., 1994), depression (Williams, Kerber, Mulrow, Medina, & Aguilar, 1995), and diabetes mellitus (Ahroni, Boyko, Davignon, & Pecoraro, 1994 [SF-20]; Bagne, Luscombe, & Damiano, 1995; Hanestad & Graue, 1995; Jacobson et al., 1994; Nerenz, Repasky, Whitehouse, & Kahkonen, 1992; Morton et al., 1996). There are now studies comparing the SF-36 with other measures of health status, including one scale of the SIP (*Kutner et al., 1994), physical performance measures (*Reuben et al., 1995), and the full SIP and other health forms (Katz et al., 1992). The SIP, QWB, and three SF-36 scales also have been compared among older adults (*Andresen, Patrick, et al., 1995). The SF-36 and QWB are used in the ongoing Beaver Dam Health Outcomes Study (*Fryback et al., 1993). The Dartmouth COOP charts were compared with an abbreviated SF-36 (McHorney, Ware, Rogers, Raczek, & Rachel-Lu, 1992). The SF-36 and SIP are used for the FICSIT Trials (Buchner et al., 1993; Cress et al., 1995), although the SF-36 is not applied in the nursing home sites of the study. The SF-36 was compared with utility measures (standard gamble and time trade-off) among cardiac patients, and the results suggest that the SF-36 does not measure patients' utilities (that is, preferences; Lalonde, Clarke, & Grover, 1995). Generally, the SF-36 fares well in terms of its ease of administration, and it may be as responsive as longer and more complex surveys in some instances. The evidence on its merits compared with other instruments for assessing older adults is limited, and most investigators still need to pilot test candidate instruments to ensure the right choice (e.g., *Fryback et al., 1993, *Kantz et al., 1992; Kurtin et al., 1992; Lubeck & Fries, 1993; Nerenz et al., 1992; Mangione et al., 1992, *1993).

Scaling Variations of SF-36

There are three groups publishing the SF-36—a situation that can be confusing. It was originally developed from the Medical Outcomes Study research by the RAND Corporation, whose scoring version is available as the RAND 36-Item Health Survey 1.0, or RAND 36 (Hays, Sherbourne, & Mazel, 1993; RAND, P.O. Box 2138, 1700 Main Street, Santa Monica, CA 90407-2138). A second scoring version (which varies only in the scoring of the Bodily Pain and General Health scales) is available from the Medical Outcomes Trust (*Ware & Sherbourne, 1992; Medical Outcomes Trust, 20 Park Plaza, Suite 1014, Boston, MA 02116-4313). The two versions are quite comparable and appear to yield similar scale results (Brazier, 1993; Hays et al., 1993). Both versions can be obtained free of charge by contacting and registering with the respective groups, although a variety of helpful publications, scoring programs, and later versions and translations may require a modest fee for copying and publication costs. A third source of information is the Health Outcomes Institute (2001 Killebrew Drive, Suite 122, Bloomington, MN 55425), which releases a hybrid scoring version of the

SF-36 as the Health Status Questionnaire (HSQ version 2.0). This institute has also developed condition-specific instruments to be used in tandem with the basic health status form (described below). This group offers a publication of population-based norms for the SF-36; these tables are useful for age-specific comparison data. Other normative data, comparing telephone and mailed modes of administering the SF-36, are given by *McHorney, Kosinski, and Ware (1994), although the results for older adults are collapsed into a single group of subjects aged 65 and older.

Subscales of the MOS have also been described by the MOS investigators. For example, the 10-item Physical Functioning Scale (the PF-10; Haley, McHorney, & Ware, 1994) might be considered a stand-alone measure for purposes other than assessing general, multidimensional health status. McHorney and Ware (1995) have published an alternative stand-alone General Mental Health Scale derived from the SF-36 and called the MHI-5. John Ware and colleagues describe a very brief screening tool of 6 items from the SF-36 (Ware, Nelson, Sherbourne, & Stewart, 1992) and a 12-item version (Ware et al., 1995). There is also, as of December 1996, a preliminary 12-item version from the Health Outcomes Institute called the Health Status Questionnaire-12 Version 2.0. Although a very brief form would be desirable in some settings, any revision will need to be tested among older adults in a variety of settings and populations before it can be embraced by either clinicians or researchers.

The Health Outcomes Institute also markets a variety of condition-specific forms (called Technology of Patient Experience, or TyPEs) to accompany its version of the SF-36 for use in an outcomes management system. These condition-specific additions may be of interest to those with very specific patient populations, but to date there is sparse evidence in the published literature regarding their use. As of December 1996, the available data protocols for TyPE forms covered angina, asthma, carpal tunnel syndrome, cataracts, chronic sinusitis, chronic obstructive pulmonary disease, depression, diabetes, hip fractures, hip replacement, hypertension and lipid disorders, low back pain, osteoarthritis of the knee, panic disorder, prostatism, rheumatoid arthritis, stroke, and substance use disorder: alcohol.

One of the drawbacks of the SF-36 is that it has eight different scale scores rather than a single multidimensional measure of health status. Investigators usually report all eight scores, although they sometimes use the General Health Status scale as a measure of outcomes, to be compared among groups or with other measures. A new pair of composite measures has been developed by the Health Institute (associated with the Health Outcomes Trust): the Physical Health Summary Scale and the Mental Health Summary Scale (Ware, Kasinski, & Keller, 1994). A manual can be purchased from the Health Institute (New England Medical Center, NEMC, Box 345, 750 Washington St., Boston, MA 02116) to assist users with the scoring programs for the two composite scales. These composite scales have been tested and appear to be useful for older adults (Aydelotte et al., 1996; Andresen, Rothenberg, et al., 1996).

QUALITY OF WELL-BEING SCALE

Background and Use

The Quality of Well-Being questionnaire was developed as a measure of health status that would include utilities (preferences) for different health states. It provides a single index score, summarizing information from multiple scale components. The development and refinement of the QWB are described by Kaplan, Patrick, and others (Kaplan, 1985; Kaplan et al., 1976; Kaplan, Bush, & Berry, 1979; Kaplan et al., 1993; Kaplan & Bush, 1982; Patrick & Erickson, 1993; *Patrick et al., 1973). The QWB has been especially useful in studies of cost utility and decision analysis (e.g., *Hornberger, Redelmeier, & Petersen, 1992; Mold et al., 1992). A very thorough review of the QWB (and similar measures) and its application to research and health-policy approaches requiring cost-utility ratios is given by Patrick and Erickson (1993). Discussion of the use of quality-adjusted life years (QALYs) in clinical trials is given by Ganiats and colleagues (1995).

The QWB in its traditional form (see "Scaling Variations," below) is administered in 15 to 30 minutes by a trained interviewer. It has two parts. In the first section, the interviewer reads a "symptom-problem complex" (SPX) list; if the person has experienced any of these items on any of the 3 to 6 days preceding the interview day (again, see "Scaling Variations," below), the item is checked for one or all of these days. The respondent is then asked to decide, for each day, which symptom was the "worst." SPX items are assigned standard weights that rank their relative severity.

The second part of the interview scores the person's level of limitation for each of three dimensions—mobility, physical activity, and social activity. Disability on each dimension is also weighted according to standardized weights. The weights assigned to the SPX items and to the levels of disabilities were derived from a ranking procedure using panels of subject "judges" and reflect, theoretically, societal preferences for different health states. The validity of these reported symptoms has been established among a variety of populations and patient groups (Kaplan, 1994; Kaplan, Anderson, et al., 1995; Squier & Kaplan, 1995). For each day, a QWB score is calculated using the algorithm: QWB Score = 1 − mobility step weight − physical activity step weight − social activity step weight − worst symptom score. The QWB score ranges, in theory, from 0 to 1, where 1 represents a state of "symptom-free" health and 0 represents death. An average QWB score is computed as the mean of the day scores. One can also use the QWB score to calculate "well years" or quality-adjusted life-years (QALYs) for each subject.

The QWB is usually given in person, sometimes using cue cards to aid subjects' responses. It has been tested and found to be acceptable as a telephone-administered interview instrument with mailed cue cards among relatively healthy, community-dwelling older adults (*Andresen et al., 1995); and it was also modified for telephone use to accommodate adult subjects with low educational levels (Patrick & Erickson, 1993, pp. 338–352). Neither mode of administration would appear to obviate the need for extensive training of interviewers (*Andresen et al., 1995; Bombardier & Raboud, 1991; *Visser et al., 1994). Kaplan, Ganiats, Rosen, Sieber, and Anderson (1995) have recently proposed a self-administered version of the QWB that is undergoing testing among older adults. This version also selects a single SPX item based on severity and does not require the subject to select a worst symptom. The QWB is available in a variety of languages (e.g., Spanish, German, French, Indo-Chinese languages).

Because of its complexity, the QWB has been applied in fewer settings than might be indicated by its careful composition and testing. It is unique among the instruments discussed here because of its application to studies of outcomes requiring a calculation of years of healthy life. This application is possible because of its preference-weighting component and the theoretical lowest-scored level (death). Research that has used the QWB includes large population-based studies such as the National Health Interview Survey (Erickson, Kendall, Anderson, & Kaplan, 1989; Patrick & Erickson, 1993, pp. 302–305), the ongoing Beaver Dam Health Outcomes Study (*Fryback et al., 1993), and a study of preventive services for Medicare recipients (*Gerrity, Gaylord, & Williams, 1993). The QWB also provided data for the formation of the Oregon Basic Health Services Act of 1989 (Patrick & Erickson, 1993, pp. 338–352). Erickson and colleagues (1989) considered the QWB the "gold standard" when they compared various health status scoring methods and concluded that other traditional indicators seemed to underestimate the level of health by about 10% to 50%.

The QWB's sensitivity and usefulness were endorsed in a pilot for a British clinical trial of angina pectoris therapies (*Visser et al., 1994), but the scale was not applied in the final study, because of practical difficulties and need for significant training of interviewers. In a comparison of the QWB, SF-36, and SIP among healthy older adults in Seattle, WA, the QWB was unique in demonstrating no problems of "ceiling" or "floor" measurement (*Andresen et al., 1995), but it was considered impractical for some applications where a brief and inexpensive measure is needed. *Ganiats, Palinkas, and Kaplan (1992) compared the QWB and the 12-item Functional Status Index (FSI) in a stroke prevention trial and found that the two measures were only moderately correlated unless the SPX section was discarded. The QWB was used successfully in a study of recovery from trauma, although the average age of this group was only 30

(Holbrook, Hoyt, Anderson, Hollingsworth-Fridlund, & Shackford, 1974); in a study of clinical decision making in older men with asymptomatic prostate nodules (Mold et al., 1992); and in a randomized trial of rehabilitation among patients with chronic obstructive pulmonary disease (Kaplan, Atkins, & Timms, 1984; *Ries, Kaplan, Limberg, & Prewitt, 1995). The QWB was used for some subjects in a study of nursing home residents (Siu et al., 1993) but was discontinued in order to ''reduce respondent burden'' (p. M10). The QWB also has been tested for use in studies of arthritis (Bombardier & Raboud, 1991; *Calfas, Kaplan, & Ingram, 1992), kidney disease (Kaplan & Mehta, 1994), and the effects of offering patients advance directives (Anderson, Kaplan, & Schneiderman, 1994); *Liang, Fossel, and Larson (1990) found it compared well with the SIP for research on joint replacement.

Scaling Variations of the QWB

An early version of the QWB that is still in use has a 22-item SPX list (e.g., Bombardier & Raboud, 1991), but this has been disaggregated into a list of 36 items for some uses (e.g., *Andresen et al., 1995) and augmented with new SPX items for other uses, for example, in nursing homes (Hays et al., 1996). Investigators have changed the wording of items and simplified or revised interviewing formats for specific uses (e.g., Hays et al., 1996; Patrick & Erickson, 1993). The current QWB version and foreign language versions are available from Kaplan (Robert M. Kaplan, Division of Health Care Sciences, Department of Community Medicine, School of Medicine, M-022, University of California, San Diego, La Jolla, CA 92093) or the Medical Outcomes Trust (20 Park Plaza, Suite 1014, Boston, MA 02116-4313). Another version, combining a 32-item SPX list over 4 days plus an independent list of 16 current symptoms, is available from the National Center for Health Statistics (Pennifer Erickson, Clearinghouse on Health Indexes, Centers for Disease Control, Room 1070, National Center for Health Statistics, 6525 Belcrest Road, Hyattsville, MD, 20782).

The developers of the QWB have responded to concerns that it is difficult to administer and is too sparse on mental health measurement by developing an enhanced, self-administered version called the QWB-SA (Kaplan, Ganiats, et al., 1995). Pilot tests suggest that this version can be completed in about 10 minutes, and larger field studies are under way to test it. If successful, the QWB-SA would prove to be a viable alternative to other generic health status measures and would be preferable whenever investigators need to use QALYs as a measure of outcomes. The QWB would then be equivalent to other societal preference-weighted measures, such as the 15-question Health Utilities Index (HUI-Mark 3) used extensively in Canada (Feeny, Furlong, Boyle, & Torrance, 1995; Torrance, Furlong, Feeny, & Boyle, 1995), and the British EuroQoL/EQ-5D (Dolan, Gudex, Kind, & Williams, 1995).

RECOMMENDATIONS

At present, there is no single measurement tool for assessing the health status of older adults that will meet the requirements of every setting, every special group, or every application (e.g., a clinical versus a research tool). The three instruments reviewed in this chapter have different advantages and limitations. For brevity, the SF-36 and SIP-NH may be preferred. However, the SF-36 may be inappropriate for the frailest older adults, and the SIP (in all versions) is inappropriate for some applications with especially healthy individuals. In addition, the SF-36 offers only an eight-scale profile of health status and would be difficult to interpret when a single index measure is required that summarizes across health constructs. The Physical and Mental Health summary measures may alleviate some of this concern and could be used in some applications. When the SF-36 scales are used as measures of outcome in research, investigators should consider which of the eight scales are their primary end points and are "responsive"—that is, which scales represent the constructs most likely to differ among study groups. An analysis plan that seeks to measure any change using all of the scales may suffer from statistical concerns of "multiple testing"; any differences detected on single scales could be criticized as a result of increased statistical chance of a falsely significant result, because of the many tests being performed. Currently, the QWB is the best choice for applications in health services and health policy research. However, it may not be useful as a screening survey. The new self-administered version has potential if it is piloted successfully with patient groups and older adult groups.

None of the three instruments discussed here was developed exclusively for use with older adults, but all three have the advantage of being the subjects of published research that covers a broad age range. Published studies of a full spectrum of adult ages allow comparisons with results for individuals or study groups and might be used in prospective studies of the changing nature of health status in the aging process. The SIP, probably because of its long history, has the most comprehensive record of use in studies of chronic diseases and among older adults. However, the SF-36 is quickly gaining a strong published record for its use in older populations and would be well suited for some applications. The use of health status instruments as clinical tools is still exploratory (see the introduction to this book) and will require further scaling refinements or perhaps new measures (McHorney, 1996).

This chapter has suggested the various values and drawbacks of these health status instruments. An additional concern is that some of the variability in health status measures may be an artifact of cultural diversity of different groups and not health differences (Johnson & Wolinsky, 1994; Krause & Jay, 1994; Linn, Hunter, & Linn, 1980; Williams, Agha, & Kelly, 1995). There are limited formal studies that have investigated this issue across the three measures (Deyo, 1984;

*Johnson et al., 1995; Keller, Ware, & Gandek, 1995; Patrick et al., 1985; Ware, Gandek, et al., 1995). Before making a final decision, potential users would still be wise to pilot test one or more instruments in the specific setting and population for which the tool is needed.

ANNOTATED BIBLIOGRAPHY

Sickness Impact Profile (SIP)

Development and Methods

Bergner M, Bobbitt RA, Carter WB, & Gilson BS. (1981). The Sickness Impact Profile: Development and final revision of a health status measure. *Med Care, 19,* 787–805.

Design. This article describes the multifaceted testing of the final 136-item SIP question-naire. The 1976 study reported here completed 6 years of development and testing. Scores on the SIP were compared with clinical diagnoses and other self-reported measures. In addition, various psychometric tests were performed. Test-retest reliability was measured using Pearson's correlation coefficient, rather than the now preferred intraclass correlation coefficient. Internal consistency was measured by Cronbach's α. The authors report that the SIP was developed to provide a measure of perceived health status that would be sensitive to detecting change over time and between groups, and across disease types, severities of illness, and demographic and cultural subgroups. Its intended use is to measure the effects or outcomes of health care for evaluation, program planning, and policy formulation. The SIP was intended to be sensitive to low-level negative impacts on health status.

Sample. The sample included 696 enrollees in a health maintenance organization (HMO; 80% response), a sample of 199 ill persons attending one medical practice (77% response), and smaller samples of patients with hyperthyroidism ($n = 14$), rheumatoid arthritis ($n = 15$), and hip replacement ($n = 15$).

Summary. Test-retest reliability was based on 53 persons surveyed a second time within 24 hours and overall yielded an *r* of 0.92; internal consistency resulted in an overall *r* of 0.94. Three administration formats were also tested: interviewer (I); interviewer-delivered, self-administered (ID); and mail-delivered, self-administered (MD; no retest on these). A decreasing level of reliability for less personally administered formats, especially mailed surveys, is apparent in the results.

The validity of the SIP was measured against independent measures of sickness and disability, and the results were in the hypothesized direction. There was greater agreement between the SIP and subjects' perceptions than with other criteria. There was less agreement between the SIP and the National Health Interview Survey's (NHIS) index of activity limitation (disability days), which included work loss and "bed days," than with subject perceptions. A multiple regression technique (multitrait, multidimensional; Campbell & Fisk) that yielded mean correlations among measures was also used. A complex table shows the SIP and other measures behaving in the hypothesized directions; the correlations with clinical judgments about the patients were lower; the correlations with self-rated scales were higher.

The clinical validity among the samples with diseases (n = 14 to 15 in each category) was also measured. The investigators used disease-specific measures of dysfunction or illness in each group, including physical (clinical) measures and other self-assessments. Details of the SIP score profiles are shown for the group with hip replacement, and they indicate a similar pattern of scores on the SIP scales at each follow-up, even as function increases (and the SIP scores decrease). The correlations of the SIP scores and the clinical measures for all three disease groups were moderate to high.

Discussion. This article is the best reference on the final version of the SIP. It describes the 6-year research project to develop this instrument. The paper highlights some of the strengths of this instrument in a broad range of the population that includes ill persons. Less obvious are the instrument's limitations for relatively well individuals. The statistics reported here on reliability and validity, while impressive, should be tested or compared with other populations similar to the one an investigator expects to include in his or her own research.

Gerety MB, Cornell JE, Mulrow CD, Tuley M, Hazuda HP, Lichtenstein M, Aguilar C, Kadri AA, & Rosenberg J. (1994). The Sickness Impact Profile for Nursing Homes (SIP-NH). *J Gerontol*, *49*, M2–M8.

Design. Because of the length of the SIP and the inclusion of some items that do not apply to the residents of nursing homes, these authors propose a shorter version. Both expert groups and statistical processes were used to identify items to remove. Correlations between the new SIP-NH version and the longer version tested the ability of the shorter version to predict the total score, and other comparison measures (here called "validity") were tested against the original and shortened version by using Pearson correlations. Subjects were interviewed using the 15-item Geriatric Depression Scale (GDS), the Folstein Mini-Mental State Exam (MMSE), and the SIP. For subjects in physical therapy, two other measures were also applied: A medical record review was used to compute a score for the Katz Activities of Daily Living (ADL) Scale, and physical therapists scored patients on the Physical Disability Index (PDI). Construct validity was tested by comparing the ADL and PDI with the new SIP-NH Physical Dimension score and comparing the GDS and MMSE with scores of the Psychosocial Dimension of the SIP-NH.

Sample. Subjects were residents of one academic Veteran Affairs home and four community nursing homes. There were 895 residents at the study sites; 205 residents could not communicate and were excluded (31%), 27 (3%) refused to participate, and 349 did not meet other criteria for the study. Eligible and ineligible subjects were comparable on some measures (age, ADL, education) but not on others (MMSE, ethnicity). An additional 83 patients who were eligible later refused (26%); as a result, there were 231 study participants (23.8%). The subjects were 56% women and 74% white; their average age was 78.2 years. Thirty-seven percent were on Medicaid.

Summary. Sixty-six items were removed from the SIP, including all of the items in the Work and Home Management scales. Adjustment of item weights was deemed unnecessary after further testing, so that the SIP-NH uses scoring methods similar to the original SIP except for differences in the total sums (denominators) in the scoring algorithm. The original SIP and SIP-NH scale means were remarkably similar; the lowest correlation was 0.91 for the Social Interaction subscale. Correlations of the SIP and SIP-NH versions with the validating instruments were also quite similar, usually within a few hundredths of a point; for example, the correlation between the SIP-NH Psychosocial Dimension and the GDS was 0.45, whereas for the original SIP and the GDS it was 0.46.

Discussion.   This 66-item shortened version of the SIP will benefit from additional testing conducted with different populations and using various study designs, including interventions. Testing should include test-retest reliability and validity. The current sample was restricted to nursing home residents who could communicate effectively, and a test of the SIP-NH administered to a surrogate responder should be explored. However, these authors have proposed a very sensible version that measures health status among frail nursing home residents, and the resulting scores appear to be comparable to those reported in previous SIP research and for other populations. The psychometric testing of the SIP-NH supports shortening the instrument.

Applications

Callahan CM, Hendrie HC, Dittus RS, Brater DC, Hui SL, & Tierney WM. (1994). Improving treatment of late life depression in primary care: A randomized clinical trial. *J Am Geriatr Soc*, *42*, 839–846.

Design.   This article reports on a randomized clinical trial (RCT) of an intervention aimed at primary care physicians and intended to improve compliance with recommended standards of care for depression in late life. Measures include the Center for Epidemiologic Studies (CES-D, reviewed in Chapter 5) and Hamilton depression scales and the SIP. Outcomes include mean changes in patients' scores on the SIP and Hamilton, as well as physicians' practices in diagnosing and treating depression. The CES-D was used as the case-finding tool and was considered positive for depressive symptoms at 16 points. All physicians in a large, general medical practice were notified that patients ages 60 and older would be screened for depression, and half of these patients were targeted for a "physician education" intervention.

Sample.   During 29 months the investigators contacted 4,413 patients during routine clinic visits. There were 115 patients who refused, 284 who were ineligible, and 247 who could not complete the CES-D; 3,767 (86%) completed screening surveys. The mean age of the screened patients was 68 years (range, 60–102). They were 68.8% women and 63.4% African American; 43.6% had 8 years or less of education. About 80% of patients who answered the question reported monthly incomes at or below $800; however, nearly 30% refused to answer this question.

Summary.   Six hundred and twelve patients scored 16 or more points on the CES-D (16.2%). Of those, 97 received a structured psychiatric interview, and 515 were eligible for a second-stage screening of depression using the Hamilton Depression Scale, of whom 254 (49%) agreed. Those who refused were slightly older and had lower mean CES-D scores than the participants. Among RCT patients with depressive symptoms, analyses showed that physicians' care for depression improved. At the patient level, the intervention and control groups both experienced a significant improvement in depression scores over a 6-month period, with no difference between the groups. Mean SIP scores were at or above 30% at baseline, and although scores improved during the study period, they were still above 25% after 9 months; there was no difference in SIP scores between the treatment and control groups. A random sample of patients of similar ages without depression had a mean SIP score of about 15%.

Discussion. This study provides evidence that a directed intervention by a physician increased the medical care provided for depression but did not reduce patients' depressive symptoms or improve their general health status (as measured by the SIP). The SIP Psychosocial Dimension might have been a more appropriate measurement tool for this specific study, and a comparison with instruments that screen for depressive symptoms would have been interesting. The fact that no single tool for screening depression was used consistently is difficult to understand, especially as there is no comparison between the CES-D and Hamilton scales in this study.

Longstreth WT, Nelson L, Linde M, & Munoz D. (1992). Utility of the Sickness Impact Profile in Parkinson's disease. *J Geriatr Psychiatry Neurol, 5,* 142–148.

Design. The utility of the SIP was investigated by comparing patients with Parkinson's disease (PD) and age- and gender-matched controls. In addition to descriptive analyses of the SIP results, other PD-specific scales were compared with SIP using statistical correlation. Subjects were screened with the MMSE and were given Hiehn and Yahr's PD scale (five stages) and the Columbia Parkinson scale (14 items, scale range of 0 to 56 points).

Sample. Forty-four consecutive clinic patients with PD were compared with 44 age- and gender-matched control subjects. The age range of the subjects was 18 to 88 years (mean age 64 for cases, 66 for controls). Twenty-four spouses were also asked to complete the SIP on the patient's function.

Summary. Two items of the SIP were most commonly affirmed: difficulty writing or typing (75%) and decreased sexual function (61%). The greatest dysfunction for PD patients was in the Psychosocial Dimension (especially Communication, Home Management, and Recreational Activities), rather than in the Physical Dimension. Correlations with PD scale ratings (Hoehn and Yahr's scale and the Columbia Parkinson Scale) were strong for most SIP subscales. The overall SIP score was correlated with Hoehn and Yahr's scale at $r = 0.59$ and with the Columbia Scale at $r = 0.54$. Patient-spouse intraclass correlations for the SIP were generally acceptable but ranged from poor to excellent. The 24 spouses tended to overestimate the dysfunction on the SIP scales of Sleep and Rest and Body Care and Movement and to underestimate dysfunction on all other SIP scales. The correlation between the spouse's SIP score and Hoehn and Yahr's scale was lower than for the patient-scale association (0.55 versus 0.63).

Discussion. These results show the general utility of the SIP as a generic measure of health status. As one would expect, the physical dimension and component scales were correlated more strongly with PD-specific scales than the psychosocial scales. The profile of PD dysfunction is demonstrated by the common items and scale results of the SIP. Importantly, the article also yields results on potential problems with spouse-surrogate responses to the SIP.

Mulrow CD, Gerety MB, Cornell JE, Lawrence VA, & Kanten DN. (1994). The relationship between disease and function and perceived health in very frail elders. *J Am Geriatr Soc, 42,* 347–380.

Design.   This is a cross-sectional survey of residents of nine nursing homes that was designed to examine associations between disease (from a standard chart review), objective function (measured by Katz ADLs), and self-reported health status (measured by the SIP). Other measures used in the study were the GDS and the MMSE. The study is part of the National Institute on Aging (NIA) project on "Frailty and Injuries: Cooperative Studies of Intervention Techniques" (FICSIT).

Sample.   Subjects were nursing home residents in San Antonio, TX, who were dependent in at least two ADLs but had no severe cognitive impairment. There were 3,440 residents in nine institutions: 1,259 were eligible by age criteria (60 or older), and 252 were eligible after screening. One hundred and ninety-four of these (77%) consented to the study. The average age of subjects was 80.6 years, 71% were women, 20% were married, and 28% were Mexican American.

Summary.   The mean total SIP score was very high among subjects (43.5; SD = 18.3), as were mean scores for the Psychosocial and Physical Dimensions (54.8 and 37.0, respectively). The investigators used a Burden of Disease (BOD) scoring system and reported an average score of 12.2 for the study sample. The mean GDS score was 6.3 (SD = 3.5), and the MMSE mean score was 21.4 (SD = 4.2). Pearson correlation coefficients between SIP scores and the BOD scale were quite small, but the SIP and ADL association yielded modest but statistically significant correlations (r = 0.34 to 0.39). Scores on ADL and BOD were weakly correlated (r = 0.14 to 0.21). In multivariate regression models, diseases explained 26% of the variance in SIP scores and 25% of the variance in ADL scores.

Discussion.   These authors conclude that disease, objective function, and self-perceived health status are interrelated but somewhat distinct constructs. The disease measure was strongly weighted toward chronic and medical diagnoses, and neither the BOD nor ADL measures included psychosocial and social health measures. Not surprisingly, the SIP was not strongly related to either measure, and the authors do not report relationships between the SIP and the GDS.

Rothman ML, Hedrick S, & Inui T. (1989). The Sickness Impact Profile as a measure of the health status of noncognitively impaired nursing home residents. *Med Care*, 27, S157–S167.

Design.   The purpose of the study was to assess the feasibility, reliability (via internal consistency), and validity of the SIP as a health status measure for residents of long-term care (LTC) facilities. Subjects were interviewed using the SIP, ADLs, the Barthel Index, the Life Satisfaction Index Z (LSIZ), and the Philadelphia Geriatric Center Morale Scale (PGCMS). The six characteristics the investigators considered important for an instrument were: (1) sensitivity to small but clinically important changes in moderate to severe dysfunction, (2) a multidimensional definition of health, (3) capacity for administration by the interviewer, (4) minimal burden on the respondent, (5) a reasonable administration time, and (6) adequate reliability and validity.

Sample.   There were 168 male veterans housed in veteran and community nursing homes from four Veteran Medical Centers. Subjects were selected by social workers. The mean age of the subjects was 68.

Summary.   The administration time for the SIP varied between 20 and 65 minutes (mean = 35). Internal consistency was fairly good, and α, alpha, coefficients varied from 0.60

to 0.84; most exceeded the original SIP development reports. The SIP scores were higher for LTC residents when compared with a prior published report on patients with chronic obstructive pulmonary disease (COPD). A matrix of correlation coefficients showed high correlations between the SIP and the ADL ($r = 0.74$). The LSIZ ($r = -0.31$) and PGCMS ($r = -0.40$) yielded lower but still substantial correlations. Both of these latter scales measure more psychological well-being, so this lower association makes some sense. Mean scores for dimensions and selected categories of the SIP were as follows: Psychosocial Dimension (27.1), Physical Dimension (37.3), Recreation and Pastimes (57.1), Sleep and Rest (42.5), Eating (14.1).

Discussion. The report is interesting in that it indicates some success at interviewing residents of LTC facilities, even those with substantially abnormal MMSE scores. The estimates of health status from this study provide comparative data on the SIP for investigators using either the full SIP or the briefer nursing home version (SIP-NH; *Gerety et al., 1994).

Weinberger M, Samsa GP, Tierney WM, Belyea MJ, & Hiner SL. (1992). Generic versus disease specific health status measures: Comparing the Sickness Impact Profile and the Arthritis Impact Measurement scales. *J Rheum, 19,* 543–546.

Design. The SIP and the Arthritis Impact Measurement Scale (AIMS) were administered to subjects in a longitudinal study of patients with osteoarthritis (OA) of the knee or hip. The similar dimensions common to the two scales (physical, psychological, and total health) were compared using correlation coefficients. The SIP and AIMS were administered three times to patients over 12 months. Correlations were based on change scores within measures (SIP and AIMS at different points in time) and on regressions between measures (SIP and AIMS at baseline).

Sample. A university-affiliated hospital database was used to identify patients with OA. Of 193 eligible patients, 150 agreed to participate (77.7%). Data were complete for 115 (59.6% of those eligible), and these were the study population. They were 87.0% women and 84.3% African Americans; mean age was 66.0 years. The sample was financially poor, with 63.2% reporting an annual income under $6,000.

Summary. Mean SIP total scores as well as the Psychosocial and Physical Dimension scores showed consistent decrements over the year. The AIMS scores showed less consistent changes. The SIP scores at baseline were high, indicating that the patients had considerable disability. The mean scores were 23.3 for the SIP total score, and 17.5 and 25.6 for the Psychosocial and Physical Dimensions, respectively. The SIP and AIMS were significantly ($p < 0.001$) correlated for the physical scales (0.75 to 0.76) and total health measures (0.70 to 0.73). Correlations for psychological health were statistically significant but smaller (0.37 to 0.40).

Discussion. The two scales gave similar descriptions of the health status of this patient group. However, the SIP seemed to show a greater decrement in health over 12 months than the AIMS. This may be evidence of the SIP's greater sensitivity to health status if these patients' health actually worsened, but there are no independently valid health measures with which to compare it. If the health status of patients with arthritis were to be compared with that of other patients with chronic diseases or the general population, the generic SIP would offer an obvious advantage over the disease-specific AIMS.

Short-Form 36 (SF-36)

Development and Methods

Ware JE, & Sherbourne CD. (1992). The MOS 36-Item Short-Form Health Survey (SF-36): I. Conceptual framework and item selection. *Med Care*, *30*, 473–483.

Design.   A 36-item short-form health survey instrument (SF-36) was constructed for the Medical Outcomes Study and was intended to meet the need for a brief, comprehensive, and psychometrically sound instrument to measure health status. The SF-36 was designed for use in clinical practice and research, evaluation of health policy, and surveys of the general population. It was intended for self-administration by persons 14 years of age and older or for administration by a trained interviewer in person or by telephone. The rationale for items is discussed in this publication (it is mostly based on the prodigious experience and expertise of these researchers). The history of the development of the SF-36, the origin of specific items, and the logic underlying their selection are summarized here. Ware and Sherbourne describe the content and features of the SF-36 and compare it with the earlier 20-item MOS short form.

Summary.   The resulting SF-36 is a multiscale survey that assesses eight health concepts: (1) limitations in physical activities because of health problems, (2) limitations in social activities because of physical or emotional problems, (3) limitations in usual role activities because of physical health problems, (4) limitations in usual role activities because of emotional problems, (5) bodily pain, (6) general mental health (psychological distress and well-being), (7) vitality (energy and fatigue), and (8) general perceptions of health. In addition, the SF-36 has one question about change during the last year, although that item does not add to the score of any of these scales. The previous SF-20 was limited to six health concepts.

Discussion.   This is the basic reference on the SF-36 and provides a concise review of its development. Among possible problems suggested by the authors are a lack of questions with enough detail about health, which may result in both "ceiling" and "floor" effects for persons who tend toward the extremes of health. They suggest that adding items may be desirable in some populations to make the SF-36 more sensitive. As the authors point out, a brief survey has to trade off between breadth and depth. In addition, the scoring yields in eight distinct scores rather than a single, summary measure of health status. These results make comparisons among groups complex because of multiple potential tests. An investigator should use the SF-36 scales with some a priori hypothesis as to the dimension (among the eight scales) that would be expected to differ among groups.

Andresen EM, Bowley N, Rothenberg B, Panzer R, & Katz P. (in press). Test-retest performance of a mailed version of the SF-36 among older adults. *Med Care*.

Design.   The authors describe the test-retest reliability and internal consistency of a mailed version of the SF-36 among community-living older adults and report on practical measurement issues associated with the use of a mailed instrument in an older population. A reminder postcard was used, and surveys were remailed to nonrespondents after 3 weeks. In addition to the SF-36, a computerized database on clinic visits was used to compute a comorbidity scale (Deyo/Charlson) to characterize subjects' medical conditions.

Sample.   Subjects were randomly selected from the patient lists of two clinics in Rochester, New York, overselecting those with higher comorbidity scores. A total of 253 of 422 older adults returned baseline surveys (60.0% of the original sample). Overall, usable test-retest responses were returned by 186 individuals. Of the 253 who returned baseline surveys, 62.8% were women, 55.4% were married, and 92.8% were white. Forty percent had not completed high school. The subjects were, on average, 76.5 years old ($SD = 6.8$).

Summary. SF-36 scale scores were not available for 2% to 5% of subjects, because of missing data. The mean SF-36 scale scores decreased significantly with increasing age and with increasing levels of the comorbidity score. The mean score for the General Health scale was 58.8 ($SD = 21.3$). Test-retest correlations for all eight SF-36 scales ranged from 0.65 to 0.87, and internal consistency (Cronbach's α) for scales ranged from 0.80 to 0.92.

Discussion. The internal consistency reported here duplicates or exceeds that found in other studies of older adults. The test-retest estimates are high, especially in light of the long 1-month repeated mailing. The fairly selected nature of the sample may lead to overestimation of reliability for other applications among older adults.

McHorney CA, Ware JE, Lu JFR, & Sherbourne CD. (1994). The MOS 36-Item Short-Form Health Survey (SF-36): III. Tests of data quality, scaling assumptions, and reliability across diverse patient groups. *Med Care, 32,* **40–66.**

Design. This is a report of the psychometric properties of the eight scales of the SF-36 using data from the Medical Outcomes Study, with specific comparisons among population groups defined by disease, age, and other sociodemographic parameters. The SF-36 was self-administered. A clinician form was also used to identify several medical conditions. A brief composite version of the Center for Epidemiologic Studies Depression survey (CES-D, reviewed in Chapter 5) was also used; those with positive responses were called to complete the National Institute of Mental Health's Diagnostic Interview Schedule (DIS). The authors report data completion and internal measures of item consistency, validity, and reliability of the SF-36. "Floor" and "ceiling" effects were defined using statistical tests of skewness.

Sample. Data are from subjects who visited medical clinics in three cities (Boston, Chicago, and Los Angeles) during nine days in 1986. A total of 22,462 patients completed the survey (70%). Patients ($n = 4,842$) selected for their medical conditions were enrolled in a longitudinal study, and 3,445 were available for analysis (71%). Twenty-four subgroups were identified by disease and other characteristics among those in the longitudinal study. There were 987 subjects aged 65 and older (28.6%). Overall, the group was 61.7% women and 76.2% white, and 7.3% were defined as being "in poverty."

Summary. Specific items were missed by as many as 5.9% subjects (for a Physical Function scale item on vigorous activities) to as few as 1.1 % subjects (for the General Health scale question on general health status, which is question number one of the SF-36; on average, 3.9% of responses were missing for individual items. Completeness of data varied by subgroup. It was inversely related to age and was lower for women (possibly owing to their older ages), for minority groups, and for those with less education or in poverty (the latter three factors may be interrelated). Scores could be computed for about 90% or more of subjects in specific subgroups, and completeness of the scale varied by subgroup. The authors reported that most subgroups showed the full range of item responses; but formal tests of skewness implicated the Role-Physical and Role-Emotional scales for both "floor" and "ceiling" effects and the Social Functioning, Physical Functioning, and Bodily Pain scales as showing some "ceiling" effects. As expected, "ceiling" effects were more problematic in healthy young patients, and "floor" effects were more pronounced in the oldest patients and among those with medical conditions. The authors summarized various psychometric tests by specifying cutoffs for acceptable levels of test statistics and noted that for the entire sample, each test yielded impressive results. Analyses of subgroups suggested that item discrimination was lower among those with low education and among some patient groups; psychometric tests tended to be lower among the oldest patients (aged 75 and older), nonwhites, those with less education, and those in poverty.

Discussion.   This report is important, as it describes the performance of the SF-36 among different groups. The results are good for older adults, but some limitations are suggested, including lower response and the potential for "floor" effects for older adults due to age, medical problems, or both. The authors tested multiple psychometric properties across 24 subgroups; the article can be used as a basic reference, but specific groups should be tested again to confirm that the findings reported here are not a statistical artifact of conducting numerous tests.

McHorney C, Kosinski M, & Ware JE. (1994). Comparisons of the costs and quality of norms for the SF-36 Health Survey collected by mail versus telephone interview: Results from a national survey. *Med Care, 32,* 551–567.

Design.   Computer-assisted telephone interviews were compared with mailed surveys of the SF-36 in terms of quality of responses and of data. Subjects were selected from the General Social Survey (GSS) of the 1990 National Survey of Functional Health Status (NSFHS) to provide population norms for the SF-36. Eighty percent were chosen randomly to receive the mail survey, which included a $2 incentive, a mailed postcard reminder, and follow-up to nonrespondents by mail at 2 weeks and by telephone after 1 month. Computer-assisted telephone interviews (CATI) were preceded by a mailed letter, but no incentive was offered. Subjects selected for telephone interviews who had no telephones or who requested it were sent surveys by mail. The surveys contained 104 items, including the SF-36, a checklist of standardized chronic medical conditions, and indicators of social support and quality of life.

Sample.   Subjects were selected by a two-stage probability sample resulting in 2,909 households in the United States. Older adults were oversampled, and the final sample had 3,252 individuals. Ten percent of subjects from the mailed survey arm were not located, versus 12% of those selected for telephone surveys.

Summary.   Surprisingly, response was higher for the mailed surveys than the telephone surveys (79.2% versus 68.9%, $p < 0.05$), although it is not clear what role the incentive or the fact that the telephone surveys were computer-assisted may have played in this increased response. Costs for telephone surveys were higher than for mailed surveys ($47.86 versus $27.07 per completed written survey). However, mailed surveys suffered from having more missing items (mean of 1.59 items versus 0.49), and they may have been biased by age (more nonresponse among young subjects by mail). Alpha (α) coefficients for internal consistency were equal overall for the two modes (median = 0.85), but there were some differences, possibly random, for individual scales. Mean scores for the SF-36 were lower among mailed respondents, and there were "floor" and "ceiling" effects for mailed, but not telephone, respondents. There were also differences in chronic conditions, with mailed survey subjects listing more conditions. Normative data are presented by broad age groupings for both modes of administration.

Discussion. This manuscript is crucial as a general guide to SF-36 scale norms. Of particular interest is the breakdown of scale norms by mode of administration. Older adults are collapsed into a single category aged 65 and older, and more finely defined age and gender groups would be needed for some users of the SF-36 with older adult populations. Despite the sparse information about older adults, trade-offs between the two modes of administration are well defined by the authors, and this should help investigators make a choice. The lower cost and greater response with mailed surveys are encouraging.

Reuben DR, Valle LA, Hays RD, & Siu AL. (1995). Measuring physical function in community-dwelling older persons: A comparison of self-administered, interviewer-administered, and performance-based measures. *J Am Geriatr Soc*, *43*, 17–23.

Design. The investigators compared the performance of several measures of health status among older adults as part of a program designed to recruit frail older adults for a consulting geriatric assessment program. Subjects self-administered the Functional Status Questionnaire (FSQ), Basic and Intermediate Activities of Daily Living scales, and the SF-36; and they were interviewed using the Katz Activities of Daily Living (ADL) and the Older Americans Resources and Services Instrumental Activities of Daily Living (OARS-IADL). They also completed the Physical Performance Test (PPT) and were observed by a trained interviewer. Instruments were (1) compared for correlations among similar measures; (2) "validated" against the performance-based measure, the PPT; and (3) submitted to psychometric tests, including principal components analysis and internal consistency (Cronbach's α).

Sample. Eighty-three older adults were recruited for a geriatric assessment program from community service sites; only 72 returned the SF-36, which could be taken home and returned by mail, but all other measures were complete. The mean age of subjects was 76 (range, 64–92), and 54% were women. The majority were white (90%), and 75% had at least a high school education.

Summary. Mean SF-36 scores are given for all eight scales and ranged from a low of 63.5 (General Health) to a high of 74.8 (Role-Emotional). Despite the fact that the population was supposed to consist of frail older adults, over half of the subjects received scores of 100 (perfect health) on the SF-36 Role-Emotional and Physical scales, as well as the Katz ADL, OARS IADL, and FSQ Basic Activities of Daily Living scales. The only scale that might be considered to have any problem with "floor" effects was the SF-36 Physical-Role scale, where 20% of subjects received scores of zero. Estimates of internal consistency were good for the SF-36 scales and ranged from 0.84 (General Health) to 0.93 (Role Functioning-Physical); these were higher than all of the other measures used in the study. Correlations among similar measures were high; for example, between the SF-36 Physical Functioning and FSQ-IADL, $r = 0.76$. All six measures of physical function demonstrated unidimensionality on principal components analysis (i.e., each scale represented a single dimension). When these researchers used a technique to explore answers to items in different scales that measured similar tasks, most responses were consistent for self-administered measures. However, answers about similar tasks differed for some subjects between interviews or performance measures and self-administered items. Compared with an objective measure, i.e., performance-based assessment of function, the SF-36 scales were poorly or minimally correlated ($r < 0.25$) except for the Role-Physical scale ($r = 0.50$). The Physical Functioning scale was weakly correlated with the performance-based PPT ($r = 0.26$).

Discussion.   This is a good example of assessing the relative merits of different potential measures in a study. The authors were specifically interested in physical function and, not surprisingly, found that the more global measures of health status (e.g., the SF-36 General Health scale) and other constructs (e.g., SF-36 Energy/Fatigue scale) measured something different. The PPT performance-based measure, when time and money allow, is clearly a very effective measure of the single construct of physical function, but its usefulness would be limited if a more global measure of health status was required.

Weinberger M, Nagle B, Hanlon JT, Samsa GP, Schmader K, Landsman PB, Uttech KM, Cowper PA, Cohen HJ, & Feussner JR. (1994). Assessing health-related quality of life in elderly outpatients: Telephone versus face-to-face administration. *J Am Geriatr Soc*, *42*, 1295–1299.

Design.   As part of a randomized trial, the investigators compared two modes of administering the SF-36. Telephone and face-to-face interviews were compared for internal consistency (Cronbach's α) and systematic mean differences.

Sample.   Subjects were male veterans who were patients of an ambulatory care clinic. Only patients aged 65 and older who were prescribed at least 5 medications were eligible. Those with cognitive impairment (and no proxy to answer for them) and veterans in nursing homes were excluded. The study enrolled and randomized 208 persons for a clinical trial of a pharmacist intervention for older outpatients. At the 1-year follow-up, 173 patients were interviewed by telephone. Only 42 of these were eligible for the SF-36 face-to-face survey, and 31 completed it. The subjects had a mean age of 68.5 years; 80.7% were white. Their mean educational level was 10.9 years.

Summary.   Mean scale scores for the SF-36 were similar by telephone and face-to-face modes, but seven of the eight SF-36 scale scores were the same or higher on the latter (only the Vitality scale yielded a higher score on the telephone). Alpha coefficients (internal consistency estimates) were somewhat higher on seven of eight scales for face-to-face administration (only Role-Emotional was marginally lower, 0.82 versus 0.85). Importantly, the telephone surveys were administered in less time than the face-to-face interviews (10.2 versus 14.0 minutes).

Discussion.   If one accepts that face-to-face questionnaires are the best standard mode of administering a survey, this report is important in that it confirms the need for caution in the use of telephone administration of the SF-36. However, it is surprising that the telephone interviews, which require a good deal of communication by both parties, were briefer. The patient group studied is not representative of a general population of older adults, so that the experiences of the investigators might be viewed with some caution. The mean SF-36 scale scores provide some comparative data for male patient groups with multiple chronic conditions.

Applications

Johnson PA, Goldman L, Orav EJ, Garcia T, Pearson SD, & Lee TH. (1995). Comparison of the Medical Outcomes Study Short-Form 36-item health survey in black and white patients with acute chest pain. *Med Care*, *33*, 145–160.

Design. This is a cross-sectional survey of emergency department (ED) patients with chest pain in which baseline clinical data were collected by physicians, research nurses, or both. Nurses also collected information from medical records. Final diagnoses of acute myocardial infarction (AMI) and unstable angina were determined by a study protocol. Interviews were conducted within about 48 hours of hospital admission or by telephone for discharged persons and included the SF-36 and the Specific Activity Scale (SAS), a four-class scale of cardiovascular function. The SF-36 scores of African American and white patients were compared before and after adjustment for confounding variables. The potential for different scaling of the SF-36 by race was checked by comparing white and African American patients' correlations among the eight SF-36 scales and scale internal consistency (Cronbach's α).

Sample. Persons age 30 and older with a complaint of acute chest pain were eligible; 1,903 were identified, and 1,286 (68%) consented. Of the latter, 10% were dropped because they were not members of one of the two racial groups of interest, and 1,160 made up the final sample. Sixty-nine percent ($n = 803$) were white and 31% (357) were African American. White patients were older than African American patients (mean age = 59 versus 52 years, $p < 0.05$), and there were more men among the white patients (59% versus 33%).

Summary. White patients had more extensive histories of prior clinically identified cardiovascular disease (e.g., prior myocardial infarction, angina) but better Specific Activity Scale class profiles. African Americans had more diabetes and hypertension. Fifty-three percent of African American patients were admitted to the hospital versus 69% of white patients; of those admitted, slightly more white patients were diagnosed as having AMI (15% versus 11%) and significantly more were diagnosed as having acute ischemic heart disease (61% versus 36%; $p < 0.05$). African American patients had lower SF-36 scores for all scales. In multivariate linear regression models, adding demographic and comorbidity variables reduced this difference between the patient groups to statistically insignificant levels. Correlations among scales showed similar patterns of magnitude for both patient groups, and internal consistency for all scales was also similar between groups. Medical and demographic variables were also correlated in similar patterns with SF-36 scale scores for African American and white patients, with the exception of male gender, which correlated with lower scores in African American patients and higher scale scores in white patients.

Discussion. This study is an important addition to our understanding of the performance of the SF-36 among culturally and racially diverse patient groups. Using psychometric analyses similar to those used in the development and testing of the SF-36, the authors found that the SF-36 provides similar information for African American and white ED patients with chest pain. The many exploratory analyses might be viewed with some caution and interpreted as a descriptive process until other research confirms similar patterns. See, for example, Johnson and Wolinsky (1994) for an in-depth analysis of the SF-36 scaling results among older whites and African-Americans.

Kantz ME, Harris WJ, Levitsky K, Ware JE, & Ross Davies A. (1992). Methods for assessing condition-specific and generic functional status outcomes after total knee replacement. *Med Care, 30,* MS240–MS252.

Design. The generic SF-36 and a modified SF-36 were compared with the Knee Society's Clinical Rating System (KSCRS) for 66 patients undergoing total knee replacement.

Analyses were conducted of the correlations among the generic SF-36, condition-specific scales based on the SF-36, and the condition-specific measures based on the KSCRS. The authors repeated some of SF-36 specifically expected to be related to knee problems: the Physical Functioning, Role-Physical, and Bodily Pain scales. Various psychometric tests were conducted on the SF-36 as well.

Sample.   Of 125 potential patients from one practice, 80 were eligible for the survey and were mailed the SF-36; 66 of the forms (82.5%) were returned. Those who returned the forms were a mean 7.5 years postsurgery, with a mean age of 77 years, and about half were women. Nonrespondents were older and further postsurgery (mean =10 years).

Summary.   Of the eight SF-36 scales, the lowest mean score was reported for the Role-Physical scale (51.1). Cronbach's α was high (0.77 to 0.90) for internal reliability for all scales of the SF-36. Correlations were high among the SF-36 scales, but the modified Knee Society score was correlated at only $r = 0.02$ with the generic SF-36 Physical Functioning score, at only $r = 0.05$ with the generic SF-36 Role-Physical score, and at only $r = 0.01$ with the Bodily Pain score. It appeared that the condition-specific SF-36 battery and the condition-specific Knee Society scales were more highly correlated. If patients also had back problems, the regression results showed significant relationships with the SF-36 physical scale scores, but not so for other comorbidities; however, other comorbidities had a significant impact on the generic Role-Physical SF-36 scale score. The results include complete correlations tables with patients split into two groups, with and without comorbidities; they showed stronger relationships among the latter.

Discussion.   Clinical indicators based on X-rays and range of motion were only weakly related to all measures of function, a finding that is consistent with other studies of health status in patient groups (e.g., Deyo et al., 1982, 1983). The article provides evidence of the benefit of using more global ratings of health status to study the outcomes of patient groups. The decision of any investigator to use a standard SF-36 or a disease-specific modification may rely on the ability to compare the former with external population norms.

Mangione CM, Marcantonio ER, Goldman L, Cook EF, Donaldson MC, Sugarbaker DJ, Poss R, & Lee TH. (1993). Influence of age on measurement of health status in patients undergoing elective surgery. *J Am Geriatr Soc*, *41*, 377–383.

Design.   The authors report on the cross-sectional measurement of preoperative health status among older patients in a teaching hospital. In addition to the SF-36, the study measures included the Specific Activity Scale (SAS) for ranking subjects on four levels of function and a rating question ranking global health on a scale of 1 to 100. The study also collected data from a history and physical for the Charlson Comorbidity Index and ranked patients using the American Society of Anesthesiologist's Physical Status Class (ASA Class). Mean scores on the SF-36 were compared across seven procedure groups using Pearson product-moment correlation coefficients. Linear regression was also performed with SF-36 scores as the outcome and age as the independent variable, after controlling for other covariates. Internal consistency (by Cronbach's α) was also calculated for each subscale for two age groups.

Sample.   Patients admitted to a single hospital who were aged 50 or older were eligible. Subjects were selected from among admissions for major, elective, noncardiac operations. Subjects were excluded if they were not able to speak English or had other cognitive or communication problems. A total of 818 eligible subjects gave consent, and 745 (91%)

were available for the analyses reported here. The patient group was 54% women and 96% white. The mean age was 67 years (range, 50–89); 37% were older than 70.

Summary.   Subjects were grouped by age (≤ 70, > 70) for comparison. Older subjects had significantly worse ASA Class scores and somewhat poorer Charlson Comorbidity Scale scores. Scale scores for the SF-36 demonstrated sensible differences across procedure groups on the Physical Function and Pain scales. Older age was associated with lower SF-36 scores on some subscales (e.g., Pain, Role-Physical, Physical Function, Energy and Fatigue) but not on the more global and psychosocial scales. In a multivariate regression analysis, adjusting for comorbidity and procedure, older age retained a significant association with the Pain subscale of the SF-36 and was associated with a significantly better score on the Mental Health scale. Alpha (α) coefficients for subscales were similar and high older and younger subjects were compared (0.82 to 0.96). The global health score (0 to 100) was strongly correlated with the SF-36 Health Perception scale ($r = 0.60$), and other correlations were lower between measures purporting to measure different underlying constructs (e.g., Physical Function and Mental Health, $r = 0.19$). Correlations tended to be weaker for older subjects.

Discussion.   The study is important in verifying the good internal consistency of the SF-36 scales for the oldest people (over age 70). The less potent correlations among health constructs for the older subjects is intriguing and suggests that self-reported health may take on a different meaning at older ages or that the relationships are more complex than among younger subjects. Studies on the ability of the SF-36 scales to demonstrate change over time would be important in following up on these observations.

Quality of Well-Being Scale (QWB)

Development and Methods

Patrick DL, Bush JW, & Chen MM. (1973). Methods for measuring levels of well-being for a health status index. *Health Serv Res*, 8, 228–245.

Design.   This is the primary reference for the psychometric scaling methods used in the Quality of Well-Being Scale (QWB). The aim of this research was to obtain social preference ratings for a disability continuum. An earlier article (Patrick et al., 1973) had developed a matrix of 29 function levels, 5 age classes, and 42 "symptom-problem complexes" describing a universe of possible functional states. A single trait—level of well-being—is measured by this index. For this study, "judges" were graduate students and health field leaders who were asked to rate 50 case descriptions of functional status that ranged from complete well-being to death. Three psychometric scaling procedures were used: (1) category rating, a difference or partition measure whereby each judge rated health states on a scale of 1 to 11 points; (2) magnitude estimation, a ratio measure; and (3) equivalence rating, a method of adjustment to utility analysis representing trade-offs in health resource allocation and quantifying compromises. This third method asks subjects—the judges—to adjust variable comparison stimuli until they are subjectively equal to a standard stimulus on a defined continuum; it is a very complex method. Convergent validity was tested by the (statistical) similarity with which the different methods came to the same conclusion about the social preference ratings of different health states.

Summary. The results indicated no dramatic differences among methods or groups of judges, so that category rating, which is the simplest, was considered valid and was adopted. *Discussion.* The results suggested to the authors that it is feasible to measure the social values associated with health status in household interviews. The resulting QWB scale would have to be tested for feasibility in a more general population before this could be accepted as true. The judges differed greatly from the general population in education (and motivation), and health states may not be similarly ranked among other groups; however, Squier and Kaplan (1995) subsequently validated rankings among patient groups.

Applications

Calfas KJ, Kaplan RM, & Ingram RE. (1992). One-year evaluation of cognitive-behavioral intervention in osteoarthritis. *Arthritis Care Res, 5,* 202–209.
Design. This was a randomized trial of an educational intervention among osteoarthritis (OA) patients comparing traditional lectures by health professionals and a cognitive-behavioral intervention for coping with pain and disability. Participants were interviewed before the study and at 2, 6, and 12 months using QWB, Arthritis Impact Measurement Scales (AIMS), and Beck Depression Inventory (BDI, reviewed in Chapter 5).
Sample. There were 40 adult subjects (of 79 inquiries), recruited as volunteers in response to advertisements and physician referrals from the San Diego area. Two subjects in each group dropped out before completing the intervention, and additional subjects dropped out before the 12-month follow-up interview. The study sample was 72% women, and the average age was about 67 years. There was only one nonwhite participant.
Summary. Both groups showed some improvement in their QWB scores immediately following the intervention, although the improvement was more dramatic in those receiving the cognitive intervention. This improvement reversed for both groups, and by 12 months the QWB scores of the two groups were indistinguishable. Multivariate regression analysis using the 12-month QWB as the outcome variable showed that baseline physical measures and social support were the primary predictors.
Discussion. This was a very small and highly selected sample, and the intervention was largely unsuccessful. The study is interesting because of its use of multiple measures for a relatively homogeneous patient group. A comparison of the measures would also be instructive.

Ganiats TG, Palinkas LA, & Kaplan RM. (1992). Comparison of Quality of Well-Being scale and Functional Status Index in patients with atrial fibrillation. *Med Care, 30,* 958–964.
Design. As part of a large randomized trial, two instruments were tested as potential outcome measures of health status: the QWB and the Functional Status Index (Jette FSI). The modified FSI had 12 items asking subjects about their level of difficulty in the past month with performing activities of daily living and physical tasks, including vigorous activities. Responses were scaled from 0 to 4 (higher numbers indicating less difficulty). The QWB used a 27-item "symptoms-problems complex," including such items as "excessive worry or anxiety" and "intoxication." The authors provide a list of the items and their weights for this version of the QWB. Analyses compared correlations between

the two instruments and their ability to detect a difference (improved health) in the treatment arm subjects.

Sample.   The patients were in the NIH Stroke Prevention of Atrial Fibrillation study, a multicenter, placebo-controlled trial of stroke prophylaxis with aspirin or warfarin in patients with nonvalvular atrial fibrillation. The analyzed sample included 664 subjects out of a total of 1,135 enrolled. Seventy percent were men, and 82% were white. The average ages were 65.4 years for men and 67.8 years for women.

Summary.   The mean QWB score was 0.699 (*SD* = 0.105), and the modified FSI mean was 44.23 (*SD* = 5.24). The correlation between the two instruments was moderate, with *r* = 0.46. There was a weak positive correlation between treatment and the QWB score (i.e., better health), after adjustment for FSI (as a baseline measure of health) and other variables. The FSI and QWB scores were compared using a scatter plot. The QWB had the least variation with low FSI scores, and FSI had the least variation with high QWB scores. Removing the SPX component (symptoms-problems list) of the QWB made it more of a functional assessment tool, and the FSI and QWB were then found to have larger statistical correlations.

Discussion.   These two tools produced somewhat similar results in this population, although the QWB was subjected to an unusual rescoring to make it equivalent to the FSI. By removing the SPX section, the authors also withdrew an important measurement component of the QWB. However, the authors do provide some support for use of the shorter FSI as an outcome measure for these patients, in light of the long and complex administration of this version of the QWB.

Ries AL, Kaplan, RM, Limberg TM, & Prewitt LM. (1995). Effects of pulmonary rehabilitation on physiologic and psychosocial outcomes in patients with chronic obstructive pulmonary disease. *Ann Intern Med, 122,* 823–832.

Design.   This is a randomized trial comparing patient education (usual care) to rehabilitation for patients with chronic obstructive pulmonary disease (COPD). Both groups received 8 weeks of intervention. Education was provided, consisting of videos, lectures, and discussion sessions. The intervention group received individualized education, psychosocial support, exercise, and monthly reinforcement sessions. Subjects received baseline physiologic and other evaluations, and outcomes were assessed after the intervention and regularly during 72 months of follow-up. Psychosocial measures included a self-efficacy questionnaire for walking, the QWB, and the Centers for Epidemiologic Studies Depression scale (CES-D, reviewed in Chapter 5). Self-reported hospitalizations and visits to an emergency department were also recorded. Investigators compared the groups by analyzing the change from baseline at four time intervals.

Sample.   Subjects were stable COPD patients recruited to an academic center by advertisements to the general public and to physicians. During 18 months, 352 patients were screened for eligibility and 128 met the study criteria; 9 of these dropped out before completing the intervention, leaving a study group of 119. Seventy-three percent (*n* = 87) were men; mean ages were 61.5 years for the rehabilitation intervention group and 63.6 years for the control group.

Summary.   Baseline QWB scores for these patients were 0.67 (*SD* = 0.10) for the intervention group and 0.65 (*SD* = 0.07) for the control group. QWB scores decreased throughout the study for both groups (incorporating death into the scale for patients who died) and were not different between groups. The number of hospital days, CES-D scores, and pulmonary function outcomes were also similar between the two groups. Other measures of pulmonary and physical health were significantly improved with the rehabilitation intervention, and the improvements persisted for 6 months (for perceived muscle fatigue) to 24 months (perceived breathlessness during exercise).

Discussion.   This is a good example of using the QWB as a measure of health status, but the authors did not measure and incorporate cost into an outcome measure, as the QWB is well suited to do. While the results demonstrate some benefits of intensive rehabilitation (especially specific to the exercise intervention), the QWB and the CES-D, both non–disease-specific measures, showed no improvement in overall health-related quality of life as an outcome.

Comparisons among Instruments

Andresen EM, Patrick DL, Carter WB, & Malmgren JA. (1995). Comparing the performance of health status measures for healthy older adults. *J Am Geriatrics Soc*, **43, 1–5.**

Design.   This study compared the performance of the SIP, the QWB, and three scales of the SF-36 among community-living older adults. Specifically, the authors compared correlations among similar scales, looked for potential extreme scaling problems ("floor" and "ceiling" effects), and reported on practical problems of administration and response. Enrollees from a health maintenance organization were randomly selected for a health promotion intervention. The baseline survey contained three SF-36 scales; the Positive Affect Scale, a measure of life stress; and the Chronic Disease Score (CDS), a measure computed from automated pharmacy records. This was followed with the SIP (mailed) and QWB (administered by telephone with mailed cue cards). Some measures were repeated at a 1-year follow-up mailing.

Sample.   Subjects were 200 of 283 older adults (68.2% response) selected from those who had responded to the mailed baseline survey. The mean age of the sample was 72.5 years.

Summary.   The SIP and two SF-36 scales (Physical Functioning and Role-Physical) were skewed toward scores indicating perfect health (scores of 0 on the SIP, 100 on the SF-36). The SIP had a mean of 3.4% ($SD = 4.4$). The QWB scores were well distributed and ranged from 0.50 to 0.90 (mean = 0.729, $SD = 0.87$). The MOS SF-36 General Health scale was normally distributed, with a mean of 77.1 ($SD = 22.4$). The SIP, QWB, and MOS SF-36 scales were moderately to strongly correlated among similar scale constructs, and the SIP Psychosocial Dimension was correlated with the independent measure of stress. The 1-year intraclass correlation coefficient for the Physical Functioning scale of the SF-36 was $r = 0.61$.

Discussion.   Because the sample of older adults was relatively healthy, on the basis of all measures of health status, the SIP suffered from a "ceiling" effect, as did the two physical scales of the SF-36. While the QWB demonstrated an acceptable distribution of scale scores, it was the most complex of the three measures to administer. Each of these three scales may be appropriate in different studies and populations.

Fryback DG, Dasbach EJ, Klein R, Klein BEK, Dorn N, Peterson K, & Martin PA. (1993). The Beaver Dam Health Outcomes Study: Initial catalog of health-state quality factors. *Med Decis Making, 13,* 89–102.

Design. Interviews were completed for a population-based study of nutrition and eye disease in a small town in rural Wisconsin. In-person interview protocols were extensive and included 13 sections, with a concentration on the measures of vision, but also including both the QWB and the SF-36 measures of health status, a measure of recent life stress, and two time trade-off measures to assess preferences for different health states. Twenty-eight different health problems are reported here, of over 300 elicited. The entire interview averaged 56 minutes. The QWB and SF-36 were administered in random order.

Sample. The subjects were part of the Beaver Dam Eye Study cohort and were drawn from the city and township of Beaver Dam, Wisconsin. Residents aged 45 and older were eligible (5,584), and only 6.8% refused. This paper reports on 1,356 interviews completed during 19 months in 1991 and 1992. The sample was 58.7% women, and the mean ages were 64.8 years ($SD = 11.0$) for women and 63.0 years ($SD = 10.5$) for men. The residents of Beaver Dam are predominantly white (over 99%), and only four study subjects were nonwhite. Twenty-six percent of subjects had not completed high school.

Summary. Overall, scores on the QWB and the General Health Perceptions scale of the SF-36 decreased significantly ($p < 0.001$) with increasing age; they also decreased with increasing numbers of reported medical conditions. The decrease in health status with increasing numbers of medical conditions was not explained by increasing age. The authors also report age-adjusted mean scores for specific conditions and compare them with those of individuals unaffected by the same condition; as expected, those affected by a disease scored lower on both the SF-36 and the QWB. The correlation between the SF-36 General Health Perceptions scale and the QWB was $r = 0.52$. Tables of these results are helpful in showing comparison scores for multiple instruments.

Discussion. This very important population-based study is unique for its impressive scale and its use of multiple measures of health status. Future publications related to it will be important in assessing both practical and statistical properties of the QWB and SF-36. The results are interesting for comparisons among older adults, because the large sample included 650 persons aged 65 and older. The results are somewhat limited because the sample was racially homogeneous. The ongoing study represents an important potential source of comparative data on subjects, but in this publication only the results of one SF-36 scale (General Health) are shown.

Hornberger JC, Redelmeier DA, & Petersen J. (1992). Variability among methods to assess patients' well-being and consequent effect on a cost-effectiveness analysis. *J Clin Epidemiol, 45,* 505–512.

Design. The authors wished to measure quality of life in a study of the cost-effectiveness of in-center hemodialysis (in quality-adjusted life-years, or QALYs). They compared six methods: the SIP, two Index of Well-Being scales (Campbell IWB and Kaplan/Bush IWB; the latter is an early QWB), categorical scaling, standard gamble, and time trade-off techniques. Patients self-administered the instruments unless they were blind ($n = 6$). All scores were computed on a scale of 0 to 100; higher numbers indicate greater well-being. Responses were compared using paired t tests for differences at two time points during a 1-year period.

Sample.   The results are reported for 58 patients with chronic renal failure at one site. Some patients were excluded because they did not meet study criteria (they did not speak English, the duration of their treatment was too short, etc.). A total of 110 patients were initially eligible; 21 were excluded and 5 refused. The total number is confusing, as it appears that only 58 of the resulting 84 were assessed, for a response proportion of 69%. Little information is given on the general demographics of these subjects, although their average age was 53 (versus 63 among nonparticipants).

Summary.   The results of the six methods varied remarkably, and there was a special problem with a narrow distribution using the SIP and the QWB. There were low correlations among measures at baseline for the 58 assessed subjects. The SIP/QWB correlation was modest at $r = 0.44$. For the cost-QALY analysis, the SIP produced the lowest estimate, and the standard gamble produced the highest estimate ($34,893 versus $45,254). The authors conclude that this wide variation precludes the use of any one measure for similar research.

Discussion.   The results are disappointing and fail to recommend a single, or best, outcomes measure for QALY outcomes research.

Kutner NG, Schechtman KB, Ory MG, & Baker DI. (1994). Older adults' perceptions of their health and functioning in relation to sleep disturbance, falling, and urinary incontinence. *J Am Geriatr Soc*, 42, 757–762.

Design.   This is a multicenter prospective study of the relationship between the self-reported health status of older adults and self-reported problems in sleep, falling, and urinary incontinence. The data presented here are from cross-sectional baseline surveys. Measures included the Mini-Mental State Exam (MMSE, reviewed in Chapter 4), the Center for Epidemiologic Studies Depression scale (CES-D, reviewed in Chapter 5), one scale of the SIP (Ambulation), and four of the SF-36 scales (General Health, Role-Physical, Role-Emotional, and Social Functioning). The SF-36 scales were used as outcome (dependent) variables in regression models that are used to examine the predictive nature of other measures, including demographic variables.

Sample.   The overall study population is from Frailty and Injuries: Cooperative Studies of Intervention Techniques (FICSIT). The subjects in this paper were recruited and studied at academic institutions in Seattle, WA; Atlanta, GA; and Farmington, CT. Exclusions and recruitment methods are not discussed, but the sample of 352 included in this paper was reported to be about two-thirds women, primarily white (98%), averaging 77.1 years of age and 14.7 years of education.

Summary.   The authors confirmed prior research on the high prevalence of recent sleep disturbances (68%), recent falls (3%), and urinary incontinence (14%) among adults aged 65 and older. All three problems were more common among women. Correlations among the SF-36 measures and sleep, falling, and incontinence were negligible or modest (0.25 or lower), although, because of the sample size, modest correlations reached statistical significance. There was a general trend toward lower SF-36 scale scores for those reporting any of the health problems. Correlations among SF-36 scores and the SIP were somewhat higher (for SIP Ambulation and the SF-36 scales, they ranged from 0.24 to 0.34), and they were highest between the CES-D and SF-36 Role-Emotional scale ($r = 0.45$). In multivariate models, depression (measured by the CES-D) and ambulation (measured by the SIP) were strongly related to all SF-36 scale scores. The pattern of predictors varied among the SF-36 scales. The explanatory ability of these models in predicting SF-36 scale scores ranged from an $R^2 = 0.12$ to $R^2 = 0.26$.

Discussion. The study is unusual in its choice of selected components of health status and other measures and allows comparison among these scales. Several sensible and expected correlations are reported, including an association between the SF-36 Role-Emotional and CES-D scales. The generalizability of these results is somewhat limited because of the relatively good health and high socioeconomic status of the group. In addition, these are cross-sectional analyses; the associations will be more persuasive with longitudinal data.

Liang MH, Fossel AH, & Larson MG. (1990). Comparisons of five health status instruments for orthopedic evaluation. *Med Care*, 28, 632–642.

Design. This is a longitudinal methods study to evaluate outcome measures for patients undergoing total joint arthroplasty. The candidate instruments include the Arthritis Impact Measurement Scales (AIMS), Functional Status Index (FSI), Health Assessment Questionnaire (HAQ), Index of Well-Being (Kaplan QWB), and SIP. Patients were interviewed 2 weeks before hip or knee arthroplasty and 3, 12, and 15 months after surgery. Response of the measures to clinical change was judged for four constructs: global health, pain, mobility, and social function (neither the SIP nor the QWB has a pain scale). All scales were transformed to linear scores of 0 to 100, with 0 representing no dysfunction and 100 maximum dysfunction. Using actual improvements measured by each scale, the authors estimated sample sizes that would be needed to assess therapies in future studies.

Sample. There were 38 subjects, followed for at least 1 year (of 50 recruited); 58% were women, 87% had osteoarthritis. Hip replacement surgery was under way for 55%; the remainder were receiving knee replacement surgery. The average age at surgery was 67.4 years. Subjects of the longitudinal study were older but were in better health than the 12 who were not followed.

Summary. Early response to treatment was measured as significantly improved for all constructs, with the greatest gains in mobility and reduction of pain. There were strong correlations among all of the constructs except the QWB. Distinct scales from different measures that purport to measure similar components of health status were moderately correlated. A complex and competent statistical yardstick for size of effect was applied to all of the instruments. Three instruments produced "large" response sizes and were also deemed suitable for sample size estimates: the HAQ, QWB, and SIP.

Discussion. This is a very competent methods investigation of health status measures for a homogeneous patient group. The sample size for the comparison is quite small but serves as a thoughtful statistical guide to investigators of similar patient populations. Three instruments were judged appropriate for future outcomes research, so that investigators might consider the practical advantages of the surveys before making a selection.

Visser MC, Fletcher AE, Parr G, Simpson A, & Bulpitt CJ. (1994). A comparison of three quality of life instruments in subjects with angina pectoris: The Sickness Impact Profile, the Nottingham Health Profile, and the Quality of Well Being Scale. *J Clin Epidemiol*, 47, 157–163.

Design. This was a cross-sectional pilot for a clinical trial of the benefits or adverse effects of transdermal glyceryl trinitrate. The three instruments examined here are the

Nottingham Health Profile (NHP), the SIP, and the QWB. They were compared with the New York Heart Association (NYHA) classification for severity of angina. The NYHA has only four categories and was suspected of being insensitive to changes in quality of life. However, none of the three instruments had been tested among persons with angina pectoris. The SIP, QWB, and NHP, plus the Symptom Rating Test (SRT; a psychological measure of distress), were correlated with NYHA categories 1 to 3. The QWB was interviewer-administered; the SIP, NHP, and SRT were self-administered.

Sample.   The subjects were 59 British patients (43 men) aged 46 to 79 with stable angina.

Summary.   The 136-item SIP showed a strong expected positive association with increasing NYHA scores. The associations were stronger for scales representing areas sensibly expected to differ with increasing symptoms of angina—for example, the Ambulation scale—rather than for scales like Eating or Sleep and Rest. The QWB was deemed less practical, since it required 7 days of training for the interviewers. The QWB score demonstrated a slight but nonsignificant association with increasing symptoms of angina. When broken down into components, the Physical Activity and Symptoms parts of the QWB had somewhat stronger correlations with increasing NYHA categories. The 45-item NHP showed increasing scores with increasing NYHA categories in the six domains of experience (Part 1), but not in Part 2, which asks about interference with seven usual life activities. Symptom Rating Test (SRT) scores also increased with NYHA categories. The NHP and SIP were highly correlated with each other, as were similar dimensions among the SIP, SRT, and NHP. Both the SIP and the NHP were skewed toward lower scores; zero scores were especially a problem with the NHP. The SIP was chosen for the final trial, and while no treatment benefits were detected, the SIP results suggested an adverse effect of the drug in the psychosocial dimension, possibly due to headaches.

Discussion.   This article adds to the understanding of the utility of three health status measures for one chronic-disease patient population, those with angina pectoris. It is one of very few studies comparing the performance of different methods. The results suggest the importance of considering the specific needs of each research effort, especially given the spectrum and impact of chronic diseases and practical considerations of research with older adults.

Weinberger M, Samsa GP, Hanlon JT, Schmader K, Doyle ME, Cowper PA, Uttech KM, Cohen HJ, & Feussner JR. (1991). An evaluation of a brief health status measure in elderly veterans. *J Am Geriatr Soc, 39*, 691–694.

Design.   This was a small cross-sectional study of male veterans with random-order, interviewer-administered SIP and SF-36 surveys. The authors compared the practical administration of and the associations between the two measures of health status. The SIP scores were subtracted from 100 to make comparison with the SF-36 easier; both scales thus have higher scores for better health status.

Sample.   A "convenience" sample of 29 regularly scheduled clinic patients (ages 65 and older) were invited to participate, and 25 completed both instruments. The mean age of subjects was 73.5 years; 68% were white, 44% had at least a high school degree, and their mean annual income was $7,024.

Summary.   Administration time was shorter for the SF-36 than the SIP; the means were 14 to 15 minutes versus 21 to 33 minutes in two settings. The SIP showed consistently higher functioning than the SF-36 for three comparisons (physical function, social function, and overall function). However, correlations were high between similar constructs of the two instruments: For physical function, $r = 0.78$; for social function, $r = 0.67$; and for overall function, $r = 0.73$.

Discussion. The authors do not report the range of scores of the SIP and SF-36 subscales but suggest that the SIP demonstrates a "ceiling" effect and thus would not be sensitive to real improvements. A summary of maximum scores (perfect health) would have made it easier to examine this problem. The patients may have been relatively healthier than some older veterans. Nevertheless, the results support the potential use of the SF-36 in such subjects by virtue of its relative brevity for in-person administration. Weinberger et al. continued these reports of health status measures among veterans (1994, 1996).

REFERENCES

Aaronson NK. (1988). Quality of life: What is it? How should it be measured? *Oncology*, 2, 69–76.

Adams PC, Ghent CN, Grant, DR, & Wall WJ. (1995). Employment after liver transplantation. *Hepatology*, *21*, 140–144.

Ahroni JH, Boyko EJ, Davignon DR, & Pecoraro RE. (1994). The health and functional status of veterans with diabetes. *Diabetes Care*, *17*, 318–321.

Alonso J, Prieto L, & Antó JM. (1995). La versión Española del "SF-36 Health Survey" (Cuestionario de Salud SF-36): Un instrumento para la dedida de los resultados clínicos [Spanish version of SF-36 Health Survey: An instrument for clinical use.], *Med Clin*, *104*, 771–776.

Anderson JP, Kaplan RM, & Schneiderman LJ. (1994). Effects of offering advance directives on quality adjusted life expectancy and psychological well-being among ill adults. *J Clin Epidemiol*, *47*, 761–772.

Anderson S, Abdellatif M, Schreiner S, McDonell M, Reda D, & Fihn S. (1995). Information system for a multi-hospital study using optical scanning and hospital database downloads [Abstract]. *Controlled Clin Trials*, *16*(Suppl. 3s), 76S.

*Andresen EM, Bowley N, Rothenberg B, Panzer R, & Katz P. (1996). Test-retest performance of a mailed version of the SF-36 among older adults. *Med Care, 34*, 1165–1170.

*Andresen EM, Patrick DL, Carter WB, & Malmgren JA. (1995). Comparing the performance of health status measures for healthy older adults. *J Am Geriatr Soc*, *43*, 1–5.

Andresen EM, Rothenberg BM, Panzer R, Katz P, & McDermott MP. (1997). Comparison of mailed versions of the SF-36 and SIP questionnaires among older adults. Submitted for publication.

Anonymous. (1993). Study protocol for the World Health Organization project to develop a Quality of Life assessment instrument (WHOQOL). *Qual Life Res*, *2*, 153–159.

Anonymous. (1995). The World Health Organization Quality of Life assessment (WHO-QOL): Position paper from the World Health Organization. *Soc Sci Med*, *41*, 1403–1409.

Anthonisen NR, Wright EC, & Hodgkin JE. (1986). Prognosis in chronic obstructive pulmonary disease. *Am Rev Respir Dis*, *133*, 14–20.

Aydelotte ME, Andresen EM, & Podgorski CA. (1997). Test characteristics of the Short-Form 36 (SF-36) in a nursing home population. Submitted for publication.

Bagne CA, Luscombe FA, & Damiano A. (1995). Relationships between glycemic control, diabetes-related symptoms, and SF-36 scales scores in patients with non-insulin dependent diabetes mellitus [Abstract]. *Qual Life Res*, *4*, 392–393.

Beaton D, Erdeljan S, Hogg-Johnson S, & Bombardier C. (1995). Comparison of performance of generic and disease-specific measures of health status in injured workers [Abstract]. *Qual Life Res*, *4*, 395.

Beaton DE, & Richards RR. (1995). Selecting a measure of disease-specific health related quality of life in shoulder patients [Abstract]. *Qual Life Res*, *4*, 395–396.

Bendtsen P, & Hörnquist JO. (1993). Severity of rheumatoid arthritis, function and quality of life: Sub-group comparisons. *Clin Exp Rheumatol*, *11*, 495–502.

Bergner L, Bergner M, Hallstrom AP, Eisenberg M, & Cobb LA. (1984). Health status of survivors of out-of-hospital cardiac arrest six months later. *Am J Public Health*, *74*, 508–510.

Bergner L, Hallstrom AP, Bergner M, Eisenberg MS, & Cobb LA. (1985). Health status of survivors of cardiac arrest and of myocardial infarction controls. *Am J Public Health*, *75*, 1321–1323.

*Bergner M, Bobbitt RA, Carter WB, & Gilson BS. (1981). The Sickness Impact Profile: Development and final revision of a health status measure. *Med Care*, *19*, 787–805.

Bergner M, Bobbitt RA, Kressel S, Pollard WE, Gilson BS, & Morris JR. (1976). The Sickness Impact Profile: Conceptual formulation and methodology for the development of a health status measure. *Int J Health Serv*, 6, 393–415.

Bergner M, Bobbitt RA, Pollard WE, Martin DP, & Gilson BS. (1976). The Sickness Impact Profile: Validation of a health status measure. *Med Care*, *14*, 57–67.

Bergner M, Hudson LD, Conrad DA, Patmont CM, McDonald GJ, Perrin EB, & Gilson BS. (1988). The cost and efficacy of home care for patients with chronic lung disease. *Med Care*, *26*, 566–579.

Bindman AB, Keane D, & Lurie N. (1990). Measuring health changes among severely ill patients: The floor phenomenon. *Med Care*, *28*, 1142–1152.

Bombardier C, & Raboud J. (1991). A comparison of health-related quality-of-life measures for rheumatoid arthritis research: The Auranofin Cooperating Group. *Controlled Clin Trials*, *12*, 243S–256S.

Bousquet J, Bullinger M, Fayol C, Marquis P, Valentin B, & Burtin B. (1994). Assessment of quality of life in patients with perennial allergic rhinitis with the French version of the SF-36 Health Status Questionnaire. *J Allergy Clin Immunol*, *94*, 182–188.

Bousquet J, Knani J, Dhivert H, Richard A, Chicoye A, Ware JE, & Michel FB. (1994). Quality of life in asthma: 1. Internal consistency and validity of the SF-36 questionnaire. *Am J Respir Crit Care Med*, *149*, 371–375.

Brazier J. (1993). The SF-36 Health Survey Questionnaire: A tool for economists. *Health Econ*, *2*, 213–215.

Brazier JE, Harper R, Jones NMB, O'Cathain A, Thomas KJ, Usherwood T, & Westlake L. (1992). Validating the SF-36 health survey questionnaire: New outcome measure for primary care. *BMJ*, *305*, 160–164.

Breslow L. (1989). Health status measurement in the evaluation of health promotion. *Med Care*, *27*(Suppl. 3), S205–S216.

Buchner DM, Hornbrook MC, Kutner NG, Tinetti ME, Ory MG, Mulrow CD, Schechtman KB, Gerety MB, Fiatarone MA, Wolf SL, Rossiter J, Arfken C, Kanten K, Lipsitz

LA, Sattin RW, & DeNino LA. (1993). Development of the common data base for the FICSIT trials. *J Am Geriatr Soc, 41,* 297–308.

Bullinger M. (1995). German translation and psychometric testing of the SF-36 Health Survey: Preliminary results from the IQOLA project (International Quality of Life Assessment). *Soc Sci Med, 41,* 1359–1366.

Bullinger M, & Heidrich H. (1995). Testing the performance of generic vs. disease-specific HRQOL measures: The example of peripheral arterial occlusive disease (PAOD) [Abstract]. *Qual Life Res, 4,* 403.

*Calfas KJ, Kaplan RM, & Ingram RE. (1992). One-year evaluation of cognitive-behavioral intervention in osteoarthritis. *Arthritis Care Res, 5,* 202–209.

*Callahan CM, Hendrie HC, Dittus RS, Brater DC, Hui SL, & Tierney WM. (1994). Improving treatment of late life depression in primary care: A randomized clinical trial. *J Am Geriatr Soc, 42,* 839–846.

Campell A, & Converse PE. (1976). The quality of American life: Perceptions, evaluations, and satisfactions. New York: Russell Sage Foundation.

Carter WB, Bobbitt RA, Bergner M, & Gilson BS. (1976). Validation of an interval scaling: The Sickness Impact Profile. *Health Serv Res, 11,* 516–528.

Carter WB, & Deyo R. (1981). The impact of questionnaire research on clinical populations: A dilemma in review of human subjects research resolved by a study of a study. *Clin Res, 29,* 287–295.

Centers for Disease Control and Prevention. (1994). Quality of life as a new public health measure: Behavioral risk factor surveillance system, 1993. *MMWR, 43,* 375–380.

Centers for Disease Control and Prevention. (1995). Health-related quality-of-life measures: United States, 1993. *MMWR, 44,* 195–200.

Clark NM, Janz NK, Becker MH, Schork MA, Wheeler J, Liang J, Dodge JA, Keteyian S, Rhoads KL, & Santinga JT. (1992). Impact of self-management education on the functional health status of older adults with heart disease. *Gerontologist, 32,* 438–443.

Cress ME, Schechtman KB, Mulrow CD, Fiatarone MT, Gerety MB, & Buchner DM. (1995). Relationship between physical performance and self-perceived physical function. *J Am Geriatr Soc, 43,* 93–101.

DeBruin AF, Buys M, De Witte LP, & Diederiks JPM. (1994). The Sickness Impact Profile: SIP-68, a short generic version. First evaluation of the reliability and reproducibility. *J Clin Epidemiol, 47,* 863–871.

DeBruin AF, Diederiks JPM, De Witte LP, & Stevens FCJ. (1994). The development of a short generic version of the Sickness Impact Profile. *J Clin Epidemiol, 47,* 407–418.

de Haan R, Horn J, Limburg M, & Van Der Meuien J. (1993). A comparison of five stroke scales with measures of disability, handicap, and quality of life. *Stroke, 24,* 1178–1181.

Dela Cruz, FA. (1995). Validating a Tagalog (Philipino) version of the RAND 36-item Health Survey 1.0 [Abstract]. *Qual Life Res, 4,* 418.

Deyo RA. (1984). Pitfalls in measuring the health status of Mexican Americans: Comparative validity of the English and Spanish Sickness Impact Profile. *Am J Public Health, 74,* 569–573.

Deyo RA. (1986). Comparative validity of the Sickness Impact Profile and shorter scales for functional assessment in low-back pain. *Spine, 11,* 951–954.

Deyo RA, & Centor RM. (1986). Assessing the responsiveness of functional scales to clinical change: An analogy to diagnostic test performance. *J Chron Dis, 39*, 897–906.

Deyo RA, Inui TS, Leininger J, & Overman S. (1982). Physical and psychosocial function in rheumatoid arthritis: Clinical use of a self-administered health status instrument. *Arch Intern Med, 142*, 879–882.

Deyo RA, Inui TS, Leininger JD, & Overman SS. (1983). Measuring functional outcomes in chronic disease: A comparison of traditional scales and a self-administered health status questionnaire in patients with rheumatoid arthritis. *Med Care, 21*, 180–192.

Dolan P, Gudex C, Kind P, & Williams A. (1995). A social tariff for EuroQol: Results from a UK general population survey. (Discussion paper 138). National Health Service Center for Reviews and Dissemination, York Health Economics Consortium, Center for Health Economics, University of York, England.

Epstein AM, Hall JA, Fretwell M, Fieldstein M, DeCiantis ML, Tognetti J, Cutler C, Constantine M, Besdine R, Rowe J, & McNeil BJ. (1990). Consultive geriatric assessment for ambulatory patients: A randomized trial in a health maintenance organization. *JAMA, 263*, 538–544.

Epstein AM, Hall JA, Tognetti J, Son LH, & Conant L. (1989). Using proxies to evaluate quality of life: Can they provide valid information about patients' health status and satisfaction with medical care? *Med Care, 27*(Suppl. 3), S91–S98.

Erickson P, Kendall EA, Anderson JP, & Kaplan RM. (1989). Using composite health status measures to assess the nation's health. *Med Care, 27*, S66–S76.

Feasley JC (Ed.). (1996). *Health outcomes of older people. Questions for the coming decade*. Washington, DC: National Academy.

Feeny D, Furlong W, Boyle M, & Torrance GW. (1995). Multi-attribute health status classification systems: Health Utilities Index. *PharmacoEconomics, 7*, 490–502.

Feio ALJ, Batel Marques FJ, Borges Alexandrino M, & Salek MS. (1995). Portuguese cultural adaptation and linguistic validation of the Sickness Impact Profile (PSIP) [Abstract]. *Qual Life Res, 4*, 424–425.

Fillenbaum G, & Smyer MA. (1981). The development, validity, and reliability of the OARS Multidimensional Functional Assessment Questionnaire. *J Gerontol, 36*, 428–434.

Fletcher AE, Dickinson EJ, & Philp I. (1992). Review: Audit measures: Quality of life instruments for everyday use with elderly patients. *Age Ageing, 21*, 142–150.

Follick MJ, Smith TW, & Ahern DK. (1985). The Sickness Impact Profile: A global measure of disability in chronic low back pain. *Pain, 21*, 67–76.

Fortrin PR, Neville C, & Abrahamowicz M. (1995). Health status measure used to validate research in chronic diseases [Abstract]. *Qual Life Res, 4*, 427–428.

Fowler FJ, Cleary PD, Magaziner J, Patrick DL, & Benjamin KL. (1994) Methodological issues in measuring patient-reported outcomes: The agenda of the work group on outcomes assessment. *Med Care, 32*, JS65–JS76.

*Fryback DG, Dasbach EJ, Klein R, Klein BEK, Dorn N, Peterson K, & Martin PA. (1993). The Beaver Dam Health Outcomes Study: Initial catalog of health-state quality factors. *Med Decis Making, 13*, 89–102.

Gafni A. (1994). The standard gamble method: What is being measured and how it is interpreted. *Health Serv Res, 29*, 207–224.

Ganiats TG, Miller CJ, & Kaplan RM. (1995). Comparing the quality-adjusted life-year output of two treatment arms in a randomized trial. *Med Care, 33,* AS245–AS254.

*Ganiats TG, Palinkas LA, & Kaplan RM. (1992). Comparison of Quality of Well-Being Scale and Functional Status Index in patients with atrial fibrillation. *Med Care, 30,* 958–964.

Garratt AM, Ruta DA, Abdalla MI, Buckingham JK, & Russell IT. (1993). The SF-36 Health Survey Questionnaire: An outcome measure suitable for routine use within the NHS? *BMJ, 306,* 1440–1444.

George LK. (1994). Multidimensional assessment instruments: Present status and future prospects. In MP Lawton & JA Teresi (Eds.), *Annual review of gerontology and geriatrics.* Vol. 13: *Focus on assessment techniques* (pp. 353–375). New York: Springer.

*Gerety MB, Cornell JE, Mulrow CD, Tuley M, Hazuda HP, Lichtenstein M, Aguilar C, Kadri AA, & Rosenberg J. (1994). The Sickness Impact Profile for Nursing Homes (SIP-NH). *J Gerontol, 49,* M2–M8.

*Gerrity MS, Gaylord S, & Williams ME. (1993). Short versions of the Timed Manual Performance Test: Development, reliability, and validity. *Med Care, 33,* 617–628.

Gill TM, & Feinstein AR. (1994). A critical appraisal of the quality of quality-of-life measurements. *JAMA, 272,* 619–626.

Gilson BS, Gilson JS, Bergner M, Bobbitt RA, Kressel S, Pollard WE, & Vesselago M. (1975). The Sickness Impact Profile: Development of an outcome measure of health care. *Am J Publ Health, 65,* 1304–1310.

GIVIO. (1994). Impact of follow-up testing on survival and health-related quality of life in breast cancer patients: A multi-centered randomized controlled trial. The GIVIO Investigators. *JAMA, 271,* 1587–1592.

Goethe JW, & Fischer EH. (1995). Functional impairment in depressed inpatients. *J Affect Disord, 33,* 23–29.

Granger CV, Cotter AC, Hamilton BB, & Fiedler RC. (1993). Functional assessment scales: A study of persons after stroke. *Arch Phys Med Rehabil, 74,* 133–138.

Gurland B, Goldon RR, Teresi JA, & Challop J. (1984). The SHORT-CARE: An efficient instrument for the assessment of depression, dementia and disability. *J Gerontol, 39,* 166–169.

Haley SM, McHorney CA, & Ware JE. (1994). Evaluation of the MOS SF-36 Physical Functioning Scale (PF-10): I. Unidimensionality and reproducibility of the Rasch item scale. *J Clin Epidemiol, 47,* 671–684.

Hall JA, Milburn MA, & Epstein AM. (1993). A causal model of health status and satisfaction with medical care. *Med Care, 31,* 84–94.

Hanestad BR, & Graue M. (1995). To maintain quality of life and satisfactory metabolic control in Type II diabetes patients: One and the same? [Abstract]. *Qual Life Res, 4,* 436–437.

Hart LG, & Evans RW. (1987). The functional status of ESRD patients as measured by the Sickness Impact Profile. *J Chron Dis, 40,* 117S–136S.

Hasley PB, Brancati FL, Rogers J, Hanusa BH, & Kapoor WN. (1993). Measuring functional change in community-acquired pneumonia: A preliminary study using the Sickness Impact Profile. *Med Care, 31,* 649–657.

Hayes V, Morris J, Wolfe C, & Morgan M. (1995). The SF-36 health survey questionnaire: Is it suitable for use with older adults? *Age Aging*, *24*, 120–125.

Hays RD, Sherbourne CD, & Mazel RM. (1993). The RAND 36-Item Health Survey 1.0. *Health Econ*, *2*, 217–227.

Hays RD, Siu AL, Keeler E, Marshall GN, Kaplan RM, Simmons S, El Mouchi D, & Schnelle J. (1996). Long-term care residents' preferences for health states on the Quality of Well-Being Scale. *Med Decis Making*, *16*, 254–261.

Hendricson WD, Russell IJ, Prihoda TJ, Jacobson JM, Rogan A, & Bishop GD. (1989). An approach to developing a valid Spanish language translation of a health-status questionnaire. *Med Care*, *27*, 959–966.

Hennessy CH, Moriarty DG, Zack MM, Scherr PA, & Brackbill R. (1994). Measuring health-related quality of life for public health surveillance. *Public Health Rep*, *109*, 665–672.

Holbrook TL, Hoyt DB, Anderson JP, Hollingsworth-Fridlund P, & Shackford SR. (1974). Functional limitation after major trauma: A more sensitive assessment using the Quality of Well-Being Scale: The trauma recovery pilot project. *J Trauma*, *36*, 74–78.

*Hornberger JC, Redelmeier DA, & Petersen J. (1992). Variability among methods to assess patients' well-being and consequent effect on a cost-effectiveness analysis. *J Clin Epidemiol*, *45*, 505–512.

Hunskaar S, & Vinsnes A. (1991). The quality of life in women with urinary incontinence as measured by the Sickness Impact Profile. *J Am Geriatr Soc*, *39*, 378–382.

Idler EL. (1993). Age differences in self-assessments of health: Age changes, cohort differences, or survivorship? *J Gerontol*, *48*, S289–S300.

Intermittent Positive Pressure Breathing Trial Group. (1983). Intermittent positive pressure breathing therapy of chronic obstructive pulmonary disease: A clinical trial. *Ann Intern Med*, *99*, 612–620.

Jacobson AM, Samson JA, & De Groot M. (1994). The evaluation of two measures of quality of life in patients with type I and type II diabetes. *Diabetes Care*, *17*, 267–274.

Jette AM. (1987). The Functional Status Index: Reliability and validity of a self-report functional disability measure. *J Rheum*, *14*(Suppl), 15ff (as cited by Ganiats et al.).

Jette AM. (1980). Health status indicators: Their utility in chronic-disease evaluation research. *J Chron Dis*, *33*, 567–579.

Jette DU, & Downing J. (1994). Health status of individuals entering a cardiac rehabilitation program as measured by the Medical Outcomes Study 36-Item Short Form Survey (SF-36). *Phys Ther*, *74*, 521–527.

*Johnson PA, Goldman L, Orav EJ, Garcia T, Pearson SD, & Lee TH. (1995). Comparison of the Medical Outcomes Study Short-Form 36-Item Health Survey in black and white patients with acute chest pain. *Med Care*, *33*, 145–160.

Johnson RJ, & Wolinsky FD. (1994). Gender, race, and health: The structure of health status among older adults. *Gerontologist*, *34*, 24–35.

Jones PW, Baveystock CM, & Littlejohns P. (1989). Relationship between general health measured with the Sickness Impact Profile and respiratory symptoms, physiological measures, and mood in patients with chronic airflow limitation. *Am Rev Respir Dis*, *140*, 1538–1543

Juniper EF, Guyatt GH, Ferrie PJ, & Griffith LE. (1983). Measuring quality of life in asthma. *Am Rev Respir Dis*, *147*, 832–838.

*Kantz ME, Harris WJ, Levitsky K, Ware JE, & Ross Davies A. (1992). Methods for assessing condition-specific and generic functional status outcomes after total knee replacement. *Med Care, 30,* MS240–MS252.

Kaplan RM. (1985). Quality-of-life measurement. In P Karoly (Ed.), *Measurement strategies in health psychology* (pp. 115–146). New York: Wiley.

Kaplan RM. (1994). Value judgement in the Oregon Medicaid experiment. *Med Care, 32,* 975–988.

Kaplan RM, Anderson JP, & Ganiats TG. (1993). The Quality of Well-Being Scale: Rationale for a single quality of life index. In SR Walker & RM Rosser (Eds.), *Quality of life assessment: Key issues in the 1990s* (pp. 65–94). London: Kluwer Academic.

Kaplan RM, Anderson JP, Patterson TL, McCutchan JA, Weinrich JD, Heaton RK, Atkinson JH, Thal L, Chandler J, & Grant I. (1995). Validity of the Quality of Well-Being Scale for persons with human immunodeficiency virus infection. *Psychom Med, 57,* 138–147.

Kaplan RM, Atkins CJ, & Timms R. (1984). Validity of a quality of well-being scale as an outcome measure in chronic obstructive pulmonary disease. *J Chron Dis, 37,* 85–95.

Kaplan RM, & Bush JW. (1982). Health related quality of life measurement for evaluation of research and policy analysis. *Health Psychol, 1,* 61–80.

Kaplan RM, Bush JW, & Berry CC. (1976). Health status: Types of validity and the Index of Well-Being. *Health Serv Res, 11,* 478–507.

Kaplan RM, Bush JW, & Berry CC. (1979). Health Status Index: Category rating versus magnitude estimation for measuring levels of well-being. *Med Care, 27,* 501–525.

Kaplan RM, Ganiats TG, Rosen P, Sieber W, & Anderson JP. (1995). Development of a self-administered quality of well-being scale (QWB-SA): Initial studies [Abstract]. *Qual Life Res, 4,* 443–444.

Kaplan RM, & Mehta R. (1994). Outcome measurement in kidney disease. *Blood Purif, 12,* 20–29.

Karlsson J, Sjostrom L, & Sullivan M. (1995). Swedish obese subjects (SOS)—An intervention study of obesity: Measuring psychosocial factors and health by means of short-form questionnaires. Results of a method study. *J Clin Epidemiol, 48,* 817–823.

Katz JN, Larson MG, Phillips CB, Fossel AH, & Liang MH. (1992). Comparative measurement sensitivity of short and longer health status instruments. *Med Care, 30,* 917–925.

Keller SD, Ware JE, & Gandek B. (1995). Equivalence of translations of response choices widely used in health questionnaires: Comparison of results from nine countries in the IQOLA project [Abstract]. *Qual Life Res, 4,* 445.

Kirshner B, & Guyatt G. (1985). A methodological framework for assessing health indices. *J Chron Dis, 38,* 27–36.

Kosorok MR, Omenn GS, Diehr P, Koepsell TD, & Patrick DL. (1992). Restricted activity days among older adults. *Am J Public Health, 82,* 1263–1267.

Krause NM, & Jay GM. (1994). What do global self-rated health items measure? *Med Care, 32,* 930–942.

Krenz C, Larson EB, Buchner DM, & Canfield CG. (1988). Characterizing patient dysfunction in Alzheimer's-type dementia. *Med Care, 26,* 453–461.

Krumholz HM, McHorney CA, Clark L, Levesque M, Baim DS, & Goldman L. (1996). Changes in health after elective percutaneous coronary revascularization. A comparison of generic and specific measures. *Med Care, 34,* 754–759.

Kurtin PS, Davies AR, Meyer KB, DeGiacomo JM, & Kantz ME. (1992). Patient-based health status measures in outpatient dialysis: Early experiences in developing an outcomes assessment program. *Med Care, 30*, MS136–MS149.

*Kutner NG, Schechtman KB, Ory MG, & Baker DI. (1994). Older adults' perceptions of their health and functioning in relation to sleep disturbance, falling, and urinary incontinence. FICSIT Group. *J Am Geriatr Soc, 42*, 757–762.

Lalonde L, Clarke AE, & Grover SA. (1995). Comparing a health status instrument with conventional utility instruments [Abstract]. *Qual Life Res, 4*, 451.

Lansky D, Butler LBV, & Waller FT. (1992). Using health status measures in the hospital setting: From acute care to "outcomes management." *Med Care, 30*, MS57–MS73.

Liang MH, Cullen K, & Larson M. (1982). In search of a more perfect mousetrap (health status or quality of life instrument). *J Rheumatol, 9*, 775–779.

*Liang MH, Fossel AH, & Larson MG. (1990). Comparisons of five health status instruments for orthopedic evaluation. *Med Care, 28*, 632–642.

Lichtenstein MJ, Bess FH, Logan SA, & Burger MC. (1990). Deriving criteria for hearing impairment in the elderly: A functional approach. *J Am Academ Audiol, 1*, 11–22.

Linn MW, Hunter KI, & Linn BS. (1980). Self-assessed health, impairment and disability in Anglo, black and Cuban elderly. *Med Care, 28*, 282–288.

Litaker DG, Bronson DL, & Solomon GD. (1995). Correlating quality of life and costs of care: The SF-36 Health Survey as triage tool for cost containment [Abstract]. *Qual Life Res, 4*, 456.

*Longstreth WT, Nelson L, Linde M, & Munoz D. (1992). Utility of the Sickness Impact Profile in Parkinson's disease. *J Geriatr Psychiatry Neurol, 5*, 142–148.

Lubeck DP, & Fries JF. (1993). Health status among persons infected with human immunodeficiency virus. *Med Care, 31*, 269–276.

Lyons RA, Perry HM, & Littlepage BNC. (1994). Evidence for the validity of the Short-Form 36 Questionnaire (SF-36) in an elderly population. *Age Ageing, 23*, 182–184.

MacKenzie CR, Charlson ME, DiGioia D, & Kelley K. (1986). Can the Sickness Impact Profile measure change? An example of scale assessment. *J Chron Dis, 39*, 429–438.

Maitland ME, & Mandel, AR. (1994). A client-computer interface for questionnaire data. *Arch Phys Med Rehabil, 75*, 639–642.

*Mangione CM, Marcantonio ER, Goldman L, Cook EF, Donaldson MC, Sugarbaker DJ, Poss R, & Lee TH. (1993). Influence of age on measurement of health status in patients undergoing elective surgery. *J Am Geriatr Soc, 41*, 377–383.

Mangione CM, Phillips RS, Seddon JM, Lawrence MG, Cook EF, Dailey R, & Goldman L. (1992). Development of the 'Activities of Daily Vision Scale': A measure of visual functional status. *Med Care, 30*, 1111–1126.

Martin C, Marquis P, & Bonfils S. (1994). A 'quality of life questionnaire' adapted to duodenal ulcer therapeutic trials. *Scand J Gastroenterol, 29*(Suppl. 206), 40–43.

Mathias SD, Fifer SK, & Patrick DL. (1994). Rapid translation of quality of life measures for international clinical trials: Avoiding errors in the minimalist approach. *Qual Life Res, 3*, 403–412.

McCallum J. (1995). The SF-36 in an Australian sample: Validating a new, generic health status measure. *Aust J Public Health, 19*, 160–166.

McCusker J, & Stoddard AM. (1984). Use of a surrogate for the Sickness Impact Profile. *Med Care, 22*, 789–795.

McDowell I, & Newell C. (1987). *Measuring health: A guide to rating scales and questionnaires.* New York: Oxford University Press.

McHorney C, & Ware JE. (1995). Construction and validation of an alternate form general mental health scale for the Medical Outcomes Study Short-Form 36-Item Health Survey. *Med Care, 33,* 15–28.

*McHorney C, Kosinski M, & Ware JE. (1994). Comparisons of the costs and quality of norms for the SF-36 Health Survey collected by mail versus telephone interview: Results from a national survey. *Med Care, 32,* 551–567.

McHorney, CA. (1996). Measuring and monitoring general health status in elderly persons: Practical and methodological issues in using the SF-36 Health Survey. *Gerontologist, 36,* 571–583.

*McHorney CA, Ware JE, Lu JFR, & Sherbourne CD. (1994). The MOS 36-Item Short-Form Health Survey (SF-36): III. Tests of data quality, scaling assumptions, and reliability across diverse patient groups. *Med Care, 32,* 40–66.

McHorney CA, Ware JE Jr, & Raczek AE. (1993). The MOS 36-Item Short-Form Health Survey (SF-36): II. Psychometric and clinical tests of validity in measuring physical and mental health constructs. *Med Care, 31,* 247–263.

McHorney CA, Ware JE Jr, Rogers W, Raczek AE, & Rachel-Lu JF. (1992). The validity and relative precision of MOS Short- and Long-Form health status scales and Dartmouth COOP Charts: Results from the Medical Outcomes Study. *Med Care, 30*(Suppl. 5), MS253–MS265.

McSweeny AJ, Grant I, Heaton RK, Adams KM, & Timms RM. (1982). Life quality of patients with chronic obstructive pulmonary disease. *Arch Intern Med, 142,* 473–478.

Meyer KB, Espindle DM, DeGiacomo JM, Jenuleson CS, Kurtin PS, & Davies AR. (1994). Monitoring dialysis patients' health status. *Am J Kidney Dis, 24,* 267–279.

Mold JW, Holtgrave DR, Bisonni RS, Marley DS, Wright RA, & Spann SJ. (1992). The evaluation and treatment of men with asymptomatic prostate nodules in primary care: A decision analysis. *J Fam Pract, 34,* 561–568.

Morton AR, Singer MA, Meers C, Lang C, McMurray M, Hopman WM, & MacKenzie TA. (1996). Assessment of health status in peritoneal dialysis patients: A potential outcome measure. *Clin Nephrol, 45,* 199–204.

*Mulrow CD, Gerety MB, Cornell JE, Lawrence VA, & Kanten DN. (1994). The relationship between disease and function and perceived health in very frail elders. *J Am Geriatr Soc, 42,* 374–380.

Muller MJ, Aaronson NK, te Velde A, Sprangers MAG, Buitelaar AC, & Abbonk EM. (1995). Psychometric properties of the MOS SF-36 health survey in a population of patients with cancer [Abstract]. *Qual Life Res, 4,* 465.

Mutchler JE, & Burr JA. (1991). Racial differences in health and health care utilization in later life: The effect of socioeconomic status. *J Health Soc Behav, 32,* 342–356.

Nelson LM, Longstreth WT, Koepsell TD, & van Belle G. (1990). Proxy respondents in epidemiologic research. *Epidemiol Rev, 12,* 71–86.

Nerenz DR, Repasky DP, Whitehouse FW, & Kahkonen DM. (1992). Ongoing assessment of health status in patients with diabetes mellitus. *Med Care, 30*(Suppl), MS112–MS124.

Nocturnal Oxygen Therapy Trial Group. (1980). Continuous or nocturnal oxygen therapy in hypoxemic chronic obstructive pulmonary disease: A clinical trial. *Ann Intern Med, 93,* 391–398.

Noonan M, Chervinsky P, Busse WW, Weisberg SC, Pinnas J, DeBoisblanc BP, Boltansky H, Pearlman D, Repsher L, & Kellerman D. (1995). Fluticasone propionate reduces oral prednisone use while it improves asthma control and quality of life. *Am J Respir Crit Care Med, 152,* 1467–1473.

Nydevik I, & Hulter-Asberg K. (1991). Subjective dysfunction after stroke: A study with Sickness Impact Profile. *Scand J Prim Health Care, 9,* 271–275.

Nydevik I, & Hulter-Asberg K. (1992). Sickness impact after stroke: A 3-year follow-up. *Scand J Prim Health Care, 10,* 284–289.

O'Brien BJ, Buxton MJ, & Patterson DL. (1993). Relationship between functional status and health-related quality-of-life after myocardial infarction. *Med Care, 31,* 950–955.

Okamoto LJ, Noonan M, DeBoisblanc BP, & Kellerman DJ. (1996). Fluticasone propionate improves quality of life in patients with asthma requiring oral corticosteroids. *Ann Allergy Asthma Immunol, 76,* 455–461.

Ott CR, Sivarajan ES, Newton KM, Almes MJ, Bruce RA, Bergner M, & Gilson BS. (1983). A controlled randomized study of early cardiac rehabilitation: The Sickness Impact Profile as an assessment tool. *Heart Lung, 12,* 162–170.

*Patrick DL, Bush JW, & Chen MM. (1973). Methods for measuring levels of well-being for a health status index. *Health Serv Res, 8,* 228–245.

Patrick DL, & Deyo R. (1989). Generic and disease-specific measures in assessing health status and quality of life. *Med Care, 27,* S217–S232.

Patrick DL, & Erickson P. (1993). *Health status and health policy: Allocating resources to health care.* New York: Oxford University Press.

Patrick DL, Sittampalam Y, Somerville SM, Carter WB, & Bergner M. (1985). A cross-cultural comparison of health status values. *Am J Public Health, 75,* 1402–1407.

Perenger TV, Leplège A, Etter J-F, & Rougemont A. (1995). Validation of a French-language version of the MOS 36-Item Short Form Health Survey (SF-36) in young healthy adults. *J Clin Epidemiol, 48,* 1051–1060.

Persson LO, Karlsson J, Bengtsson C, Steen B, & Sullivan M. (1995). Psychometric and clinical validity of the Swedish version of the SF-36 [Abstract]. *Qual Life Res, 4,* 472.

Pierre U, Korner-Bitensky N, Hanley J, & Wood-Dauphinee S. (1995). Proxy use of the SF-36 in rating health status of the elderly [Abstract]. *Quality Life Res, 4,* 473.

Pocock SJ. (1991). A perspective on the role of quality-of-life assessment of clinical trials. *Controlled Clin Trials, 12,* 257S–265S.

Pollard WE, Bobbitt RA, Bergner M, Martin DP, & Gilson BS. (1976). The Sickness Impact Profile: Reliability of a health status measure. *Med Care, 14,* 146–155.

Reimer M, Thurston WE, & Russell M. (1995). Issues in measuring quality of life in cognitively impaired adults [Abstract]. *Qual Life Res, 4,* 477.

Revicki DA. (1992). Relationship between health utility and psychometric health status measures. *Med Care, 30,* MS274–MS282.

*Reuben DB, Valle LA, Hays RD, & Siu AL. (1995). Measuring physical function in community-dwelling older persons: A comparison of self-administered, interviewer-administered, and performance-based measures. *J Am Geriatr Soc, 43,* 17–23.

*Ries AL, Kaplan, RM, Limberg TM, & Prewitt LM. (1995). Effects of pulmonary rehabilitation on physiologic and psychosocial outcomes in patients with chronic obstructive pulmonary disease. *Ann Intern Med, 122,* 823–832.

Roland M, & Morris R. (1983). A study of the natural history of back pain: Part I. Development of a reliable and sensitive measure of disability in low-back pain. *Spine*, *8*, 141–144.

Rothman ML, Diehr P, Hedrick SC, Erdly WW, & Nickinovich DG. (1993). Effects of contract adult day health care on health outcomes and satisfaction with care. *Med Care*, *31*(Suppl.), SS75–SS83.

*Rothman ML, Hedrick S, & Inui T. (1989). The Sickness Impact Profile as a measure of the health status of noncognitively impaired nursing home residents. *Med Care*, *27*, S157–S167.

Rubenstein LV, Calkins DR, Greenfield S, Jette AM, Meenan RF, Nevins MA, Rubenstein LZ, Wasson JH, & Williams ME. (1988). Health status assessment for elderly patients: Report of the Society of General Internal Medicine Task Force on Health Assessment. *J Am Geriatr Soc*, *37*, 562–569.

Ruta DA, Garratt AM, Leng M, Russell IT, & MacDonald, LM. (1994). A new approach to the measurement of quality of life: The Patient Generated Index. *Med Care*, *32*, 1109–1126.

Schneider JR, McHorney CA, Malenka DJ, McDaniel MD, Walsh DB, & Cronenwett JL. (1993). Functional health and well-being in patients with severe atherosclerotic peripheral vascular occlusive disease. *Ann Vas Surg*, *7*, 419–428.

Schoenfeld DE, Malmrose LC, Blazer DG, Gold DT, & Seeman TE. (1994). Self-rated health and mortality in the high-functioning elderly—A closer look at healthy individuals: MacArthur Field Study of Successful Aging. *J Gerontol*, *49*, M109–M115.

Schrier AC, Dekker FW, Kaptein AA, & Dijkman JH. (1990). Quality of life in elderly patients with chronic nonspecific lung disease seen in family practice. *Chest*, *98*, 894–899.

Schuling J, Greidanus J, & Meyboom-de Jonghe B. (1993). Measuring functional status of stroke patients with the Sickness Impact Profile. *Disabil Rehabil*, *15*, 19–23.

Shaw LJ, Miller DD, Romeis JC, Kargl D, Younis LT, & Chaitman BR. (1994). Gender differences in noninvasive evaluation and management of patients with suspected coronary artery disease. *Ann Intern Med*, *120*, 559–566.

Sherbourne CD, & Meredith LS. (1992). Quality of self-report data: A comparison of older and younger chronically ill patients. *J Gerontol*, *47*, S204–S211.

Shiely J-C, Bayliss MS, Keller SD, Tsai C, & Ware JE. (1996). *SF-36 Health Survey annotated bibliography: First Edition (1988–1995)*. Boston, MA: Health Institute.

Siu AL, Hays RD, Ouslander JG, Osterwell D, Valdez RB, Krynski M, & Gross A. (1993). Measuring functioning and health in the very old. *J Gerontol*, *48*, M10–M14.

Squier HC, & Kaplan RM. (1995). Validation of symptom reporting in different patient populations on the Quality of Well-Being Scale [Abstract]. *Qual Life Res*, *4*, 488–489.

Spilker B, Molinek FR, Johnston KA, Simpson RL, & Tilson HH. (1990). Quality of life bibliographies and indexes. *Med Care*, *28*(Suppl.), DS1–DS77.

Steinberg EP, Tielsch JM, Schein OD, Javitt JC, Sharky P, Cassard S, Legro MW, Diener-West M, Bass EB, Damiamo AM, Steinwachs DM, & Sommer A. (1994). The VF-14: An index of functional impairment in patients with cataract. *Arch Ophthalmol*, *112*, 630–638.

Stewart AL, Greenfield S, Hays RD, Wells K, Rogers WH, Berry SD, McGlynn EA, & Ware JE. (1989). Functional status and well-being of patients with chronic conditions: Results from the Medical Outcomes Study. *JAMA*, *262*, 907–913.

Stewart AL, Hays RD, & Ware JE. (1988). The MOS Short-Form General Health Survey: Reliability and validity in a patient population. *Med Care*, *26*, 724–735.

Stewart AL, & Ware JE. (Eds). (1992). *Measuring functioning and well-being: The Medical Outcomes Study approach.* Durham, NC: Duke University Press.

Stucki G, Liang MH, Lipson SJ, Fossel AW, & Katz JN. (1994). Contribution of neuromuscular impairment to physical functional status in patients with lumbar spinal stenosis. *J Rheumatol*, *21*, 1338–1343.

Sullivan M, Ahlmen M, Archenholtz B, & Svensson G. (1986). Measuring health in rheumatic disorders by means of a Swedish version of the Sickness Impact Profile: Results from a population study. *Scand J Rheumatol*, *15*, 193–200.

Sullivan M, Karlsson J, Persson L-O, & Steen B. (1995). Self-rated health in 92 year olds: How reliable? [Abstract.] *Qual Lif Res*, *4*, 493–494.

Sullivan M, Karlsson J, Sjostrom L, Backman L, Bengtsson L, Dahlgren S, Jonsson E, Larsson B, Lindstedt S, Naslund I, Olbe L, & Wedel H. (1993). Swedish obese subjects (SOS)—An intervention study of obesity. Baseline evaluation and health and psycholosocial functioning of the final 1743 subjects examined. *Intl J Obesity*, *17*, 503–512.

Sullivan M, Karlsson J, & Ware JE Jr. (1995). The Swedish SF-36 Health Survey—I. Evaluation of data quality, scaling assumptions, reliability, and construct validity across general populations in Sweden. *Soc Sci Med*, *41*, 1349–1358.

Swanink CMA, Vercoulen JHHM, Bleijenberg G, Fennis JFM, Galama JMD, & Van Der Meer JWM. (1995). Chronic fatigue syndrome: A clinical and laboratory study with a well matched control group. *J Intern Med*, *237*, 499–506.

Tarlov AR, Ware JE, Greenfield S, Nelson EC, Perin E, & Zubkoff M. (1989). The Medical Outcomes Study: An application of methods for monitoring the results of medical care. *JAMA*, *262*, 925–930.

Temkin NR, Dikman S, Machamer J, & McLean A. (1989). General versus disease-specific measures: Further work on the Sickness Impact Profile for head injury. *Med Care*, *27*, S44–S53.

Tennant A, Fear J, Hillman M, & Chamberlain MA. (1995). Missing values and the MOS SF-36: An over 55 year-old sample with arthritis [Abstract]. *Qual Life Res*, *4*, 495–496.

Torrance GW, Furlong W, Feeny D, & Boyle M. (1995). Multi-attribute preference functions: Health Utilities Index. *PharmacoEconomics*, *7*, 503–519.

van Tulder MW, Aaronson NK, & Bruning PF. (1994). The quality of life of long-term survivors of Hodgkin's disease. *Ann Oncology*, *5*, 152–158.

van Zanten SJOV. (1991). Quality of life as outcome measures in randomized clinical trials. *Controlled Clin Trials*, *12*, 234S–242S.

*Visser MC, Fletcher AE, Parr G, Simpson A, & Bulpitt CJ. (1994). A comparison of three quality of life instruments in subjects with angina pectoris: The Sickness Impact Profile, the Nottingham Health Profile, and the Quality of Well Being Scale. *J Clin Epidemiol*, *47*, 157–163.

Wagner EH, LaCroix AZ, Grothaus LC, & Hecht JA. (1993). Responsiveness of health status measures to change among older adults. *J Am Geriatr Soc*, *41*, 241–248.

Ware JE. (1987). Standards for validating health measures: Definition and content. *J Chron Dis*, *40*, 473–480.

Ware JE, Gandek B, Kosinski M, Aaronson N, Apoline G, Bech P, Brazier J, Bullinger M, & Sullivan M. (1995). The factor structure and factor content of the SF-36 health status scales in seven countries: Results from the IQOLA project [Abstract]. *Qual Life Res, 4*, 501–502.

Ware JE, Keller SD, Gandek B, Brazier JE, Sullivan M, and the IQOLA Project Group. (1995). Evaluating translations of health status questionnaires: Methods from the IQOLA Project. *Int J Technol Assess Health Care, 11*, 525–551.

Ware JE, Kosinski M, Bayliss MS, McHorney CA, Rogers WH, & Raczek A. (1995). Comparison of methods for the scoring and statistical analysis of the SF-36 Health Profile and Summary Measures: Summary of results from the Medical Outcomes Study. *Med Care, 33*, AS264–AS279.

Ware JE, Kosinski M, & Keller SD. (1994). *SF-36 Physical and Mental Health Summary Scales: A user's manual.* Boston, MA: The Health Institute.

Ware JE, Kosinski M, & Keller SD. (1995). *SF-12: How to score the SF-12 Physical and Mental Health Summary Scales.* Boston, MA: The Health Institute.

Ware JE, Nelson EC, Sherbourne CD, & Stewart AL. (1992). Preliminary tests of a 6-item General Health Survey: A patient application. In AL Stewart & JE Ware (Eds.), *Measuring functioning and well-being* (pp. 291–303). Durham, NC: Duke University Press.

*Ware JE, & Sherbourne CD. (1992). The MOS 36-Item Short-Form Health Survey (SF-36): I. Conceptual framework and item selection. *Med Care, 30*, 473–483.

*Weinberger M, Nagle B, Hanlon JT, Samsa GP, Schmader K, Landsman PB, Uttech KM, Cowper PA, Cohen HJ, & Feussner JR. (1994). Assessing health-related quality of life in elderly outpatients: Telephone versus face-to-face administration. *J Am Geriatr Soc, 42*, 1295–1299.

Weinberger M, Oddone EZ, Samsa GP, & Landsman PB. (1996). Are health-related quality of life measures affected by the mode of administration? *J Clin Epidemiol, 49*, 135–140.

*Weinberger M, Samsa GP, Hanlon JT, Schmader K, Doyle ME, Cowper PA, Uttech Km, Cohen HJ, & Feussner JR. (1991). An evaluation of a brief health status measure in elderly veterans. *J Am Geriatr Soc, 39*, 691–694.

*Weinberger M, Samsa GP, Tierney WM, Belyea MJ, & Hiner SL. (1992). Generic versus disease specific health status measures: Comparing the Sickness Impact Profile and the Arthritis Impact Measurement scales. *J Rheumatol, 19*, 543–546.

Wiklund I, & Karlberg J. (1991). Evaluation of quality of life in clinical trials: Selecting quality of life measures. *Controlled Clin Trials, 12*, 204S–216S.

Williams JI, Agha M, & Kelly J. (1995). Societal and ethnic variations in self-ratings of health [Abstract]. *Qual Life Res, 4*, 504.

Williams JW, Kerber CA, Mulrow CD, Medina A, & Aguilar C. (1995). Depressive disorders in primary care: prevalence, functional disability, and identification. *J Gen Intern Med, 10*, 7–12.

Wu AW, Damiamo AM, Lynn J, Alzola C, Teno J, Landefeld CS, Desbiens N, Tsevat J, Mayer-Oakes A, Harrell FE, & Knaus WA. (1995). Predicting future functional status for seriously ill hospitalized adults: The SUPPORT Prognostic Model. *Ann Intern Med, 122*, 342–350.

Zeldow PB, & Pavlou M. (1988). Physical and psychosocial functioning in multiple sclerosis: Descriptions, correlations and a tentative typology. *Br J Med Psychol, 61*, 185–195.

3

Measures of Severity of Illness and Comorbidity

Barbara M. Rothenberg, Cathleen Mooney,
Lesley Curtis

OVERVIEW

Over the last decade, there has been a proliferation of measures developed to adjust for severity of illness or for comorbidity. This growth has been spurred by a variety of factors, including (1) the desire to control for these factors adequately in clinical studies; (2) interest in developing alternatives to fee-for-service payments adjusted for the complexity of care required; (3) increased interest in comparing "performance," as measured by mortality rates, for example, across providers; and (4) the growing popularity of outcome studies, particularly those that use nonrandom designs or rely on large administrative data sets. It is undeniable that severity of illness and comorbidity can be important determinants of outcomes, whether measured in terms of mortality, functional status, or utilization of health care. The debate centers on how to measure and control adequately for these factors.

The distinction between severity of illness and comorbidity is not always clear. *Severity of illness* can be used to refer to the severity of a specific illness, including the diagnosis of primary interest in a study, or to the severity of the overall burden of illness for an individual. *Comorbidity* refers to all conditions other than the diagnosis of primary interest. In practice, many measures of severity of illness (defined in terms of overall "disease burden") are readily converted into comorbidity measures simply by omitting the diagnosis of primary interest from the comorbidity score. For ease of presentation, in this chapter the term *severity of illness* will be used in the broad sense to encompass both severity of illness and comorbidity, unless something else is clearly indicated.

All of these measures are intended to control for "legitimate" variability among patients that is independent of the process being examined (e.g., the care provided by a hospital or physician or a specific type of procedure or treatment). What is legitimate depends upon the purpose of the analysis. For example, if one is comparing providers' performance or setting reimbursement levels, a good measure of severity of illness should control for severity that is beyond the provider's control—typically, the burden of illness that the patient brings to the encounter—but not illness induced by error on the part of the provider. Similarly, in clinical studies or outcomes studies, an ideal measure of severity of illness should account for variability in illness before initiation of the intervention of interest. It should not be correlated with response to treatment, however, or else it will not be possible to discern the impact of treatment.

In selecting an appropriate measure of severity of illness, a variety of factors need to be taken into account:

- Outcome or outcomes of interest
- Type of data available (e.g., prospectively gathered data, information from retrospective reviews of medical records, administrative databases)
- Cost of acquiring and administering the instrument or system
- Credibility and relevance among the intended audience (e.g., physicians)
- Time frame of interest (e.g., in-hospital outcomes versus those that occur within 1 year of discharge)
- Need for disease-specific versus generic instruments

(For an excellent discussion of many of the issues involved in adjustment for severity, see Iezzoni, 1994.)

It is not possible to design a generic severity-of-illness measure that will encompass all outcomes or serve all purposes. Not surprisingly, the factors that best predict mortality, for example, are different from or may be weighted differently from those that predict length of stay in the hospital. Thus, instruments are usually developed to adjust for the impact of patients' conditions on specific outcomes. The Charlson comorbidity index, for example, is intended to adjust for the burden of illness that a patient brings to a hospital admission when comparing 1-year mortality; the Index of Coexistent Disease (ICED) is designed to adjust for a baseline severity of illness when comparing functional status after 1 year. However, the instruments are sometimes used with alternative outcome measures (e.g., *Deyo, Cherkin, & Ciol, 1992), in part because there often are no instruments available for the specific outcome of interest using the type of data available.

The types of risk adjustment measures that can be used vary greatly with the type of data available, for example, whether data are gathered prospectively or retrospectively, and whether the measures rely on reviews of medical records or administrative data sets. Administrative data sets provide information on a large number of individuals and are usually relatively inexpensive, but they are limited in the types of data they provide and in the accuracy of the data (see the discussion below). More information can be garnered from medical records, but this is more costly to acquire and therefore the sample size is usually much more limited. Medical records also suffer from problems of data quality, but to a lesser degree than administrative data.

Many of the severity-of-illness instruments are proprietary and costly to acquire (e.g., they may cost over $10,000). They are often marketed to hospitals and insurance companies and are revised frequently to address the needs of those clients. Their cost may be prohibitive for research studies or for small-scale applications, their design and performance may not be reported in peer-reviewed journals, and their distributors may be less responsive to the needs of researchers. In this chapter, we focus on instruments that are in the public domain, but we also provide a brief overview of some of the more commonly used proprietary instruments.

In selecting an instrument, it is important to take into account the audience for whom the final product is intended. For example, there appears to be considerable skepticism among physicians about the validity of many case-mix adjustment measures, especially when they are used by insurers or regulatory agencies to compare outcomes across physicians. This problem is exacerbated by the fact that many of the proprietary instruments are "black boxes," in which the precise scoring algorithms are unclear. (For a discussion of the ethical issues involved in the use of proprietary instruments, see the February 1994 issue of *Health Services Review*.) One of the advantages of the Duke University Severity of Illness (DUSOI) checklist (discussed below), despite significant limitations in other regards, is that it relies heavily on clinical judgment. This may make it more acceptable to clinicians than some of the other statistically derived instruments. The possibility of a trade-off between statistical rigor and acceptability to an intended audience should be taken into account.

The final issue to be considered is whether or not to use disease-specific instruments. If one is examining a specific disease, then disease-specific instruments such as those that have been developed to gauge the severity of arthritis (e.g., the Arthritis Impact Measurement Scales; Meenan, Gertman, & Mason, 1980) or heart disease (e.g., the New York Heart Association classification of the severity of angina; Criteria Committee of the New York Heart Association, 1964) may be appropriate. Often, however, one is interested in comparing severity of illness across diseases or in looking at the burden of all comorbid illnesses other than the disease of primary interest. In those cases, more generic measures are required. Even among the generic measures, there are some that apply different weights depending on the patient's principal diagnosis (e.g., Disease Staging, MedisGroups), while others focus on generic dimensions of any disease (e.g., the functional scale of the ICED) or on the risks faced by any hospitalized individual (e.g., the Charlson comorbidity index). The instruments with highly specific scoring or weighting schemes for each principal diagnosis tend to be proprietary and to be more costly to implement.

REVIEW OF INSTRUMENTS IN THE PUBLIC DOMAIN

The instruments selected for more detailed review in this chapter are generic instruments (i.e., they do not focus on a single disease) that are in the public domain. The list is not comprehensive but rather provides examples of the types of instruments that have been used in a variety of settings to predict several different outcomes. Although these instruments can be used for a number of purposes, the focus in this chapter will be on their use in studies with nonrandomized research designs. Furthermore, these instruments are meant to adjust for severity within and among groups and are seldom intended to produce predictions that can be applied to a given individual. All of these instruments focus on the patient as the unit of analysis—in contrast to various measures developed to rate the complexity of care provided during a given episode of service, which have more commonly been developed for reimbursement purposes (e.g., *diagnosis-related groups* or DRGs in the inpatient setting and *diagnosis clusters* in the outpatient setting). A brief review of a wider variety of instruments, many of them proprietary, is provided below. The final alternative is to develop a risk adjustment measure tailored to the particular population and condition being studied; a discussion of the methods for doing this is found in chapter 5 of *Risk Adjustment for Measuring Health Care Outcomes* (Iezzoni, 1994).

The following instruments were selected for detailed review in this section:

- The Charlson Comorbidity Index (*Charlson, Pompei, Ales, & MacKenzie, 1987) was originally developed to predict mortality attributable to comorbidities among inpatients using data from medical records. There have been various adaptions, including those by Deyo and his colleagues (*1992) and the Dartmouth-Manitoba group (*Romano, Roos, & Jollis, 1993a, b) for use with administrative data.
- Acute Physiology and Chronic Health Evaluation (APACHE; Knaus, Draper, Wagner, & Zimmerman, 1985; Knaus et al., 1991; Knaus, Zimmerman, Wagner, Draper, & Lawrence, 1981) was developed to predict mortality

caused by patients' illness and comorbidities in intensive care units. Two other instruments developed for use in intensive care units (the Simplified Acute Physiology Score or SAPS II [*Le Gall, Lemeshow, & Saulnier, 1993] and the Mortality Probability Models or MPM II [*Lemeshow, Teres, Kalr, Avrunin, Gehlbach, & Rapoport, 1993]) are also discussed briefly.

- The Index of Coexistent Disease (ICED; *Greenfield, Aronow, Elashoff, & Watanabe, 1988; Greenfield, Blanco, Elashoff, & Aronow, 1988) was developed to predict functional status one year after hospitalization using data from medical records.
- The Duke University Severity of Illness (DUSOI) scale (Parkerson, Broadhead, & Tse, 1993; Parkerson et al., 1989) was developed to measure severity of illness and comorbidity in outpatients using data either from chart reviews or from a checklist completed by physicians following an office visit.

A brief overview of each of these instruments is provided below; annotations for the relevant articles on the first three instruments are found at the end of the chapter.

Charlson Index and Modifications

The Charlson Comorbidity Index was developed to measure the impact of comorbid conditions on the risk of mortality. Although originally developed to predict 1-year mortality for a cohort of patients admitted to the medical service of a New York City hospital, the index was subsequently validated on a retrospective cohort of patients with breast cancer and was used to predict 10-year mortality.

The Charlson index uses adjusted relative risks from a proportional hazards model to create weights for each of 19 comorbid conditions. The weights range from 1, for conditions like myocardial infarction and congestive heart failure; to 6, for conditions like acquired immune deficiency syndrome (AIDS) and metastatic solid tumor. For a given patient, one simply adds the weights for each comorbidity present to arrive at the patient's composite Charlson score. A low composite score suggests little comorbid disease; a high composite score suggests significant comorbid disease.

The original index relies on data abstracted from the medical record. Because of the increasing availability of administrative data sets, Deyo and his colleagues (*1992) and Romano and his colleagues (*1993a) translated the index for use with *International Classification of Diseases, Ninth Revision, Clinical Modification* (ICD-9-CM) diagnosis codes. The scoring mechanism remains the same: The weights assigned to the various ICD-9-CM diagnoses present are summed to arrive at the composite score for a given patient.

Since its development the Charlson index has been used widely. In some cases, the Charlson index has been the focus of the study (e.g., *D'Hoore, Sicotte, &

Tilquin, 1993; *Hartz et al., 1992), that is, investigators have sought to improve the index or, in the case of Deyo and his colleagues, to translate the index for use with administrative data sets. In the majority of cases, however, the Charlson index has been used for the purpose for which it was developed—to control for the effect of comorbid conditions on outcomes. That is, the Charlson index is one of several independent variables in a multivariate model (e.g., *O'Connor et al., 1991). Although the Charlson index was developed to predict 1-year mortality, it has been used in models predicting functional status (*Dodds, Martin, Stolov, & Deyo, 1993), use of resources (*Deyo et al., 1992), and the aggressiveness of care provided to nursing home patients (*Holtzman, Pheley, & Lurie, 1994). The ease with which the index can be calculated makes its broad application tempting. It is important to note, however, that the weights and index are specific to a single outcome, 1-year mortality. Attempts have been made to apply the weights and index to a broader range of outcomes, but the results have not been very promising (e.g., *Dodds et al., 1993).

The Charlson index has been used among older populations. Deyo and his colleagues (1992), in fact, adapted it for use with administrative data using a Medicare database. Others have applied it to older populations as well (*D'Hoore et al., 1993; *Dodds et al., 1993; *Hartz et al., 1992; *Holtzman et al., 1994).

The Charlson index—both the chart abstraction version and the administrative data set versions—are straightforward to apply and interpret. As with many severity adjustment measures, however, the index is critically dependent on the quality and completeness of the data that are coded. To the extent that chronic conditions are underreported in the chart or administrative data, the index will be biased downward. In addition, the index and weights may perform differently in different populations (*Romano et al., 1993b).

Acute Physiology and Chronic Health Evaluation (APACHE)

History and Overview

The Acute Physiology and Chronic Health Evaluation (APACHE) scoring system is widely used for measuring in-hospital mortality risk in patients admitted to the intensive care unit (ICU). Given that many ICU patients are older, APACHE has been used frequently with older patients. The first version of APACHE (Knaus et al., 1981) assigned up to four points for each of 34 physiologic measurements, which had been selected by clinical judgment. The points were summed to obtain scores ranging from 0 to 50, with higher scores suggesting more severe illness and being correlated with higher mortality. APACHE did not explicitly predict mortality. Health status prior to admission was characterized with a separate four-point ranking.

The second version of APACHE (APACHE II), which was validated in a multi-institutional study, includes only 12 physiologic measurements, uses some more specific measures than the first version, and includes points based on age and presence of chronic health conditions in the overall score (*Knaus et al., 1985). The sum of the points for only the physiologic measures is referred to as the acute physiology score (APS). The choice of a minimum set of variables and weights for all candidate variables was based on clinical judgment, but the importance of additional variables was assessed using statistical analysis. The developers of APACHE II provided published equations to predict mortality on the basis of APACHE II scores for 50 disease groups.

APACHE III scores (*Knaus et al., 1991) are defined by 16 physiologic measures (some of which are in turn defined by combinations of specific laboratory measures), age, presence of any of seven comorbid conditions, and type of ICU admission (e.g., nonoperative admission from emergency room). Logistic regression was used to identify relevant variables and estimate their weights. The logic for the APACHE III score is published, but equations to predict mortality on the basis of the score and admission diagnosis are proprietary. A computerized version of APACHE III is available that obtains physiologic data from ICU equipment and automated laboratory information systems, so that staff need enter only diagnosis, age, comorbidity, and neurological status.

APACHE is one of three major systems developed for assessing severity of illness in ICU patients. The Simplified Acute Physiology Score (SAPS II) (*Le Gall et al., 1993) and the Mortality Probability Models (MPM II) (*Lemeshow et al., 1993) also were developed from statistical analyses of large data sets drawn from many institutions. SAPS II has some advantages over the most recent version of APACHE. Most notably, it can be used to predict mortality using a published formula, it depends upon identifying only three preexisting conditions, and its prediction of mortality does not depend upon identifying a single diagnosis that caused admission. The MPM II provides other advantages; for example, it offers specific models for ICU admission and 24-hour intervals thereafter, and some of those models are available in the published literature. It also does not depend upon identifying a single cause for ICU admission. The performance of SAPS II and MPM II in predicting mortality in large samples of ICU patients appears to be comparable to that of APACHE III (Lemeshow & Le Gall, 1994), although none of these three has been validated by researchers independent of the developers. Although APACHE III is newer, the second version of APACHE is the subject of most of the studies abstracted here because it has been independently validated, used in many clinical studies, and applied in general hospital populations.

Purposes and Applications

The APACHE system was designed specifically to predict in-hospital mortality, in part to facilitate valid comparisons of the quality of care across ICUs. To this end, APACHE III and related commercial products have been adopted in many hospital systems. The developers also suggested that the mortality predicted by APACHE II could be used in clinical trials as a historical control against which to compare new treatments (*Knaus et al., 1985). That approach is problematic, however, given that the national sample used for the development of APACHE II is undoubtedly different from the sample of patients who meet specific requirements for enrollment in a clinical trial. APACHE II has been used to document comparability of treatment and control groups (e.g., Kieft et al., 1994). The developers also suggest that the APACHE system could be used to facilitate clinical decision making, although the role of any predictive model in individual decision making is controversial. As Lemeshow and Le Gall (1994) have noted, any mortality predictor provides an estimate of the proportion of a group who will die, but it cannot predict which individuals will die.

Because APACHE II has been used in so many studies, a complete review is beyond the scope of this chapter. We mention a few of the most recent examples for illustrative purposes. The APACHE II score has been used to predict a variety of outcomes besides mortality, with performance varying among outcome measures. APACHE II was a significant predictor of response to treatment with antibiotics (Fink et al., 1994), need for long-term institutionalization (Kollef, 1993), complications after intra-abdominal aortic surgery (Martin, Atnip, Holmes, Lynch, & Thiele, 1994), use of vasopressor medications and length of stay in suspected bacteremia (Moscovitz, Shofer, Mignott, Behrman, & Kilpatrick, 1994), and 1-year mortality in patients requiring mechanical ventilation (*Papadakis et al., 1993). It was not a significant predictor of differences in the use of cardiac imaging procedures (Bearden, Allman, Sundarum, Burst, & Bartolucci, 1993). APACHE II can explain some variance in estimated costs within DRGs (Thomas & Ashcraft, 1991). A version of APACHE II based only on laboratory data was also used to predict in-hospital use of resources within DRGs, as reported in the development paper that is included in our abstracts (*McMahon, Hayward, Bernard, Rosevear, & Weissfeld, 1992). The APACHE II score has also been used to predict survival in specific patient groups, such as those receiving cardio-pulmonary resuscitation (Beer, Teasdale, Ghusn, & Taffet, 1994) or those who have sepsis (National Committee for the Evaluation of Centoxin, 1994) or suspected bacteremia (Moscovitz et al., 1994). Its performance has been inconsistent in these groups, which are more specifically defined than the broad disease groups described in the APACHE II development study. APACHE II also has been applied to general hospital admissions (*Daley et al., 1988; Iezzoni et al., 1992; Thomas & Ashcraft, 1991). APACHE II is designed to characterize severity of illness during the first 24 hours of ICU care, but changes in patients' APACHE II scores during their entire ICU stay have been proposed as an outcome measure to identify substandard care (Hayward, Bernard, Rosevear, Anderson, & McMahon,

1993). However, the validity of APACHE II for measuring changes in illness or response to care has never been documented.

Limitations

The interrater reliability of APACHE data collection is reported to be acceptable by its developers (Damiano, Bergner, Draper, Knaus, & Wagner, 1992), in a small single-institution study (Holt, Bury, Bersten, Skowronski, & Vedig, 1992), and in a larger study comparing several severity-of-illness adjustment systems (Thomas & Ashcraft, 1989). However, APACHE II is designed to be based on the "most deranged" physiologic values (Knaus, Draper, Wagner, & Zimmerman, 1985, p. 818) and, hence, should reflect the patient's worst level of severity during the first 24 hours of ICU care. The logic of the scoring system is somewhat complicated, and data collectors may need to refer to the scoring algorithm and recalculate the scores repeatedly in order to identify the "most deranged" value (Holt et al., 1992). The automated version of APACHE III would presumably improve data collection by identifying the most severe physiologic abnormalities more reliably.

Postoperative recipients of coronary artery bypass grafts were excluded from the analyses to predict mortality from the APACHE II score in the development study. Their pattern of high APACHE II scores coupled with low mortality rates may reflect a systematic difficulty in applying APACHE II to patients whose physiologic status has been significantly altered by treatment intervention before ICU admission rather than by underlying disease. This illustrates that APACHE II, like any severity-of-illness index, can be affected by treatment interventions, particularly those preceding ICU admission.

Applicability to Older Adults

Because a substantial number of ICU patients are older adults, the APACHE development studies and its applications have included a significant proportion of older individuals. The formula for the APACHE score assumes older patients are more severely ill and therefore have a higher in-hospital mortality rate. An independent study did demonstrate that age and gender can explain variance in mortality beyond that explained by the physiologic variables included in APACHE II (Iezzoni et al., 1992). However, there is some evidence that the relationship between age and in-hospital mortality is not monotonic in some disease groups (*Wu, Rubin, & Rosen, 1990), which suggests that the age component should be dropped from APACHE under some circumstances. Numerous other reports have discussed whether age is a predictor of ICU outcome, independent of severity of illness, without definitive conclusions (e.g., Kollef, 1993; *Papadakis et al., 1993).

Index of Coexistent Disease (ICED)

The Index of Coexistent Disease (ICED) was developed as an instrument to adjust for comorbidity. The primary outcomes of interest are patients' prognosis (that is, likelihood of experiencing full recovery), complications, and functioning at some interval (e.g., one year) following hospitalization. The ICED initially had three components:

1. An individual disease value, which indicates the existence and severity of a variety of conditions on a scale from zero to four. It is based on a modification of criteria developed by Gonnella, Hornbrook, and Louis (1984). Up to five conditions are rated per patient.
2. A measure of complications, which indicates the complications of the individual comorbid diseases. This component was dropped from later versions.
3. An indication of functional status, which is intended to measure the impact of all conditions on the individual's current health status; it is also called the physical impairment component. Functional status is rated from zero to two for 10 or 11 system categories (depending on the version), including circulation, respiration, neurological, mental status, urinary, fecal, feeding, vision, hearing, and speech.

Scores for each of the three components are calculated. For example, for the first dimension, patients are given the score corresponding to the highest score for any single disease; according to the developers, early analyses showed that having additional diseases at the same or lower level added no additional risk (*Greenfield, Apolone, McNeil, & Cleary, 1993).

Scores from the two or three components are then combined to produce a composite score. This score was initially graded on a three-point scale but was later changed to a four-point scale: A score of 1 indicates no comorbid disease or asymptomatic disease; 2, controlled but mildly symptomatic disease; 3, uncontrolled and severely symptomatic disease; and 4, life-threatening comorbid disease. Additional information on scoring of the ICED is available from the National Auxiliary Publications Service (*Greenfield et al., 1993).

The ICED is intended for use in retrospective studies and relies on information from a patient's medical record. The developers estimate that it takes a trained medical record abstractor 15 minutes per patient to complete the abstract.

The original instrument was developed in a cohort of 384 patients with breast cancer and was validated in a sample of 419 patients with colon cancer. Principal components analyses were performed within and between subscales of the ICED. However, these analyses have apparently been reported only in an abstract (Greenfield, Blanco, Elashoff, & Aronow, 1987), and no details were provided. Interrater reliability was examined, but the sample was small ($n = 30$; *Greenfield, Blanco, Elashoff, & Ganz, 1987). The four raters agreed on 66.7% (20/30) of the overall ICED scores (the κ value was not reported).

Most of the studies using the ICED were performed by the developers or their colleagues, and most of these articles report on different patient groups from the same two large studies. While the studies consistently demonstrate the utility of the ICED in adjusting for differences in comorbidity and functional status, the total amount of variation explained is quite low (the R^2 for the ICED alone in one study—*Greenfield et al., 1993—was 0.07). Also, in several of the studies only a single component of the ICED is examined or the scale is divided into only two categories.

One of the prime advantages of the ICED is its focus on comorbidity and on functional status, rather than on mortality or use of resources, as the outcome measure of primary interest. Because functional status is more difficult to measure than mortality, it is not surprising that the results regarding interrater reliability and the amount of variation explained are lower than for APACHE, for example. Nevertheless, it does provide an instrument that adjusts for these factors and that has a track record among patients who have several major diseases or have undergone one of several procedures. Further studies of its reliability and its performance in different populations would be useful.

Duke University Severity of Illness Scale (DUSOI)

The Duke University Severity of Illness Scale (DUSOI) is an instrument designed to measure severity of illness and comorbidity in the outpatient setting. The original version, first published in 1989, was based on a review of medical records. A revised version, published in 1993, developed a checklist that could be completed by physicians during the office visit. Scoring in both versions is based primarily on clinical judgment, with few explicit criteria. The physician or chart reviewer is asked to record all of a patient's diagnoses or health problems that are active at the time of the visit or during the preceding week. The health problems are described in the physician's own words and are later classified using the International Classification of Health Problems in Primary Care (ICHPPC). The basic approach to assessing the burden of illness was adapted from work by Horn et al. (1985). The physician or chart reviewer then scores each condition along three or four dimensions using a five-point scale from 0 to 4, where 0 represents none. The original instrument had three dimensions: (1) current symptom level, (2) current complication level (i.e., health problems secondary to another health problem that in the rater's judgment do not warrant listing as a separate problem), and (3) treatability and prognosis. The revised version split treatability and prognosis into two dimensions, prognosis without treatment and treatability, which indicate, respectively, the perceived need for treatment and the expected response to treatment if needed. The scores are combined and averaged and produce a single score for each health problem. Overall severity scores are calculated by taking the highest score and adding scores for additional conditions weighted by consecutively smaller weights (the precise formula is provided in Parkerson et al., 1993). Overall comorbidity scores are calculated simply by deleting the score for the diagnosis of primary interest and reassigning weights.

One of the primary features of this instrument is that it relies principally on clinical judgment rather than more systematic criteria in devising severity-of-illness scores. This comment is particularly true of the physician-completed checklist, and it suggests both advantages and disadvantages. On the positive side, clinical judgments can incorporate the subtle distinctions that are routinely made by clinicians and that take into account the myriad of factors that may never be noted in a medical chart. On the negative side, the checklist apparently does not establish explicit criteria for the physician to follow, potentially introducing much greater variability in scoring across patients and physicians and making interpretation of results difficult. However, the reliability of this instrument has been assessed in several of the studies. The interrater reliability for the chart-based version or between the chart-based version and the physician checklist has ranged from about 0.56 to 0.68; the intrarater reliability has ranged from 0.67 to 0.89 (Parkerson et al., 1989, 1993). The test-retest correlation ranged from 0.59 for the chart-based version to 0.65 for provider-generated scores with an average interval of 75.5 (SD = 52.4) days (Parkerson et al., 1993). One study (Parkerson et al., 1995) found that the DUSOI's predictive accuracy, as measured by the area under the receiver operating characteristic (ROC) curve, for a variety of outcomes measuring utilization and severity of illness during an 18-month follow-up period ranged from 60% to 68.9%. As the authors point out, this performance does not match that of other, more elaborate, severity adjustment measures such as APACHE, but it is better than would be predicted by chance alone.

One of the difficulties in assessing the DUSOI is that the primary outcome of interest is not completely clear. The original study (Parkerson et al., 1989) focused on the relationship between family support and stress, on the one hand, and self-reported functional health, on the other, while controlling for severity of illness, among other factors. One of the other major articles on the instrument (Parkerson et al., 1993), however, simply reports correlations with a variety of other independent variables, such as age and gender. A third study (Parkerson et al., 1995) examines the ability of the DUSOI scores to predict a variety of outcome measures: follow-up visits, referral to a specialist or hospital admission, and office charges and severity of illness during the follow-up period. The diversity of the outcome measures makes it difficult to evaluate the face validity of some of the scoring results. For example, in one study (Parkerson et al., 1993), the disease or condition with the highest score was "sprains or strains." It ranked ahead of diseases such as chronic ischemic heart disease and diabetes mellitus. The reason for this is the relative weight given to symptoms versus prognosis and complications. If the principal focus is on patients' short-term perceptions of well-being, then perhaps the current weighting system is warranted. For many of the purposes for which one might want to use a severity adjustment measure, however, these results seem questionable. The pluses and minuses of the instrument would also be more apparent if it had also been applied to a sicker population. The instrument was developed and tested among ambulatory patients from a rural primary care community health clinic in North Carolina. But in some cases patients were excluded because they were too sick to participate.

Because of some of the reservations about the DUSOI and the limited literature on this topic (in particular the absence of any studies on older populations), we have not included annotations of the literature on the DUSOI. The development and testing of the DUSOI is described primarily in Parkerson et al., 1989, 1992, 1993, and 1995. Articles about applications include a small study of the impact of comorbidities on hypertensive patients' self-assessed health status (Lahad & Yodfat, 1993) and an article in Spanish comparing patients at two types of outpatient clinics in New York City (Fernandez de Sanmamed, Fein, Morrison, & Moy, 1993). There are also two studies looking at the interaction between depression and comorbidities (Broadhead, Clapp-Channing, Finch, & Copeland, 1989; Coulehan, Schulberg, Block, Janosky, & Arena, 1990), but in these cases the DUSOI is not being used to control for comorbidity in the traditional sense.

A BRIEF REVIEW OF PROPRIETARY INSTRUMENTS

While many well-established severity adjustment tools are in the public domain, others have evolved as proprietary systems. These systems vary widely with respect to their underlying logic and associated licensing fees. Estimated fees range from $10,000 to over $50,000 per year, although fees are sometimes reduced or waived for nonprofit research. Most of these systems were developed primarily to categorize patients by the cost of their care in order to facilitate reimbursement to providers or utilization review. Like systems in the public domain, proprietary systems require either primary data abstraction from the medical record or information provided from hospital discharge data (ICD-9-CM based).

Inpatient Care

MedisGroups, marketed by MediQual System, is perhaps the most widely used severity adjustment system requiring abstraction from medical records. Medis-

Groups uses objective clinical findings to categorize patients into one of five levels of severity. Specifically, the number and type of abnormal findings are combined into an ordinal scale that ranges from 0 (no abnormal findings) to 4 (organ failure). Severity scores are based on findings documented during the first 48 hours of a patient's stay. In addition to the admission-oriented measure, MedisGroups also requires a second review for patients who stay in the hospital beyond a certain number of days. MedisGroups has been evaluated extensively in the literature. For a summary of the development of MedisGroups, see Brewster et al., 1985; for a clinical assessment of the system, see Iezzoni and Moskowitz, 1988.

The Computerized Severity Index (CSI) is a hybrid system. It relies on both ICD-9-CM-based data from discharge abstracts and clinical data abstracted from the medical record. Two severity scores are calculated from these data. The admission severity score uses data from the first 48 hours of the patient's stay. The maximum severity score uses data from the entire stay without regard to when the data were collected. For a thorough description of the system, see Horn, 1986; Horn and Horn, 1986; and Health Systems International (HSI) and Horn, 1987.

Of those systems that rely exclusively on discharge abstract data, three are perhaps most widely known. The Acuity Index Method (AIM) of Iameter, Inc., calculates severity on the basis of relative lengths of stay. The AIM divides DRGs into five subcategories that reflect the influence of several risk factors on length of stay. Little information has been published regarding AIM. Disease Staging, marketed by Systemetrics/McGraw-Hill, Inc., uses combinations of diagnoses, procedures, the patient's discharge status, and gender to determine the stage of each of the patient's conditions. Disease-specific staging information is then integrated to produce an overall severity score for each patient. Publications concerning Disease Staging are dominated by the system's developers (Gonella et al., 1984), although independent researchers have examined the system as well (Thomas & Ashcraft, 1991). The Patient Management Categories (PMC) system is quite different from the others described. Although it uses ICD-9-CM diagnosis and procedure codes, the system does not simply assign a severity score. Rather, it assigns patients to one (or more) of nearly 800 narrowly defined categories that incorporate severity of illness. Relatively few studies have been published regarding the performance of PMC (for example, Calore & Iezzoni, 1987; Charbonneau et al., 1988). For a more detailed review of proprietary inpatient instruments, see Iezzoni, 1994, chapter 1. A recent article by Iezzoni et al. (1996) also compares the performance of MedisGroups, a component of APACHE, Disease Staging, Patient Management Categories, the Deyo adaptation of the Charlson Comorbidity Index, all patient refined diagnosis-related groups (APR-DRGs), and refined diagnosis-related groups to compare hospitals' risk-adjusted mortality.

Outpatient Care

While it is challenging to devise adequate case-mix adjustment measures for the inpatient setting (discussed further below), the difficulties pale in comparison with those encountered in adjusting for severity of illness in the outpatient setting. Among the factors that make the outpatient setting particularly demanding are the numerous types of providers, settings, and services provided; the difficulty in defining the beginning and end of episodes of illness; and the prevalence of less advanced clinical information systems, which may not be computerized. (For two overviews of efforts to develop ambulatory case-mix measures, see Berlowitz, Rosen, & Moskowitz, 1995; and Weiner, 1991.) Nevertheless, there are a number of instruments for use in outpatient settings in addition to DUSOI which are based on different responses to these challenges.

The Ambulatory Care Groups system is a proprietary index available for a reduced fee for use in nonprofit academic research through the Johns Hopkins School of Hygiene and Public Health (Starfield, Weiner, Mumford, & Steinwachs, 1991; Weiner, Starfield, Steinwachs, & Mumford, 1991). This computerized system creates 34 ambulatory diagnostic groups (ADGs) from about 5,000 ICD-9-CM diagnosis codes that occur frequently in ambulatory care claims. Each patient is in turn assigned to one of 51 mutually exclusive ambulatory care groups (ACGs) based on ADGs, age, and gender. ACGs are designed to be homogeneous with respect to several dimensions of complexity, but the primary criterion for the groupings was expected persistence of the condition. This system is most useful for analyzing ambulatory care over a period of time, rather than for characterizing individual contacts between patients and providers. The authors recommend it for setting capitation rates for reimbursement, as well as for adjusting providers' utilization review measures. A study to explore the usefulness of the ACG system specifically among older adults was in progress at the time of this writing.

A second proprietary instrument, the Ambulatory Patient Severity (APS™) system, has not been documented in the literature as well as ACGs. According to marketing information distributed by its developer, International Severity Information Systems, Inc. (ISIS), of Sparks, MD, the system uses physiologic data and severity criteria similar to those used by the Computerized Severity Index (CSI). A description of the development of a predecessor to APS, the Ambulatory Severity Index, suggests that the index depends upon additional data collected at the time of a patient-provider encounter, such as the patient's compliance and the urgency of the visit (Horn, Buckle, & Carver, 1988).

Four additional indexes are designed to characterize visits or encounters, rather than assessing the severity of illness for patients, and as such are probably of limited use for clinical studies. Diagnosis Clusters were designed to collapse the ICD-9 codes noted on ambulatory claims data into broad groups that are clinically similar (Schneeweiss et al., 1986; Schneeweiss, Rosenblatt, Cherkin, Kirkwood, & Hart, 1983). The logic for the clusters is available upon request from the developers. The remaining three instruments are the Clinical Complexity Index (Perkins, 1991), Ambulatory Patient Groups (Averill et al., 1990), and Products of Ambulatory Care (Tenan et al., 1988). These were developed primarily to correlate with various proxies for the cost of care. Although these systems do not provide a summary measure of a patient's severity, the aggregate complexity of patients, as measured by the maximum or mean of the visit indexes, might be of use to some investigators.

ASSESSING THE PERFORMANCE OF SEVERITY-OF-ILLNESS INSTRUMENTS

Given the number of severity-of-illness and comorbidity instruments, it is crucial to assess which performs best for a given question. The psychometric properties (e.g., reliability, validity) discussed in the Introduction with respect to functional status instruments are relevant to severity-of-illness instruments as well. That is, one wants to be reasonably certain that a severity adjustment measure gives consistent answers for similar cases (reliability). Further, it is important that the instrument actually measures severity of illness (validity).

A specific form of validity—predictive validity—is particularly relevant, since severity-of-illness instruments are most often used to adjust for differences in case mix. Predictive validity addresses the question: How well does the severity adjustment instrument predict the outcome of interest? For example, the Charlson comorbidity index was developed to measure the impact of comorbid conditions on the risk of mortality. Its predictive validity is measured by the extent to which high Charlson scores are associated with or "predict" mortality, the outcome of interest.

The quantitative measures that assess predictive validity vary depending on the nature of the outcome of interest. When the outcome of interest is a continuous variable (e.g., length of stay or postdischarge functional status), the standard summary measure of performance is R^2. Technically, R^2 represents the proportion of variability in the outcome that is accounted for by differences in severity of illness. The R^2 ranges from 0 to 1; a higher R^2 implies that the severity-of-illness instrument accounts for a higher proportion of variation in the outcome. For dichotomous outcomes—such as death or occurrence of a specific clinical event—it is particularly important to know how well the instrument discriminates between those who experienced the outcome and those who did not. Again, using the Charlson index as an example, one would expect the actual mortality rate to be higher for patients with high Charlson scores than for those with low Charlson scores. In addition, when severity-of-illness measures explicitly estimate outcomes such as mortality rates, one wants to be certain that the actual and predicted outcome rates are nearly equal (calibration).

A thorough discussion of the statistical techniques used to assess discrimination and calibration is beyond the scope of this book. For an excellent and straightforward presentation of the statistical techniques, see chapters 8 and 9 in *Risk Adjustment for Measuring Health Care Outcomes* (Iezzoni, 1994; see also Lemeshow & Le Gall, 1994, and Daley, 1994, for briefer discussions of how to evaluate risk adjustment models).

LIMITATIONS OF ADMINISTRATIVE AND MEDICAL RECORD DATA

Most generic severity-of-illness measures rely on information either from administrative databases, essentially data collected for billing purposes, or from reviews of medical records. Both sources of information have limitations in terms of the accuracy and completeness of the data that must be taken into account when interpreting the results of severity-of-illness measures. (The following discussion relies heavily on the extensive review of this topic in Iezzoni, 1994, chapters 3 and 4.)

The primary limitations of medical records include incomplete information and variability in the amount of detail from one provider to another. For example, Iezzoni et al. (1990) found that records from academic hospitals tend to include much more information on patients' comorbidities than records from other types of hsopitals. The completeness of the information provided may also vary with the type of information being examined. For example, Iezzoni (1994) cites a number of studies demonstrating that the principal complaint is often recorded quite reliably but that often very few data are provided on functional status and social history (e.g., whether or not patients live alone). Another problem can arise if severity measures rely on the results of certain tests that are performed at varying rates across providers; a low severity-of-illness score may be the product not of less disease but simply of less use of tests for gauging severity. Some of the problems found in medical records are inherent to the practice of medicine (e.g., low levels of interrater reliability in the interpretation of results of diagnostic tests). But whereas efforts can be made to control for these factors in prospective studies or at least to measure the magnitude of the problem, studies based on retrospective chart review often accept the data as given. Finally, most studies find that some percentage of the charts simply cannot be found.

The problems encountered in dealing with medical records are compounded when one examines administrative data, since the latter rely on information summarized from the former and add a number of additional constraints of their own. One of the major concerns in using administrative data, which has been the subject of considerable study, is the accuracy and completeness of the diagnostic coding (see, for example, Fisher et al., 1992; Jollis et al., 1993; Romano et al., 1994; Roos, Sharp, & Cohen, 1991). This information is essential in measuring severity of illness, as well as for a variety of other purposes.

Most administrative databases contain diagnostic codes based on the ICD-9-CM coding system. Diagnoses are usually assigned retrospectively by abstractors of hospital medical records on the basis of the discharge summary, the entire medical record, and consultation with the physician if necessary (although this apparently does not occur frequently in practice); physicians must also sign off on all discharge diagnoses, at least for Medicare patients. A variety of potential problems exist with these data:

- The medical record itself may be incomplete or ambiguous, leading to the omission or miscoding of relevant diagnoses.
- The coding system, while extensive, does not contain explicit criteria defining the clinical terms. For example, there are 37 codes for different types of anemia but no specification of what hematocrit level justifies a diagnosis of anemia (Iezzoni, 1994). Thus, there is variation across hospitals in the codes typically assigned to patients with certain diseases.
- The potential variation in the ordering of the diagnoses and particularly the designation of the principal diagnosis, which is supposed to be the diagnosis chiefly responsible for the admission of the patient to the hospital, can make it difficult to identify a cohort of interest. Ordering can be affected by financial as well as clinical considerations, since the designation of the DRG, upon which the hospital's reimbursement is calculated, is based on the principal diagnosis. Studies have shown considerable discrepancies between the ordering found in administrative data and the judgments of independent reviewers (discussed further below). Furthermore, the accuracy of the coding varies by condition.
- The number of diagnoses and procedures allowed per record has varied. Until 1992, Medicare data included five diagnoses and three procedure codes; these data have since been expanded to nine diagnoses and six procedures. As a result, not all diagnoses could be included for individuals with complex conditions or multiple comorbidities, and that introduces an additional potential bias into the data. However, a study by Iezzoni and colleagues (1992) suggests that simply increasing the number of coding spaces will not solve the problem completely. Underreporting is likely to continue, and its severity is likely to vary by condition (but see also Romano & Mark, 1994, who find that expanding the number of coding spaces to nine represents a significant improvement).
- As with medical records, the level of detail found in discharge abstracts may vary from hospital to hospital as well; some hospitals may simply be

heavy coders, and this would make their patients appear to be sicker than those at other hospitals.

- Many of the administrative databases do not indicate whether or not a given diagnosis was present on admission. Therefore, it is difficult in some cases to distinguish between preexisting risk factors and complications encountered during the hospitalization.

All of these potential limitations need to be taken into account in using severity-of-illness measures with administrative data. In particular, one needs to investigate what is known about the relative accuracy of coding for the disease or diseases of primary interest and also make decisions about how many diagnoses to include, given the purposes of the study. For example, in defining a cohort, will a study include only individuals with the disease of interest listed as the principal diagnosis or also incorporate those with this disease listed as a secondary diagnosis?

Despite all of these caveats, administrative data provide extensive information on whole populations of individuals at relatively low cost, so they will continue to be used. The challenge is to design studies that will limit the influence of the potential biases introduced by these limitations. For example, linkage of hospital claims data with outpatient data can provide confirmation that certain conditions were present before a given hospitalization.

EVALUATION: CURRENT STATE OF THE ART
AND FUTURE DIRECTIONS

There are clearly a number of alternative methods available for adjusting for case mix and comorbidity, and each of them has its own advantages and limitations. This is a relatively new field that has grown quite rapidly during the last decade. Much progress has been made, yet definitive solutions remain elusive in a number of areas. Nevertheless, the importance of adjusting for severity of illness or comorbidity in comparing groups of individuals, particularly in nonrandomized studies, cannot be overestimated. Therefore, the only reasonable option is to continue to use less-than-ideal tools selected on the basis of the characteristics of the specific study, while remaining fully cognizant of their limitations and of the fact that they are unlikely to have adjusted completely for differences in case mix.

Given the increasing emphasis on monitoring severity-adjusted outcomes, one expects the number and variety of severity of illness measures to grow. While refined and expanded tools will add to the existing body of knowledge about measuring severity of illness, choosing among measures will become increasingly difficult. That is, a researcher must confront the fundamental question: Given my hypothesis, which severity-of-illness measure should I use? The literature is surprisingly sparse with respect to direct comparisons of severity-of-illness measures for defined patient populations. These direct comparisons are needed if researchers and clinicians are to make educated decisions about the measures. In addition, even for some widely used tools, there are surprisingly few independent assessments of their performance. Again, this type of research is crucial if we are to make informed decisions.

ANNOTATED BIBLIOGRAPHY

Charlson Index and Modifications

Development and Methods

Charlson ME, Pompei P, Ales KL, & MacKenzie CR. (1987). A new method of classifying prognostic comorbidity in longitudinal studies: Development and validation. *J Chron Dis*, 40, 373–383.

Design. The paper reports the development and validation of a weighted index of comorbidity that quantifies the impact of prognostically important comorbidities on short-term mortality. Data collected for the study include the admitting residents' assessments of severity of illness, reasons for admission, demographic and clinical characteristics, number and severity of comorbid diseases, and the subsequent course of the patient. Proportional hazards models are used in the statistical analysis.

Sample. The sample on which the index was developed consisted of 559 patients admitted to the medical service at a large teaching hospital (99.3% of intended sample). Information about the age and gender distribution of the sample is not included. Detailed information is provided about the prevalence of several comorbid diseases. Hypertension, angina, congestive heart failure, myocardial infarction (MI), arrhythmia, and mild pulmonary disease were each present in more than 10% of the sample.

The validation cohort consists of 685 women with histologically proven primary cancer of the breast who underwent their first treatment in a large teaching hospital between 1962 and 1969. Again, information about the age distribution of the sample is not included. While no detailed information about comorbid conditions is present, the authors report that the prevalence of comorbid disease was significantly lower than in the development cohort.

Summary. The Comorbidity Index was developed in three steps. First, Charlson and her colleagues assessed the prognostic impact of individual comorbid diseases at 1 year. Unadjusted relative risks were calculated as the proportion of patients with the condition who died divided by the proportion of patients without the disease who died. Adjusted relative risks were computed from the coefficients produced by a proportional hazards model and estimate the risk of death with a given comorbid condition controlling for other factors (e.g., all coexistent comorbid diseases, severity of illness, and reason for admission).

Second, the authors assessed the impact of combinations of comorbid diseases on 1-year mortality. Although the authors found that the total number of comorbid diseases did predict 1-year mortality ($p < 0.05$), the approach implausibly assumes that all comorbid diseases carry an equal burden (e.g., the presence of leukemia is equivalent to the presence of diabetes).

Third, to address the intuitive problem of equal weighting of comorbid diseases, the authors developed a weighted index that accounts for the number and severity of the comorbid conditions. Charlson and her colleagues used a proportional hazards model to predict 1-year mortality using the adjusted relative risk of individual comorbid diseases. The weighted index was a significant predictor of 1-year survival ($p < .0001$). In addition, the authors reported that the model explained a higher proportion of variance than the model based only on the number of comorbid diseases ($R^2 = 0.087$ versus $R^2 = 0.038$).

Charlson and her colleagues validate the weighted index in the retrospective cohort of patients with breast cancer. Deaths were attributed either to breast cancer or to comorbid disease. To be cited as a "comorbid death," the patient must have been free from metastatic disease at the last examination performed before the time of death.

The proportional hazards model used in the validation cohort predicted 10-year mortality using anatomic stage, nodal status, clinical rate of growth, menstrual status, age, and comorbidity. Only age and comorbidity were significant predictors. Each decade of age and rank of comorbidity added similar risk. Specifically, the relative risk for each increasing level of the comorbidity index was 7.3 (95% CI, 1.9–2.8) and 2.4 (95% CI, 2.0–2.9) for each decade of age. Although still quite low, the proportion of variance explained by the model ($R^2 = 0.091$) was comparable to that in the development data set ($R^2 = 0.087$).

The authors hypothesize that age became an important predictor of death from comorbid disease because of the length of follow-up. They suggest that the weighted index of comorbidity be modified to account for age when used in longer-term (> 5-year follow-up) studies. Specifically, they recommend adding 1 point to the total comorbidity score for each decade of age over 40.

Discussion.   The paper provides a thorough description of the analytical process used to arrive at the weighted comorbidity index. Furthermore, the weighted index itself, which is presented in the paper, is simple to use. The total comorbidity score is calculated by summing the weights of all comorbid illnesses present. Detailed definitions for each of the comorbid illnesses are provided in an appendix.

Limitations exist, however, with the weighted index. First, as the authors point out, the development and validation samples are relatively small, given the low prevalence of many of the conditions included in the index. Second, although the comorbidity index is a significant predictor of death, the proportion of variation explained by the model (R^2) is very low. At best, the model explains 10% of the variation; 90% of the variability associated with 1-year mortality is unexplained. Finally, although the authors present a method for incorporating age into the weighted index, they do not validate the method. They report that the method performed well in predicting 10-year survival, but they do not provide additional detail to support the assertion.

Deyo RA, Cherkin DC, & Ciol MA. (1992). Adapting a clinical comorbidity index for use with ICD-9-CM administrative databases. *J Clin Epidemiol*, 45, 613–619.
Design.   Deyo and his colleagues adapted the Charlson weighted comorbidity index for use with ICD-9-CM diagnoses coded in an administrative database. The authors validated the adapted index using a Medicare data set from the Health Care Financing Administration that included detailed information on claims for beneficiaries who underwent lumbar spine

surgery in 1985. The data set included linked data for all previous hospitalizations for 1 year prior to the index hospitalization.

Sample.   Claims data from 27,111 index hospitalizations for unique patients were included in the study. Excluded from the sample were (1) patients not continuously eligible for Medicare for at least 1 year prior to the index admission; (2) patients who were Medicare beneficiaries because of end-stage renal disease or Social Security Disability Insurance (SSDI); (3) patients with a diagnosis during the index admission which indicated a neoplasm, spinal infection, or spine fracture; and (4) patients with a second major surgical procedure during the index admission (e.g., coronary artery bypass graft—CABG—surgery or prostatectomy). The mean age of the patients included in the sample was 71.8 years; 57.1% were women. A Charlson index score of 0 was established for 71% of patients. The range of comorbidity scores was relatively small, and very few patients had scores above 3.

Summary.   Deyo and his colleagues began by mapping the comorbid conditions included in the Charlson index to ICD-9-CM diagnosis codes. Diagnoses that could be complications of lumbar spine surgery (e.g., MI, acute stroke) were included only if they appeared during a hospitalization that occurred in the year prior to the index admission. Other diagnoses that indicated chronic disease (e.g., diabetes or chronic obstructive pulmonary disease, COPD) were included whether they occurred during the index admission or during a previous admission.

Chi-square analyses and logistic regression were used to test for associations between the adapted comorbidity index and the dichotomous outcomes (mortality, complications, blood transfusion, and nursing home discharge). Analysis of variance and multiple linear regression were used to test for associations between the index and continuous outcomes (mean length of stay—LOS—and total hospital charges). The analysis suggests that, in fact, the index can be successfully applied to administrative databases. Specifically, as index scores increased, so did the likelihood of poor outcomes (in-hospital complications, blood transfusions, discharge to nursing home, and mortality) and increased resource consumption (LOS and total hospital charges). Since cross-sectional data are frequently the only data available to researchers, the investigators repeated the analysis using only those comorbid diagnoses recorded during the index 1985 hospitalization. The associations between the comorbidity score and outcomes persisted, although the distribution of overall scores shifted downward.

Discussion.   The Charlson index was designed for use with data abstracted from medical records. Because of the increasing use of administrative databases in health services research, Deyo and his colleagues adapted the index for use with the ICD-9-CM diagnoses recorded in administrative databases. The results of the study are encouraging for a variety of reasons. First, the index was related to several short-term outcomes of lumbar spine surgery and to use of resources even in a sample with limited variation in the key predictor variables (e.g., age and comorbidity score). Second, the relationship between the comorbidity index and the outcomes of interest persisted even when only cross-sectional data from the index hospitalization were used. Third, because the study uses a Medicare database, the applicability of the results to an older population is clear. Finally, it is relatively inexpensive to use administrative databases, in comparison with collecting data via medical record abstraction.

As Deyo and his colleagues point out, however, the value of this adaptation of the index depends on the completeness and accuracy of the coding. As they suggest, chronic conditions are likely to be underreported in patients undergoing surgery, when the surgical diagnoses and complications must be reported. On the other hand, reimbursement incentives could result in excessive "up-coding" to include relatively trivial diagnoses.

Romano PS, Roos LL, & Jollis JG. (1993a). Adapting a clinical comorbidity index for use with ICD-9-CM administrative data: Differing perspectives. *J Clin Epidemiol,* **46, 1075–1079.**

Design.   The paper presents the Dartmouth-Manitoba adaptation of the Charlson Comorbidity Index and discusses the limitations of the index and its adaptations for use with administrative databases.

Sample.   No data are analyzed in this paper.

Summary.   The Dartmouth-Manitoba adaptation of the Charlson index was developed independently of—but in a similar fashion to—the Deyo adaptation of the index. The authors note that the mapping of the Charlson-defined comorbidities to ICD-9-CM codes is not straightforward and that different investigators working independently assigned different sets of ICD-9-CM codes to the same comorbidities. The impact of these differences in interpretation can range from negligible to significant. There are three central differences between the Dartmouth-Manitoba adaptation and the Deyo adaptation.

1.   The Dartmouth-Manitoba adaptation includes conceptually similar conditions that were not explicitly described by Charlson. The Deyo adaptation, in general, represents a stricter interpretation of the Charlson-defined comorbidities. For example, the Deyo adaptation translates "dementia" into ICD-9-CM codes 290–290.9 ("senile and presenile dementias"). The Dartmouth-Manitoba adaptation also includes ICD-9-CM code 3310 ("Alzheimer's disease") in the definition.

2.   The Dartmouth-Manitoba adaptation treats malignancies as chronic conditions that can be identified from either index or prior admissions. The Deyo adaptation treats malignancies as chronic conditions only if they were present on prior admissions.

3.   The Dartmouth-Manitoba adaptation attempts to broaden definitions in ways consistent with ICD-9-CM coding guidelines. For example, ICD-9-CM coding guidelines include both "peripheral vascular disease, unspecified" (443.9) and "arterial embolism and thrombosis" (444.x) under the definition of peripheral vascular disease; the Dartmouth-Manitoba adaptation includes the latter while the Deyo adaptation excludes it.

The authors also discuss general concerns about the application of the Charlson index to administrative data sets. First, because the weights reported by Charlson were estimated using a sample of patients admitted to the medical service of one hospital, the authors express doubt that the weights apply to patients admitted for elective or emergency surgery in different geographic areas in subsequent years. Second, the authors raise concerns about the methodological techniques used to develop the index. Specifically, Charlson and her colleagues *add* weights derived from a relative hazards model to estimate composite scores for individuals with multiple comorbidities. The authors note that the proportional hazards model does not yield hazards that are additive. Intuitively, a patient with leukemia may not have any additional risk of dying if he or she also has ulcer disease, for example. Finally, because the weights were estimated to predict 1-year mortality, they are unlikely to apply to markedly different outcomes like length of stay and hospital charges.

Discussion. The authors raise important suggestions for and concerns about the adaptation of the Charlson index for use with different cohorts of patients and with administrative data sets. Unfortunately, no data are presented or analyzed, and the suggestions or concerns cannot be tested or assessed empirically. Intuitively, however, the cautions make sense. Depending on the cohort of interest, the precise definitions of the Charlson-defined comorbidities may need to change. Similarly, the index may apply less well to studies that are dramatically different from the one in which it was developed.

Applications

Romano PS, Roos LL, & Jollis JG. (1993b). Further evidence concerning the use of a clinical comorbidity index with ICD-9-CM administrative data. *J Clin Epidemiol,* **46, 1085–1090.**

Design. The paper reports the results of a head-to-head comparison of the Dartmouth-Manitoba and Deyo translations of the Charlson index. The authors use two administrative data sets for the comparison: (1) discharge abstract data from hospitalizations for coronary artery bypass graft (CABG) from Manitoba and (2) discharge abstract data from discectomy hospitalizations in California.

Sample. Two samples were analyzed in this study. The first, derived from Manitoba Health Services Commission files, included 4,121 patients who had undergone CABG surgery in Manitoba hospitals between April 1980 and March 1992. No details are provided regarding the age and gender distribution of the sample. The presence of in-hospital complications, identified in collaboration with an expert panel, was the outcome of interest. The second sample, derived from the California Office of Statewide Health Planning and Development (OSHPD) Hospital Discharge Data set, included all records of adults over the age of 18 who were discharged from an acute care hospital between January 1988 and December 1990 after undergoing nonemergency intervertebral disk excision. The sample included 55,407 lumbar and 14,898 cervical operations. Only the lumbar discectomy data are presented, and no information is given about the age and gender distribution of the sample. In-hospital mortality was the outcome of interest.

Summary. Romano and his colleagues begin by comparing the prevalence estimates for the Charlson-defined comorbidities using the Dartmouth-Manitoba and Deyo translations. Although the two generate similar prevalence estimates, the Dartmouth-Manitoba translation generates higher estimates for the prevalence of peripheral vascular disease, diabetes with complications, and malignancy. Second, the authors compare measures of relative risk for each comorbidity between the two test data sets. While the two translations result in modest differences, the measures of association between comorbidities and outcomes are very different in the two data sets. For example, complicated diabetes and chronic pulmonary disease have a greater impact on the risk of postdiscectomy complications than on the risk of death after CABG surgery. Similarly, if Charlson and her colleagues had used Manitoba CABG data to develop their comorbidity index, the weight assigned to congestive heart failure would have been 3 instead of 1.

Discussion.   This head-to-head comparison of the Dartmouth-Manitoba and Deyo translations of the Charlson index suggests that modest differences exist between the two. In
fact, although the two translations do generate markedly different estimates for peripheral
vascular disease, diabetes with complications, and malignancy, the differences have little
impact on the multivariate risk models that include all comorbidities.

Perhaps the most important finding of this paper is that data for different cohorts of
patients generate very different estimates of the Charlson comorbidity weights. Congestive
heart failure and peripheral vascular disease conferred much greater risk in this analysis
than in the original Charlson paper (Charlson et al., 1987). Romano, Roos, and Jollis
point out that the difference may reflect underreporting of comorbidities in administrative
data, differences between surgical and medical patients, temporal changes in the impact
of comorbidities, geographic variation, or differences in the outcome variable. Whatever
the cause of the difference, they encourage investigators to reestimate the weights assigned
to various comorbidities, especially if a dependent variable other than 1-year mortality
is used.

**D'Hoore W, Sicotte C, & Tilquin C. (1993). Risk adjustment in outcome assessment:
The Charlson Comorbidity Index. *Methods Inf Med, 32*, 382–387.**
Design.   The paper reports the findings of an application of the Charlson Comorbidity
Index in a multivariate model to predict in-hospital mortality. The source of data is an
administrative database (MED-ECHO), which covers all hospitalizations in the province
of Quebec.
Sample.   The sample consisted of 62,456 patients in hospitals in Quebec, Canada, from
1989 to 1990 who were diagnosed with ischemic heart disease, congestive heart failure,
stroke, or bacterial pneumonia. The sample was selected from 78 hospitals in Quebec
having at least 100 acute care beds and at least 50 medical or surgical beds. The mean
age of the sample was 64.1 years.
Summary.   The authors use the Charlson index to control for risk in an analysis of in-
hospital mortality. Because the data are based on ICD-9-CM codes, the authors translate
the Charlson-defined comorbidities into ICD-9-CM codes using a map similar to the one
developed by Deyo. The resulting composite comorbidity scores ranged from 0 to 38,
with a mean of 1.14. The score was transformed into a five-level scale similar to the one
validated by Charlson (0, 1, 2, 3, and 4 respectively, for scores 0, 1–2, 3–4, 5–6, and > 6).

The authors used logistic regression techniques to examine the relationship between
comorbidity and in-hospital mortality, controlling for age and gender. First, two models
were fitted. The first used the ordinally scaled comorbidity index (0–4); the second used
four dummy variables to represent the five-level comorbidity scale. The second model
had a significantly better fit than the first (likelihood ratio χ^2 = 18.0, 3 *df*, *p* < 0.001).
Second, principal diagnoses were introduced into the model. The authors report that the
addition of principal diagnoses significantly improved the model (as measured by a
significant difference between the areas under the ROC curves for the models with and
without the principal diagnoses).
Discussion.   The paper presents encouraging findings concerning the use of an ICD-9-
CM version of the Charlson index. Specifically, the authors find a significant relationship
between the Charlson comorbidity score and in-hospital mortality, and they generate a
model that performs as well as other commonly used models. Although the authors report

impressive results, the findings were apparently derived from a single data set. Without replicating the model on another data set, it is impossible to assess how good the model truly is.

Dodds TA, Martin DP, Stolov WC, & Deyo RA. (1994). A validation of the functional independence measurement and its performance among rehabilitation inpatients. *Arch Phys Med Rehabil, 74,* 531–536.

Design. The paper presents multifaceted tests of the Functional Independence Measurement (FIM). Internal consistency, responsiveness over time, and construct validity of the measure are tested. To test the construct validity, the authors hypothesize that a negative relationship between increasing comorbidity and FIM scores exists. The Charlson index is used to test the hypothesis.

Sample. All patients ($n = 11,102$) who underwent inpatient rehabilitation in a rehabilitation facility during the 3-year period 1988–1990 were included. The mean age was 65, and the most common impairments were stroke (52%), orthopedic conditions (10%), and brain injury (10%).

Summary. The FIM is a functional status instrument for use among rehabilitation inpatients. To test the construct validity of the tool, the authors examine the relationship between the FIM and several variables including the Charlson Comorbidity Index. The index was calculated using Deyo and colleagues' (1992) translation of the index to ICD-9-CM codes. Because some comorbid conditions included in the index are also used in the primary impairment categories, the index was modified to exclude conditions that overlapped with the primary condition.

The results suggest that the presence of any coexisting comorbidity, as measured by the Charlson index, modestly depressed FIM discharge scores. On average, patients with comorbid conditions scored 2 points lower on discharge FIM than those without a comorbid illness (95 versus 97, $p < 0.005$). In general, patients with higher comorbidity scores had lower discharge FIM scores than those with lower comorbidity scores.

Discussion. As the authors note, the application of the Charlson index to test the construct validity of a functional status instrument has serious limitations. First, the Charlson index is unlikely to be the best measure of comorbidity in a rehabilitation population. The index was developed to predict mortality, so the conditions included are those likely to affect mortality. A different set of conditions would probably have emerged if the index had been developed to predict functional status. Second, the majority of rehabilitation patients had no recorded comorbidities. This may reflect coding techniques or the fact that comorbidities relevant to rehabilitation patients were excluded from the Charlson index. The paper provides an excellent example of the range of ways the Charlson index has been used in practice. Unfortunately, the index was developed for use in predicting mortality in the inpatient setting and may have limited applicability in other settings.

Hartz AJ, Kuhn EM, Kayser KL, Pryor DP, Green R, & Rimm AA. (1992). Assessing providers of coronary revascularization: A method for peer review organizations. *Am J Public Health, 82,* 1631–1640.

Design. The paper reports the development of a method for assessing the quality of care by comparing complication rates adjusted for patients' characteristics. Two models are compared with respect to their ability to predict complications. The first model, derived from data abstracted from the medical record, relies on detailed clinical data (e.g., mitral insufficiency, enlarged heart on X-ray) to predict complications. The second model, which is derived from administrative data, uses the Charlson Comorbidity Index to predict complications.

Sample.   The sample consisted of 2,086 patients from 19 hospitals who had undergone angioplasty and 1,998 patients from 18 hospitals who had undergone CABG surgery. The average ages of the patients who had angioplasty and CABG surgery were 71.0 years and 71.4 years, respectively. Forty percent of the angioplasty patients and 36% of the CABG surgery patients were female.

Summary.   Methods to assess the quality of hospital care are often limited to comparisons of hospital mortality rates. The authors describe an alternative method that uses complications rates adjusted for patients' characteristics as a means of assessing quality of care. Nine adverse outcomes of interest were identified for patients undergoing CABG surgery and an additional four for patients undergoing angioplasty. Stepwise logistic regression techniques were used to predict adverse outcomes using detailed information abstracted from patients' medical records. Independently, the authors calculated the Charlson index based on up to five comorbidities listed in the Uniform Billing (UB82) data. The two severity-of-illness measures are then compared with respect to their ability to risk-adjust in-hospital complication rates for patients having a coronary artery revascularization procedure.

The results suggest that the model derived from detailed clinical information is able to stratify patients according to risk. That is, as predicted values of an adverse outcome increase, observed values of an adverse outcome also increase. The authors quantify this ability to stratify using the overlap index. The overlap index ranges from 0 (the predicted values of an adverse outcome are higher for all patients who had an adverse outcome than for all patients who did not have an adverse outcome) to 1 (the predicted values of an adverse outcome were similar for patients who had an adverse outcome to the predictions for those who did not have an adverse outcome). The overlap index was 0.62 for the patients undergoing CABG surgery and 0.64 for the patients undergoing angioplasty. The Charlson index, to the contrary, was only weakly associated with adverse outcomes. In fact, the overlap index exceeded 0.90 for both types of patients (CABG surgery and angioplasty). This suggests that patients with and without adverse outcomes had similar Charlson scores. The authors conclude that the Charlson index does not stratify patients or hospitals with respect to risk.

Discussion.   Although the results support the authors' conclusions, the paper highlights the potential problem of using a limited number of diagnoses to calculate the Charlson score. Only five diagnoses were available in the UB-82 administrative data that the authors used to calculate the score. Iezzoni and others (Iezzoni, 1994; Jencks, Williams, & Kay, 1988) have found that the coding of secondary diagnoses may be biased because of the limited number of spaces. Specifically, chronic diagnoses, which make up the Charlson index, are more likely to be omitted from the list of diagnoses. These omissions, in turn, are likely to bias the Charlson scores downward and decrease the variability of the scores. These biases limit the usefulness of the index as an independent variable in this multivariate model.

Holtzman J, Pheley AM, & Lurie N. (1994). Changes in orders limiting care and the use of less aggressive care in a nursing home population. *J Am Geriatr Soc*, 42, 275–279.

Design. Holtzman and his colleagues report the results of a retrospective chart review to examine what kinds of nursing home patients receive orders limiting care, including "do not resuscitate" (DNR) orders. Data were collected through chart review, and the Charlson index was used as a predictor of orders limiting care.

Sample. The sample consisted of 1,605 residents of nursing homes in Hennepin County, MN, from 1984 to 1988; a total of 1,405 charts (85%) were reviewed. The mean age of the sample was 83, and 78% were female.

Summary. The study examines patients' characteristics and other factors that are associated with DNR orders, orders limiting care, and the provision of less aggressive care. The presence of a DNR order was defined as the reviewer's finding a DNR order in effect but no other orders limiting care. The presence of other orders limiting care was defined as the reviewer's finding orders limiting care beyond DNR (e.g., "do not hospitalize," "supportive care only"). "Less aggressive care" was found to exist when cardiopulmonary resuscitation (CPR) was not performed when the patient had a cardiopulmonary arrest, and when the reviewer judged that the care delivered to the resident was less aggressive than care usually given to a person of that age. Data regarding demographic information, diagnoses, severity of illness, and functional status were also collected through chart review. The diagnoses were combined in two ways. First, the diagnoses were weighted and summed to create a Charlson comorbidity score for each patient. Second, the presence of dementia and the presence of cancer were used as separate dummy variables in the analysis. Severity of illness was assessed by the reviewer on the basis of severity of symptoms and complications.

The authors included the following variables in the prediction models: severity of illness, functional status, year of admission to nursing home, age, gender, presence of cancer, presence of dementia, and Charlson index. The results suggest that the severity score and functional status are significant predictors of DNR orders, orders limiting care, and less aggressive care. Year of admission, age, and presence of dementia were significant in some of the models. Gender, the presence of cancer, and the Charlson index were not significant in any of the prediction models.

Discussion. The prediction models include variables that are potentially highly correlated with one another. The severity score, for example, reflects the reviewer's assessment of the severity of the patient's symptoms and medical complications. If conditions like diabetes, heart failure, and gangrene were considered complications, the severity index might strongly resemble the Charlson index. If, in fact, the two scores are highly correlated, the effect would be to bias the effect toward zero, to create unstable estimates of effect, or both. The authors do not provide details about the correlation among variables included in the model, so it is difficult to assess the impact of multicollinearity. In addition, the model is not validated on a separate set of data, so it is not possible to assess the stability of the estimates of effect.

O'Connor GT, Plume SK, Olmstead EM, Coffin LH, Morton, JR, Maloney CT, Nowicki ER, Tryzelaar JF, Hernandex F, Adrian L, Casey KJ, Soule DN, Marris CAS, Nugent WC, Charlesworth DC, Clough R, Katz S, Leavitt BJ, Wennberg JE, & Northern New England Cardiovascular Disease Study Group. (1991). A regional prospective study of in-hospital mortality associated with coronary artery bypass grafting. *JAMA, 266,* 803–809.

Design. O'Connor and his colleagues report the results of a prospective regional study to determine whether differences in mortality rates following CABG surgery were solely the result of differences in the mix of patients undergoing the procedures. The authors use data collected prospectively regarding demographics of patients, indications for revascularization, priority of surgery, and results of cardiac catheterization. Discharge data are used to determine discharge status and to calculate the Charlson Comorbidity Index.

Sample. The sample included 3,055 patients who underwent CABG between July 1, 1987, and April 15, 1989, in five regional medical centers in northern New England. Data were collected from all consecutive CABG surgery patients during the study period. The mean age of the sample was 63 years, and 73.2% were male.

Summary. The study began with the stated hypothesis that much of the observed difference in crude in-hospital mortality rates following CABG surgery resulted from differences in the mix of patients undergoing the procedure. Logistic regression analysis was used to examine the relationship between patients' characteristics and mortality, and to adjust mortality rates for potentially confounding variables.

Univariate analyses suggested that age, female gender, smaller body surface area, higher comorbidity scores, prior CABG, poor ejection fraction, and priority of surgery were among the significant predictors of in-hospital mortality. To determine the variables that independently predict in-hospital mortality, multivariate analyses were used. The results were similar to those of the univariate analyses. Again, comorbidity score was a significant predictor of in-hospital mortality. None of the independent predictors, however, substantially confounded the interpretation of crude in-hospital mortality rates. Significant variability persisted in the risk-adjusted mortality rates. The authors conclude by rejecting the hypothesis that much of the observed difference in crude in-hospital mortality rates is due to differences in case mix.

Discussion. Unlike other studies described previously, this article finds the Charlson Comorbidity Index to be a significant, independent predictor of in-hospital mortality. The way in which the index is used may explain the difference in findings. Specifically, in this study the Charlson index is transformed into a dichotomous variable: 0 if the Charlson score is less than or equal to 2; 1 if the Charlson score is greater than 2. The interpretation of the finding, then, is that the presence of several comorbidities (e.g., diabetes, congestive heart failure, and acute myocardial infarction) or one major comorbidity (e.g., moderate liver disease) is a significant, independent predictor of in-hospital mortality.

Acute Physiology and Chronic Health Evaluation (APACHE)
Development and Methods

Knaus WA, Draper EA, Wagner DP, & Zimmerman JE. (1985). APACHE II: A severity of disease classification system. *Crit Care Med*, *10*, 818–828.

Design. This paper reports on the validation of APACHE II for stratifying acutely ill patients by risk of in-hospital mortality and compares the performance of APACHE II with the first version of APACHE. The authors collected information on age, diagnosis, indication for ICU admission, surgical status, preadmission history, physiologic variables required by the first APACHE classification, presence of chronic disease, and in-hospital survival for a series of consecutive ICU patients in each of 13 hospitals in the United

States who were admitted from 1979 to 1982. Scores were based on the most deranged physiologic measurements observed in the first 24 hours after admission to the ICU. Patients were assigned to 1 of 50 disease categories or 1 of 5 categories of organ system failure. The criteria for inclusion in these categories were not defined. Cross-tabulations between APACHE II scores and mortality were reported overall and within disease categories. Patients admitted after CABG surgery were excluded; then the risk of death for the remaining patients was predicted with logistic regression using the components of APACHE II, age, surgical status, and diagnosis. The accuracy of the logistic model was assessed using an ROC curve.

Sample. Data were collected for 5,815 ICU patients, 87% of whom had complete data on all 12 physiologic measurements. Between 25% and 54% of the patients from each institution were over 65 years of age. The proportion of postoperative patients varied from 2% to 89% among the institutions. Conditions of the cardiovascular system were the most frequent cause for admission to the ICU, although sepsis, intracranial hemorrhage, trauma, pneumonia, and gastrointestinal neoplasms were also frequent in some institutions.

Summary. As expected, higher APACHE II scores were associated with higher death rates in all disease groups, although absolute mortality depended on the reason for admission to the ICU. The APACHE II scores of nonsurgical patients exhibited a wider variance than those of postoperative patients. Patients undergoing CABG had high APACHE II scores coupled with low mortality, presumably because their physiologic derangements were secondary to surgical and anesthetic interventions prior to ICU admission rather than to underlying disease; hence they were excluded from the multivariate analyses. A logistic regression equation based on APACHE II components, surgical status, and admission diagnosis correctly predicted death in 85.5% of patients, assuming that all of those with at least a 50% predicted risk of death would die. The multivariate analysis is the basis for an index that predicts the risk of death for groups of patients on the basis of APACHE II and categorization of the patients into one of 50 disease categories. Interrater reliability was mentioned only briefly.

Discussion. This article provides a clear description of APACHE II and is the first article to describe its development. Although histograms of mortality rates within some disease categories are displayed, there is no assessment of how homogeneous the mortality rates are within strata. The authors report that APACHE II "performs well in all disease categories" (p. 825), but they do not define measures of performance within categories very well or attempt to answer the question, Does this measure explain much variance within categories? The authors acknowledge that predictions of mortality are dependent on accurate classification of patients into one of the 50 disease groups that they define, but they do not provide criteria for that classification in this work. The authors recommend scoring patients on the basis of their admission values, so that scores will not depend upon treatments. However, this procedure would not control for interventions initiated prior to ICU admission. Furthermore, some information is inevitably lost by using admission values rather than worst values during the 24 hours after admission. The authors report that admission values are identical to worst values during the 24 hours after admission in one institution and that the consistency of these two methods is being investigated.

Knaus WA, Wagner DP, Draper EA, Zimmerman JE, Bergner M, Bastos P, Sirio C, Murphy DJ, Lotring T, Damiano A, & Harrell FE. (1991). The APACHE III

prognostic system: Risk prediction of hospital mortality for critically ill hospitalized adults. *Chest, 100,* 1619–1636.

Design.   The development of the third version of the APACHE system, APACHE III, is reported in this study. As with previous versions of APACHE, the goal was to develop a score that stratifies patients by their risk of in-hospital mortality. Additionally, equations that predict in-hospital mortality are derived from that score. This study also assessed how selection of patients and timing of admission to the ICU could affect scores and therefore comparisons among ICUs. Logistic regression was used to assess the relationship between in-hospital mortality and 20 physiologic variables, chronic health conditions, operative status, location prior to ICU admission, and one of 212 major disease categories. Weights were estimated on one half of the data set and validated on the other half. Some variables were combined into single measures, because results using the individual measures suggested important interactions that warranted combining the variables using a very specific logic.

Sample.   Twenty-six hospitals were randomly selected to be representative of hospitals in the United States with 200 or more beds, and an additional 14 tertiary care institutions volunteered to participate. Consecutive patients (or every second or third patient) admitted between May 1988 and November 1989 were enrolled. Those admitted to rule out MI, patients under the age of 16, or those with burn injuries were excluded. Those with coronary artery bypass grafts are not included in this report. The remaining sample included 17,440 patients, of whom 48% were over the age of 65. Fifty-eight percent had not undergone surgery, and the majority of these (61%) were admitted from the emergency room. Of nonsurgical admissions, the most common disease categories were aortic aneurysms, gastrointestinal bleeding due to ulcer or laceration, acute myocardial infarction (AMI), and drug overdose. The most common operative admissions were for elective abdominal aneurysm repair and peripheral artery bypass graft. Many other disease were included in the sample.

Summary.   Most of the analyses used scores based on the most deranged physiologic measurement during the first day in the ICU. The 17 physiologic measures included in APACHE III predict mortality reasonably well, yielding a prediction on the validation data set with an area under the ROC curve of 0.88. Significant comorbid conditions all reflect compromised immunologic status and occur so infrequently in postoperative elective-surgery cases that they are not included in the scores for those patients. The APACHE III score is associated with higher mortality rates within 78 major disease categories, as illustrated by odds ratios of more than 1 for every 5-point increase in the APACHE III score. The APACHE III score was combined with major disease categories and location prior to ICU admission to improve prediction of mortality. This yielded an R^2 of 0.41 and an area under the ROC curve of 0.90. Assuming that in-hospital death will occur when the predicted mortality is 50% or higher, the sensitivity of the system is 58.4% and its specificity is 96.3%.

Discussion.   This article provides an excellent summary of the development of APACHE III, with references to other articles that discuss the methods in even greater detail. The authors discuss the potential usefulness of APACHE III to assist with clinical decision making by assessing changes in patients' status over time, but this application seems to depend on slightly different equations that are not presented in this paper. The authors do not discuss the validity of the equations for assessing quality of care—how poor care might inflate the APACHE III scores—but they seem to assume that these physiologic measures are independent of treatment. They emphasize that the APACHE III score can be used for stratification *within* "homogeneous" disease groups. This may create some difficulties for the user who must decide how to define such groups. In a sense, just defining such groups entails some risk stratification, thus raising concerns about how much stratification is being accomplished with APACHE III and how much is accomplished simply by defining the disease groups. Similarly, risk prediction with the APACHE III system depends on assigning patients to one of 78 disease categories, but the validity of the prediction will depend on two conditions: (1) The assignment of the disease categories for patients in a given ICU must be consistent with the assignment to disease categories in this study. This will be most problematic for patients with multiple diseases, because a single cause for admission must be identified. (2) The spectrum of disease within each category must be comparable to the spectra of diseases in this database. Reliability for APACHE II (not APACHE III) is reported to be high, but the reported results did not include reliability in identifying the reason for admission.

McMahon LF, Hayward RA, Bernard AM, Rosevear JS, & Weissfeld LA. (1992). APACHE-L: A new severity of illness adjuster for inpatient medical care. *Med Care,* *30*, 445–452.

Design. This study reports the formulation of APACHE-L, a modification of APACHE II, that is based only on laboratory components of APACHE II that are recorded in a hospital's information system. The authors assessed the ability of APACHE-L to predict use of resources by all patients admitted to a single university hospital between November 1989 and October 1990 and assigned to one of 13 common DRGs. The investigators created three scores based on (1) the first posted laboratory values, (2) the most deranged values in the first 24 hours after admission, and (3) the most deranged values during the entire admission. Length of stay (LOS), a relative value unit (RVU) that reflects the direct costs of all services, and the RVU of all services except laboratory use were the measures of resource use. Multiple regression analyses were conducted for all patients and by DRG to assess the amount of variance explained by DRG indicator variables and the three versions of APACHE-L.

Sample. Of 1,939 patients admitted to the institution during the study period under one of the 13 DRGs, 73 were excluded because they were outliers or died within 24 hours of admission, leaving a sample of 1,866 admissions. The most common DRG was vascular procedures except major reconstruction without pump (DRG 112), followed by chemotherapy (DRG 410); heart failure and shock (DRG 127); circulatory disorders, excluding AMI with cardiac catheterization (DRG 124); and simple pneumonia and pleurisy, age 70 or older or with complications (CC) (DRG 89). The age distribution was not presented, but the DRGs in the analysis would presumably include some patients over 65.

Summary. Models including APACHE-L scores based on the first posted laboratory values had R^2 values 0.02 to 0.04 higher than models including DRGs alone, and models including scores based on the worst laboratory values within 24 hours of admission had R^2 values 0.04 to 0.08 higher than with DRGs alone. As expected, APACHE-L scores based on worst laboratory values observed during the entire admission explained even more variance (the R^2 was 0.09 to 0.15 higher). The performance of APACHE-L within DRGs was variable, but it again depended on whether the score was based on the first laboratory values, values from the first day after admission, or the worst values over the entire admission. For urinary tract infection, the worst APACHE-L score explained 38% of within-DRG variance. For vascular procedures except reconstruction without pump; heart failure and shock; cardiac arrhythmia and conduction disorders with CC; and esophagitis, gastroenteritis, and miscellaneous digestive disorders with CC, APACHE-L explained 25% to 30% of the variance. APACHE-L explained little or no variance for chemotherapy, nutritional disorders, esophagitis or gastritis without CC, angina, other circulatory disorders with cardiac catheterization, and bronchitis.

Discussion.   As one would expect, the highest APACHE-L for the entire admission has greater explanatory power, but it may reflect results of care as well as severity of the presenting illness. The hospital's distribution of DRGs is somewhat unusual, with a large proportion of patients admitted for vascular procedures. APACHE-L may have performed poorly for some DRGs, such as chemotherapy and angina, because those DRGs are fairly homogeneous (at least with respect to physiologic disruption indicated in laboratory values or resource use). The results suggest (although they are far from conclusive) that APACHE-L performs better within DRGs that include older patients or patients with complications and comorbidities. This is not surprising, since APACHE was developed specifically for acutely ill patients. This may be a promising method for acutely ill, hospitalized patients. APACHE-L is an alternative that includes more clinical information than the usual administrative discharge abstract, but it is less labor intensive than APACHE II for institutions that have computerized laboratory results.

Applications

Daley J, Jencks S, Draper D, Lenhart G, Thomas N, & Walker J. (1988). Predicting hospital-associated mortality for Medicare patients. *JAMA*, 24, 3617–3624.

Design.   The authors assessed the ability of the Medicare Mortality Predictor System (MMPS), of which APACHE II is a component, to predict mortality in individuals with stroke, pneumonia, MI, or congestive heart failure (CHF). In addition to the APACHE II, MMPS includes measures of functional status, do-not-resuscitate (DNR) status on admission, history of previous admissions or transfer from a long-term care facility, and selected clinical variables that are specific to each of the four conditions. Patients were drawn from a sample of Medicare records for seven states, and the sample was stratified by hospital size and teaching status to be representative of hospitals admitting Medicare beneficiaries across the United States. Ordinary regression was used to assess the variance in mortality rates explained by APACHE II, and weighted logistic regression with multiple cross-validation was used to assess the predictive performance of MMPS.

Sample.   Abstracts were made from 6,559 records, and 10.2% were excluded for a variety of reasons. Hence, the analysis was based on a sample of 5,888 admissions, which were equally distributed over the four diagnoses. Overall mortality rates by diagnosis were as follows: stroke, 0.194; pneumonia, 0.179; MI, 0.225; and CHF, 0.147.

Summary.   The means, standard deviations, and R^2 values of APACHE II for the four conditions are summarized in Table 3.1. In the multiple regression, APACHE II scores had by far the largest coefficient of any predictive variable for stroke and pneumonia. For MI and CHF, APACHE II scores had significant coefficients, although a few other variables had a larger impact on predicted mortality. The results also suggest that some

TABLE 3.1   APACHE II Scores by Disease Category

	Mean	Standard Deviation	R^2
Stroke	11.74	5.50	0.22
Pneumonia	13.89	5.80	0.141
Myocardial infarction	11.21	5.76	0.092
Congestive heart failure	12.28	4.71	0.046

components of APACHE II should be more heavily weighted for certain conditions. The MMPS had higher explanatory power than APACHE II alone, and they captured some factors that would indicate the choice to avoid aggressive intervention (e.g., DNR status).
Discussion.   This study provides a good illustration of APACHE II's performance in a national sample of four conditions, including both patients admitted to ICUs and general admissions. This analysis illustrates that the variance explained by APACHE II is quite dependent on disease and shows how selected components of APACHE II might be included in an adjustment method to overcome this limitation.

Papadakis MA, Lee KK, Browner WS, Kent DL, Matchar DB, Kagawa MK, Hallenbeck J, Lee D, Onishi R, & Charles G. (1993). Prognosis of mechanically ventilated patients. *West J Med, 159,* **659–664.**
Design.   This is a retrospective analysis of how well APACHE II, along with selected other variables, predicts mortality at discharge and at 1 year after discharge in patients requiring mechanical ventilation. Additional variables were age, use of cigarettes or alcohol, low serum albumin levels, low total lymphocyte count, initiation of mechanical ventilation after cardiopulmonary resuscitation, abnormal values of arterial blood gases after 24 hours of mechanical ventilation, prolonged mechanical ventilation, length of ICU stay, and length of hospital stay. Univariate analyses were used to identify significant independent variables that were then included in logistic regression analyses to predict vital status at discharge and in proportional hazards models to predict 1-year mortality.
Sample.   The sample included all medical patients who received mechanical ventilation in one of six Veterans Administration hospitals and excluded those with cardiac disease or HIV/AIDS. Medical records were unavailable on 12%, leaving 612 subjects. Most (97%) were men, and the average age was 63.3 years, with 23% over 70 years of age. Thirty percent had an infection or sepsis, 15% had COPD, and the remainder had a variety of other conditions.
Summary.   A 10-point increase in the APACHE II score was associated with an odds ratio of 2.7 (95% confidence interval, CI, 2.1–3.5) for in-hospital mortality and a hazard ratio of 1.8 for 1-year mortality. Similar results obtained for a modified version of APACHE II that excluded age. Age, serum albumin level, CPR, and arterial carbon dioxide pressure were also significant in univariate analyses. The APACHE II score was also significant in multivariate models, along with age and serum albumin levels. The overall hospital mortality was 64%, while the APACHE II system predicted a mortality of 55% for this

sample. Prediction of mortality was most accurate for those with higher APACHE II scores, because the APACHE II system underestimated mortality in those with scores under 20. A more accurate predictive model was obtained by including serum albumin levels as well as APACHE II for the subset ($n = 308$) of patients for whom serum albumin was available.

Discussion.   Although APACHE II was designed to predict in-hospital mortality, it is of interest to note its ability to predict 1-year survival. The actual mortality was less than predicted in patients with low APACHE II scores, possibly because this sample included more seriously ill patients than those included in the APACHE II development study. APACHE II predicts mortality based on disease category. Because these patients were all receiving mechanical ventilation, they probably represented a more seriously ill spectrum than those within each disease category who were included in the APACHE II development study.

Wu AW, Rubin HR, & Rosen MJ. (1990). Are elderly people less responsive to intensive care? *J Am Geriatr Soc*, **38,** 621–627.

Design.   This article reports on a retrospective study to identify the relationship between age and mortality in ICU patients, after controlling for severity of illness as measured by the APACHE II score. For this study, age was excluded from the APACHE II score calculation, yielding a score referred to as APACHEIIM. Additional independent variables included whether or not the patient was under the care of a private physician; whether the primary diagnosis on admission to the ICU was high or low risk; and the use of diagnostic and therapeutic interventions such as mechanical ventilation, arterial catheters, and cardiac pacemakers. Univariate analyses using the Student's t test, Wilcoxon rank-sum test, and chi-square test were followed by logistic regression to assess the influence of the independent variables on mortality.

Sample.   The sample consisted of 135 patients aged 55 to 65 and 130 patients over the age of 75 admitted to an eight-bed general intensive care unit in a tertiary care hospital between 1982 and 1984. The mean APACHEIIM score was 15.9. Forty-five percent died in the hospital, with higher crude hospital mortality and lower crude ICU mortality among those over the age of 75.

Summary.   Higher APACHEIIM scores were associated with greater mortality across the range of scores, and in most ranges patients 75 and older had greater mortality than younger patients. In univariate analyses, all independent variables except gender were statistically significantly associated with mortality. In a logistic regression including APACHEIIM, age group, gender, private physician, presence of cancer, and presence of high-risk admission diagnosis, age was not a significant explanatory variable. In most subgroup analyses by APACHEIIM score ($\leq$ 15 or > 15), private versus service status, and severity of illness, older patients did not experience greater mortality than younger patients. Older patients with pneumonia did have higher mortality; younger patients with sepsis, CHF, and COPD had higher mortality.

Discussion.   The authors argue against the routine inclusion of age in the APACHE II score and assert that APACHEIIM predicts mortality well. They acknowledge that their results may be biased by policies that lead to ICU admission only for those older adults who are most likely to benefit from ICU care and that a further study including all patients who are under consideration for ICU care would be helpful.

Ziegler EJ, Fisher CJ, Sprung CL, Straube RC, Sadoff JC, Foulke GE, Wortel CH, Fink MP, Lellinger P, Teng NNH, Allen IE, Berger HJ, Knatterud GL, LoBuglio AF, Smith CR, & HA-1A Sepsis Study Group. (1991). Treatment of gram-negative bacteremia and septic shock with HA-1A human monoclonal antibody against endotoxin. *N Engl J Med, 324,* 429–436.

Design. This study was a double-blind randomized controlled trial of HA-1A, a human monoclonal IgM antibody, in patients with sepsis and suspected gram-negative infection. Patients were excluded if they were under the age of 18; were pregnant; had a clearly irreversible course; had an organ transplant, uncontrolled hemorrhage, cardiogenic shock, or a burn injury; or if they had received monoclonal antibodies or intravenous immunoglobulins within the preceding 21 days. Mortality during the 28 days after enrollment was analyzed using Kaplan-Meier survival curves, and the two groups were compared using the Wilcoxon statistic. Survival was also compared after the researchers adjusted for prognostic factors in the two study groups, including the APACHE II score at enrollment.

Sample. Two hundred patients with gram-negative bacteremia were the subject of this analysis, although 543 patients were enrolled in the trial. Three patients were lost to 28-day follow-up, although all patients were followed for at least 14 days. The average age of the subjects was 60, and 58% were male. The most common underlying diseases were neoplasms, diabetes mellitus, recent surgery, alcoholism, and chronic liver disease. The patients were severely ill, as indicated by a high proportion of subjects with hypotension, endotracheal intubation, disseminated intravascular coagulation, adult respiratory distress syndrome, acute hepatic failure, and acute renal failure.

Summary. Infusion with HA-1A was associated with improved survival overall, as well as in subgroups defined by the presence or absence of shock. Treatment effect was significant even after adjustment for a variety of other variables, such as age, site of infection, underlying disease, and adequacy of antibiotic therapy. The average APACHE II score was 25.7 for the placebo group and 23.6 for the HA-1A group. The APACHE II score was highly correlated with survival in the placebo group ($p = 0.0001$). The study sample was stratified by APACHE II score above or below 25, and the treatment effect persisted in both groups.

Discussion. Septicemia and gram-negative bacteremia have high mortality (20%–60%), so one would expect that APACHE would perform well in this setting. Stratification by the presence of shock and APACHE II scores yielded similar results, lending further validity to APACHE II.

Simplified Acute Physiology Score (SAPS II)

Le Gall JR, Lemeshow S, & Saulnier F. (1993). A new simplified acute physiology score (SAPS II) based on a European/North American Multicenter study. *JAMA, 270,* 2957–2963.

Design. This study was undertaken to develop an alternative severity score for patients in intensive care units, the Simplified Acute Physiology Score (SAPS II). Physiologic measurements were recorded for a large sample of patients from 137 medical, surgical, or mixed ICUs in 12 countries. Multiple logistic regression was used in a development data set to identify variables and create a score that is predictive of death. The study was motivated in part by the need for a simple scoring system and in part by the desire to predict mortality without assigning patients to single, specific diagnostic categories.

Sample.   The sample consisted of 13,152 consecutive ICU admissions between September 30, 1991, and February 28, 1992, at 137 ICUs in 12 countries, including the United States. Burn patients, coronary patients, and patients who had had cardiac surgery were excluded. The average age was 57.2 (*SD* = 18.5), and 40.4% of the subjects were female. The overall mortality rate was 21.8%. Sixty-five percent of this sample were randomly selected for a developmental data set, and the remaining 35% were used as a validation data set. One hundred and fifty-five cases were excluded because of missing data.

Summary.   Of 37 candidate variables, 17 were selected for the final scoring system, including 11 laboratory or physiologic measurements; age; type of admission (scheduled surgical, unscheduled surgical, or medical); presence of HIV/AIDS; metastatic cancer; or hematologic malignancy; and the Glasgow Coma Score. An analysis of interrater reliability on a 5% sample of the subjects yielded intraclass correlations of 0.81 to 0.95 for the continuous variables in the system; the categorical variables had κ values of 0.67 to 1.00. This report presents the number of points assigned to ranges of those variables. A predicted mortality can be estimated from the sum of the variable weight using a formula presented in the text. This predicted mortality has an area under the ROC curve of 0.88 (95% confidence interval: 0.87 to 0.90), which is significantly larger than that for the original SAPS.

Discussion.   SAPS II offers two distinct advantages over APACHE III: it does not require assignment of patients to a single specific disease category in order to predict mortality, and it is relatively quick and simple to obtain. Although SAPS II does depend on ascertaining the presence of three conditions, those conditions were identified with high reliability in this study, which included many institutions in many countries. SAPS II may also be advantageous in settings in which values for arterial blood gas are not generally available. The system has yet to be evaluated or used by independent researchers.

Mortality Probability Models (MPM II)

Lemeshow S, Teres D, Kalr J, Avrunin JS, Gehlbach SH, & Rapoport J. (1993). Mortality probability models (MPM II) based on an international cohort of intensive care unit patients. *JAMA, 270,* **2478–2486.**

Design.   This study was conducted to develop and validate a simple system for estimating the probability of mortality in ICU patients, the Mortality Probability Models (MPM II). Models were developed for use at the time of admission (MPM$_0$) and at 24 hours after admission (MPM$_{24}$). The authors attempted to minimize the number of variables, the use of laboratory and radiologic variables that are not part of routine care, and the use of treatment variables. They included only well-defined variables, and did not require identification of a principal diagnosis. Candidate variables were first tested in univariate analyses for their association with mortality, and those that were significant were entered into a logistic regression model. Model performance was assessed using the area under the ROC curve and the Hosmer-Lemeshow goodness-of-fit test.

Sample.   Two data sets were used. One was an international sample as described in *Le Gall et al., 1993, and the second was obtained from four teaching hospitals in the United States. The samples were drawn from consecutive admissions of adult patients; those with burns, those receiving coronary care, and those who had had cardiac surgery were excluded. A total of 19,124 cases were included in the analysis of MPM_0, of which 12,610 were used in the development of the MPM_0, and the remainder were used as a validation set. The overall mortality rate was 20.8%. The average age was 55.4 years. Those who remained in the ICU for more than 24 hours were quite different from those who were in the ICU for less than 24 hours, and so MPM_{24} was developed using only a sample of 10,357 patients who were in the ICU for more than 24 hours.

Summary. A model for use at admission was developed that employs 15 variables, including three physiologic variables, the presence of one of three chronic diagnoses, the presence of one of five acute diagnoses, age, CPR prior to admission, use of mechanical ventilation, and nonelective surgery. The reliability of data collection was better for the physiologic variables than for the presence of some chronic and acute diagnoses. The MPM_{24} is based on 13 variables including age, presence of one of three diagnoses, medical or unscheduled surgical admission, use of mechanical ventilation or vasoactive drugs, and six physiologic variables.

Discussion. The MPM II depends upon identifying acute diagnoses, which raises concerns about the validity of this model in studies that are limited to specific disease groups rather than an overall ICU population. The authors discuss this issue and report that they are investigating the validity of the model in subgroups and in some cases are modifying the model to improve its performance in subgroups (see also Le Gall et al., 1995). It would be of interest to compare MPM II to a system such as DRGs, which also controls for severity by disease category. The authors acknowledge that none of the existing prediction models (MPM, SAPS, or APACHE) are based on entirely representative ICU patients. Additional results are forthcoming with models that predict mortality at 24-hour intervals during the ICU stay.

Index of Coexistent Disease (ICED)

There is no single methods article that describes the development and testing of the ICED. Instead, it is described in a series of articles and abstracts describing specific studies. The most comprehensive description is found in *Greenfield et al., 1993. Additional information on the ICED is available from the National Auxiliary Publications Service.

Greenfield S, Aronow HU, Elashoff RM, & Watanabe D. (1988). Flaws in mortality data: The hazards of ignoring comorbid disease. *JAMA*, *260*, 2253–2255.

Design. The objective of this study is to determine whether differences in mortality rates across hospitals can be accounted for in part by patients' differing levels of comorbidity on admission. The authors focused on incident cases of breast, colorectal, and prostate cancers and also took into account the effect of severity of the primary disease and age.

Sample. The stratified sample of 969 individuals was selected from all patients with available medical records who were located in the tumor registries of seven hospitals in southern California in order to obtain patients with comparable age and comorbidity distributions from each hospital.

Summary. The authors grouped cancer stages into early or advanced, ages into less than 75 or 75 and older, and comorbidity scores into none or mildly symptomatic versus severe or life-threatening. The percentage of patients with severe comorbidity scores ranged from 9.3% to 17.9% across the seven hospitals ($p < 0.01$); there was also a significant difference in the percentage of patients 75 years or older. Of the seven hospitals, the three with the highest comorbidity had also been pinpointed in an article in the *Los Angeles Times* as high mortality outliers for at least one disease. A subsample of patients with comparable age and comorbidity distributions across hospitals was also analyzed; the percentage with advanced cancer differed significantly across hospitals ($p < 0.01$). Finally, the ranking of hospitals varied depending on whether one grouped them by age, comorbidity level, or cancer stage. This suggests that comorbidity level needs to be included as a separate variable in risk adjustment models.

Discussion.   This study provides significant suggestive evidence of the importance of adjusting for comorbidity, and not only severity of primary illness, in risk adjustment models. However, the analysis leaves a number of questions unresolved. For example, it would be interesting to see the results of a multivariate analysis that assessed the relationship between severity of primary illness, age, and comorbidity, on the one hand, and mortality or excess mortality, on the other.

Greenfield S, Blanco DM, Elashoff RM, & Ganz PA. (1987). Patterns of care related to age of breast cancer patients. *JAMA*, *257*, 2766–2770.

Design.   A retrospective review was conducted to examine the impact of age on medical care provided to patients with breast cancer. An early version of the ICED, which these researchers call the comorbidity index, was used to control for comorbidity and functional status. Patients' patterns of care were characterized using criteria maps. These maps were based on widely accepted standards of practice and did not include controversial treatments. Their three parts dealt with the completeness of diagnostic confirmation, staging, and the appropriateness of initial therapy. The scores for each of these categories were then compared across age groups, controlling for comorbidity, functional status, stage of tumor, and hospital. The reliability of scoring patterns of care and the comorbidity index was examined by comparing the results of 30 charts, each of which was reviewed by four abstractors.

Sample.   The sample consisted of women aged 50 or older with histologically confirmed adenocarcinoma of the breast who received their primary cancer management at one of seven hospitals in southern California. The hospitals were chosen to vary in patients' socioeconomic status, number of cancer patients treated per year, and university affiliation versus no university affiliation. Eligible patients had been diagnosed between 1980 and 1982. The sample was divided by comorbidity level and age group (50–69 years old and 70 or older); the goal was to have a maximum of 10 patients in each comorbidity-age combination at each hospital. In addition, no more than 5 in each group had the same physician or group of physicians.

Summary.   In the reliability study of the criteria map and comorbidity index scoring, all four raters agreed in 22 of 30 cases (73.3%) on the overall disease value, in 17 of 30 cases (56.7%) on the overall functional status, in 20 of 30 cases (66.7%) on the overall comorbidity index score, and in 27 of 30 cases (90.0%) on the criteria map treatment score. At least two raters were in agreement on the comorbidity index component and overall scores for all 30 cases. There were no significant age differences in the stage at presentation, nor were there any age differences in the diagnosis and staging scores of the criteria mapping. There were significant age differences, however, in the treatment scores. Only 64.7% of those 70 years or older received appropriate treatment, as compared with 83.4% of those 50–69 years old ($p < 0.001$, not controlling for comorbidity). Comorbidity index levels 0 and 1 were combined in subsequent analyses because the authors did not believe that physicians' management strategies would vary between them. The level of appropriate treatment was significantly higher among those with comorbidity index scores of 0–1 versus those with a score of 2 (81.3% versus 58.9%, $p < 0.001$). The levels of inappropriate treatment also increased with the stage of cancer, even though the criteria mapping took stage into account. Finally, a logistic regression of treatment scores that included age, comorbidity level, stage of cancer, and hospital as the independent variables showed that all four were significantly associated with treatment score; furthermore, there was an interaction effect between comorbidity score and stage of cancer (i.e., patients with advanced cancer and high comorbidity scores were the least likely to receive ''appropriate'' treatment). Subgroup analyses of patients with stage I and II disease only as well as those with stage I or II disease and a comorbidity index score of 0 or 1 showed that age remained an independent predictor of the appropriateness of treatment; in the first analysis, comorbidity score also continued to be significant.

Discussion.   This study highlights the utility of a measure to adjust for comorbidity and in particular demonstrates the usefulness of an early version of the comorbidity index. A previous study had shown that the levels of appropriate cancer treatment declined with age; but without controlling for comorbidity, one could not know whether this was due to older patients' poorer overall health. The present study shows both that differences in comorbidity cannot account for the variation across ages in appropriate treatment and that the comorbidity index is a useful tool for adjusting for comorbidity. The one reservation is that the interrater reliability appears to be quite low, particularly for the functional component of the comorbidity index. Furthermore, only the percentage agreement is reported; the κ coefficient, which corrects for agreement by chance, would be more informative. Additional reliability studies of the comorbidity index would be helpful.

Bennett CL, Greenfield S, Aronow H, Ganz P, Vogelzang NJ, & Elashoff RM. (1991). Patterns of care related to age of men with prostate cancer. *Cancer, 67,* 2633–2641.
Design.   This study examines whether age affects diagnostic and treatment strategies for patients with localized prostate cancer. Using a research design similar to that of *Greenfield, Aronow, Elashoff, and Watanabe's (1988) study on breast cancer, the authors developed criteria maps that measured the appropriate diagnostic and treatment strategy and then compared those scores by age, hospital, comorbidity score (using an early version of the ICED), and presence of symptoms. Two sets of analyses were performed, one for the diagnostic score and one for the treatment score from the criteria map. Bivariate analyses of the independent predictors were followed by regression models to assess the impact of each predictor variable. Logistic regression was used to evaluate the treatment strategy, since the treatment scores followed a bimodal distribution.
Sample.   The sample consisted of 242 men from a group of 410 with histologically confirmed adenocarcinoma of the prostate. Men who were unlikely to tolerate treatment, who refused treatment, or whose cancer had spread beyond the pelvis were excluded. The patients had received their primary cancer management at 1 of 10 hospitals in southern California during 1980–1982. The 10 hospitals varied in size, occupancy rates, location,

and teaching affiliation. In the analysis, hospitals were grouped into high-, moderate-, and low-scoring groups based on the criteria map scores. The sampling was performed so that there would be a comparable distribution of patients from each hospital in terms of age and comorbid disease level and so that no single physician or practice was too heavily represented. The mean age of the entire sample was 69.9 years ($SD = 9.1$). Of the 242 in the final sample, 84% were white, 9.5% were African American, and most of the remainder were Hispanic. The older men (75 and older) were significantly more likely to have local urinary symptoms, severe obstructive symptoms, and poorly differentiated tumors than either the 65- to 74-year olds or the 50- to 64-year olds.

Summary.   Older men were more likely to receive less intensive diagnostic workups and treatment than younger men. This effect of age held up after the researchers controlled for comorbidity, hospital, and symptoms (in the diagnostic model). Age was the only significant predictor of diagnostic intensity (adjusted $R^2 = 0.11$); both comorbidity and hospital were significant predictors of treatment intensity. The invasive diagnostic test, pelvic lymphadenectomy, was less likely to be performed on individuals with high comorbidity scores (2 versus 0 or 1; the two lower scores were combined in the analysis); however, the frequency of noninvasive tests did not vary with comorbidity score. Similarly, the use of surgical or radiation therapy was considerably less likely in individuals with a higher comorbidity score, but there was no difference in the use of hormonal therapy.

Discussion.   The authors point out a number of limitations to the study, including the fact that it does not take patients' preferences into account and that decreased use of some procedures, such as pelvic lymphadenectomy, may be appropriate for older men. Nevertheless, the study does provide evidence that age affects care strategies even after controlling for comorbidity. Whether this affects outcomes is not addressed in this study. The study also indicates that comorbidity itself is an important factor in the selection of treatment strategy but does not predict diagnostic intensity. However, how well the model fits the data is not reported for the logistic regression, making it difficult to evaluate the first finding fully. It should also be noted that the measurement of comorbidity was quite limited because only two categories were used.

Cleary PD, Greenfield S, Mulley AG, Pauker SG, Schroeder SA, Wexler L, & McNeil BJ. (1991). Variations in length of stay and outcomes for six medical and surgical conditions in Massachusetts and California. *JAMA*, 266, 73–79.

Design.   This study explores the degree to which interhospital variations in length of stay are associated with differences in patients' characteristics and whether outcomes are in turn related to length of stay. Data from medical records and surveys of patients were compared for five conditions: (1) acute myocardial infarction (AMI) or rule out AMI, (2) coronary artery bypass graft (CABG), (3) total hip replacement (THR), (4) cholecystectomy, and (5) transurethral prostatectomy (TURP). Patients were sent surveys 3 to 12 months (depending on the condition) following hospitalization through which they were asked about preadmission and postadmission functional status, along with several other factors. Information about comorbidities was collected using a revised version of the ICED; the only components included were comorbid disease severity and physical (i.e., functional) impairment. The Physical Status Classification of the American Society of Anesthesiologists (ASA) was also calculated. Regression analyses of lengths of stay were performed with patients' characteristics as the independent variables. Least squares adjusted lengths of stay were then calculated for each hospital. On the patient level, the relationship between length of stay and subsequent functional status (as defined by ADLs, IADLs, and social activities), as well as the probability of readmission, was evaluated using analysis of variance and linear regression.

Sample. Data were collected on 2,484 patients receiving care at six university-affiliated hospitals (three in California and three in Massachusetts) between September 1985 and February 1987. There were a variety of exclusion criteria, including diagnosis of metastatic cancer or AIDS. Hospitals were included for each condition only if they had at least 75 patients with that condition, so the number of hospitals included ranged from four to six across conditions. The survey response rates ranged from 73.0% for patients hospitalized to rule out AMI to 84.4% for those undergoing cholecystectomy. There were few significant differences between those who did and did not return the questionnaire. The mean age ranged from 46.4 years for cholecystectomy patients to 69.0 years for TURP patients. The percentage male ranged from 26.1% for cholecystectomy patients to 85.8% of CABG patients (of course, 100% of TURP patients were male). Racial composition and education levels also varied across conditions. The ICED scores ranged from 1.6 (cholecystectomy patients) to 2.7 ("rule out AMI" patients) for the comorbid disease severity score and from 0.28 (cholecystectomy patients) to 0.92 (TURP patients) for the functional impairment score.

Summary. There was significant variation in the length of stay across the six hospitals (the results are reported by condition). Patients' characteristics (including ICED scores) accounted for from 15.4% of the variation for CABG patients to 31.4% for TURP patients. Adding the hospital as a variable explained another 2.1% to 13.1% of the variance. Unfortunately for our purposes, the amount explained by the ICED components is not presented separately. The combined ICED scores and preadmission functional status (based on patients' recall at the time of the follow-up questionnaire) accounted for from 3.9% ("rule out AMI" patients) to 13.1% (TURP patients) of the variation. The adjusted average lengths of stay were not substantially different from the unadjusted values, except for THR patients, where the difference among hospitals was no longer significant.

The second set of analyses revealed no significant association between length of stay and change in functional status, except that THR patients with longer stays experienced greater improvement in IADL scores. The strongest predictor of postadmission functional status was the retrospectively self-reported preadmission functional status, which accounted for 6.3% (THR patients) to 50.9% ("rule out AMI" patients) of the variation. Adding sociodemographic characteristics and comorbidity accounted for another 4.4% to 15.3% of the variance.

Discussion. The comorbidity index may be an independent predictor of both length of stay and postdischarge functional status, although it is difficult to separate the impact of comorbidity from other characteristics of patients because of the way the results are reported. On the other hand, the differences among hospitals persist for all but one condition, even after adjustment for comorbidity and a variety of other factors. This article thus provides an interesting example of the use of the ICED components, but it does not provide a great deal of detailed information on the performance of the ICED itself. It does report average scores for each scale for the six conditions, although the select nature of this sample must be kept in mind in comparing these results with other populations.

Cleary PD, Reilly DT, Greenfield S, Mulley AG, Wexler L, Frankel F, & McNeill BJ. (1993). Using patient reports to assess health-related quality of life after total hip replacement. *Qual Life Res*, *2*, 3–11.

Design.   This study assesses health-related quality of life 1 year after a first unilateral total hip replacement (THR). It is a more detailed examination of the data on patients undergoing total hip replacement from the Six Hospital Study, also reported in *Cleary et al., 1991 (see the abstract of that article for more details on the design). The authors estimated a series of linear regression models with measures of postdischarge quality of life as the dependent variable and admitting characteristics as the independent variables. The object was to evaluate the impact of THR. Sociodemographic characteristics, severity and comorbidity (the ICED) measures, and the preadmission measures of the outcomes variables were entered into a model first. Then other functioning and process variables were considered for addition using forward stepwise regression. Duration of surgery and use of pressor support were used to measure the process of care. The seven outcome measures used as dependent variables were (1) basic and (2) intermediate ADLs, (3) social functioning, (4) mental health, (5) pain, (6) reported use of walking supports, and (7) dislocations.

Sample.   See the abstract on *Cleary et al., 1991, for a description of the sample. Of the 356 patients who agreed to participate, 284 (79.8%) returned the questionnaire; the data reported here are on the 284. Those who did not respond had significantly higher comorbidity scores and longer stays, and were also less likely to be married.

Summary.   Results on the reliability of the outcome scales are presented, along with the changes between the preadmission and postdischarge scores. The physical (i.e., functional) impairment component of the ICED was a significant predictor in six of the seven regressions (the exception was mental health). This was true even after adjustment for self-reported preadmission functional status. However, the results for the other component of the ICED, the comorbid disease severity score, are not reported. It is not clear whether or not it was included in the model. The other significant predictors varied by outcome measure, although preadmission functioning was usually one of them. That is not surprising, particularly since this is based on a retrospective self-assessment at the time of the follow-up interview. Age was not a significant predictor of postdischarge functioning, except for mental health (older patients showed greater improvement), after controlling for preadmission functioning. Income, education, the American Society of Anesthesiologists' (ASA) classification, use of pressor supports, and duration of surgery were never significant predictors.

Discussion.   The limitations of the measure of preadmission functioning are clear, as the authors themselves point out, since the data were collected retrospectively about 1 year later. It also is not surprising that the component of the ICED that measures overall functional status during hospitalization would be a significant predictor of postdischarge functioning. It would be interesting to know whether the other component of the ICED was dropped from the model because it was insignificant and whether the composite measure would also be a significant predictor.

Another study, by Guadagnoli, Ayanian, and Cleary (1992), reports more detailed results for CABG patients from this same larger study. They examine whether there is any significant difference in functional outcomes for CABG patients over and under 65 years old. They report the ICED comorbid disease severity score by age group; the percentages scoring 0, 1, and 2 are 27.4%, 69.6%, and 2.9% for those under 65 years old and 17.2%, 74.8%, and 8.1% for patients 65 or older. The difference is not statistically significant. They found no age-related differences in functioning 6 months after discharge, except that older patients had significantly better mental health scores both before admission and after discharge. They also report that the comorbid disease severity score is one of three significant predictors of postdischarge functional status (along with preadmission functioning and marital status), but they do not report detailed results.

Greenfield S, Apolone G, McNeil BJ, & Cleary PD. (1993). The importance of co-existent disease in the occurrence of postoperative complications and one-year recovery in patients undergoing total hip replacement: Comorbidity and outcomes after hip replacement. Med Care, 31, 141–154.

Design.   This study examines the impact of comorbid disease on postoperative complications and quality of life 1 year later in patients undergoing total hip replacement (THR). It is part of the Six Hospital Study, also reported in Cleary et al., *1991, *1993, and Guadagnoli et al., 1992. (See the abstract of Cleary et al., 1991, for additional information on the design.) Data were gathered from each patient's medical record regarding characteristics of the surgery, comorbidity, sociodemographic variables, and major and minor complications. Comorbidity was measured using the ICED, from which the component measuring the acute, unstable aspect of the diseases was deleted. The ICED scores were compared with the American Society of Anesthesiologists' Physical Status score (ASA PS). One year after discharge patients were also asked to complete a questionnaire which covered quality of life, perceived improvement in health status, and satisfaction with care. In predicting complications, bivariate analyses to identify potential predictors were followed by multivariate analyses to control for potential confounders. The reports are expressed in terms of odds ratios. For the prediction of health status 1 year after hospitalization, multiple linear regression was used to estimate the relationship between the ICED scores and the dependent variables while controlling for covariates.

Sample.   The sample consisted of 356 patients who underwent THR in four academic hospitals in Massachusetts and California between September 1985 and February 1987. The mean age of the sample was 64 years ($SD = 12.9$); 43% were male; 64% were married; and 93% were white. Twenty-eight percent had had prior hip surgery; and 3% had had prior knee surgery. Thirty percent of the sample had no coexistent disease on admission, and the average number of comorbid conditions for those with at least 1 was 1.5; thus, this was a relatively healthy group. Seventy-nine percent of the sample returned the follow-up questionnaire; nonrespondents were less likely to be married, had longer stays, and had more comorbidity.

Summary.   There was a statistically significantly increased risk of serious complications ($n = 38$ or 11%) with increasing levels of both components of the ICED as well as the composite score, but not of the ASA PS score. However, the correlation between the two components of the ICED was only 0.27. In a logistic regression of the ICED scores and age, both factors were significantly associated with serious complications. (The ICED was included as a series of three dummy variables; the coefficients for levels 3 and 4 were significant, but the coefficient for level 2 was not.) The model accounted for 14% of the variance. Within each of the ASA PS strata, the likelihood of serious complications increased with increasing levels of the ICED. The Spearman rank correlation coefficients between the ASA PS score and the two components and composite score of the ICED were 0.40, 0.22, and 0.53 ($p < 0.001$).

In comparing the mean functional status scores across ICED levels, there was a large and statistically significant decline in functional status with increasing ICED scores for all three functional status outcome measures: basic ADLs, IADLs, and the social activity scale. For example, the mean IADL level fell from 80 ($SD = 21$) for those with an ICED score of 1 to 53 ($SD = 39$) for those with an ICED score of 4. The ICED level remained a significant predictor of IADL level after controlling for age, sex, education, and marital status ($R^2 = 0.13$). Finally, there was a statistically significant difference among the four hospitals in the 1-year IADL scores. Adjusting for sociodemographic variables and the baseline IADL measure accounted for 16% of the variance, but the difference between two of the hospitals remained statistically significant. Adding the ICED score to the model accounted for another 3% of the variance, but there was no longer any statistically significant difference among hospitals. The ICED score when entered alone accounted for 7% of the variance.

Discussion. This article provides the most complete data on the performance of the ICED and compares it with the ASA PS score. It suggests that the ICED is a useful measure for adjusting for comorbidity in predicting posthospital functional status. However, the results of this study should be extrapolated to other settings or populations with caution. As the authors point out, the study was designed to maximize internal validity, that is, to minimize interinstitutional variation in the process of care, and this reduces its generalizability. It should also be noted that the total amount of variation explained by these models is quite low, although this is true of many severity adjustment measures. The limitations of retrospective reporting of preadmission functional status are discussed by Katz et al. (1994). In a sample of 31 patients they found that the Pearson correlation coefficient for preoperative functional status measured prospectively versus retrospectively was only 0.36. Despite these caveats, the ICED clearly did perform better than the ASA PS score and had a significant impact on the interpretation of interhospital differences in postsurgical functional outcomes. The importance of properly adjusting for comorbidity in comparing outcomes across patients and institutions is highlighted once again.

Krousel-Wood MA, Re RN, & Abdoh A. (1994). The use of three comorbidity indices in predicting mortality from TURP versus open prostatectomy [Abstract]. *Clin Res*, 42, 248A.

Design. This abstract reports on a study comparing the ability of three comorbidity indices—the Charlson, the Kaplan-Feinstein, and the ICED—in adjusting for comorbidity among patients with benign prostatic hypertrophy (BPH). The study compared 5-year mortality following TURP and open prostatectomy.

Sample. The sample consisted of 302 men undergoing prostatectomy for BPH at a large hospital between 1979 and 1984.

Summary. According to the authors, all three measures of comorbidity were shown to be relatively sensitive and specific using ROC analysis. However, neither the Charlson nor the Kaplan-Feinstein was significantly associated with the type of procedure performed. After adjustment for comorbidity using the ICED, however, the significant difference in mortality between the two procedures (16% for TURP and 4% for open prostatectomy) disappeared.

Discussion. This study reports interesting comparative data on the ICED and also shows its utility in predicting a different type of outcome measure, namely, mortality. Unfortunately, however, this is only an abstract, so many of the relevant details are omitted.

REFERENCES

Averill RF, Goldfield NI, McGuire TE, Bender JA, Mulin RL, & Gregg LW. (1990). *Design and evaluation of a prospective payment system for ambulatory care.* Wallingford, CT: 3M Health Information Systems.

Bearden DM, Allman RM, Sundarum SV, Burst NM, & Bartolucci AA. (1993). Age-related variability in the use of cardiovascular imaging procedures. *J Am Geriatr Soc, 41,* 1075–1082.

Beer RJ, Teasdale TA, Ghusn HF, & Taffet GE. (1994). Estimation of severity of illness with APACHE-II: Age-related implications in cardiac arrest outcomes. *Resuscitation, 27,* 189–195.

*Bennett CL, Greenfield S, Aronow H, Ganz P, Vogelzang NJ, & Elashoff RM. (1991). Patterns of care related to age of men with prostate cancer. *Cancer, 67,* 2633–2641.

Berlowitz DR, Rosen AK, & Moskowitz MA. (1995). Ambulatory care case mix measures. *J Gen Intern Med, 10,* 162–170.

Brewster AC, Karlin BG, Hyde LA, Jacobs CM, Bradbury RC, & Chae YM. (1985). MEDISGRPS: A clinically based approach to classifying hospital patients at admission. *Inquiry, 22,* 377–387.

Broadhead WE, Clapp-Channing NE, Finch JN, & Copeland JA. (1989). Effects of medical illness and somatic symptoms on treatment of depression in a family medicine residency practice. *Gen Hosp Psychiatry, 11,* 194–200.

Calore KA, & Iezzoni L. (1987). Disease staging and PMCs: Can they improve DRGs? *Med Care, 25,* 724–735.

Charbonneau C, Ostrowski C, Poehne ET, Lindsay P, Panniers TL, Houghton P, & Albright J. (1988). Validity and reliability issues in alternative patient classification systems. *Med Care, 26,* 800–810.

*Charlson ME, Pompei P, Ales KL, & MacKenzie CR. (1987). A new method of classifying prognostic comorbidity in longitudinal studies: Development and validation. *J Chron Dis, 40,* 373–383.

*Cleary PD, Greenfield S, Mulley AG, Pauker SG, Schroeder SA, Wexler L, & McNeil BJ. (1991). Variations in length of stay and outcomes for six medical and surgical conditions in Massachusetts and California. *JAMA, 266,* 73–79.

*Cleary PD, Reilly DT, Greenfield S, Mulley AG, Wexler L, Frankel F, & McNeill BJ. (1993). Using patient reports to assess health-related quality of life after total hip replacement. *Qual Life Res, 2,* 3–11.

Coulehan JL, Schulberg HC, Block MR, Janosky JE, & Arena VC. (1990). Medical comorbidity of major depressive disorder in a primary medical practice. *Arch Intern Med, 150,* 2363–2367.

Criteria Committee of the New York Heart Association. (1964). *Diseases nomenclature and criteria for diagnosis.* Boston: Little Brown.

Daley J. (1994). Criteria by which to evaluate risk-adjusted outcomes programs in cardiac surgery. *Ann Thorac Surg, 58,* 1827–1835.

*Daley J, Jencks S, Draper D, Lenhart G, Thomas N, & Walker J. (1988). Predicting hospital-associated mortality for Medicare patients. *JAMA, 24,* 3617–3624.

Damiano AM, Bergner M, Draper EA, Knaus WA, & Wagner DP. (1992). Reliability of a measure of severity of illness: Acute physiology of chronic health evaluation-II. *J Clin Epidemiol, 45,* 93–101.

*Deyo RA, Cherkin DC, & Ciol MA. (1992). Adapting a clinical comorbidity index for use with ICD-9-CM administrative databases. *J Clin Epidemiol, 45,* 613–619.

*D'Hoore W, Sicotte C, & Tilquin C. (1993). Risk adjustment in outcome assessment: The Charlson Comorbidity Index. *Methods Inf Med, 32,* 382–387.

*Dodds TA, Martin DP, Stolov WC, & Deyo RA. (1993). A validation of the functional independence measurement and its performance among rehabilitation inpatients. *Arch Phys Med Rehabil, 74,* 531–536.

Fernandez de Sanmamed MJ, Fein O, Morrison A, & Moy E. (1993). Limitaciones de los sistemas *case-mix* en atencion primaria: Comparacion de la gravedad de los pacientes atendidos en un centro ubicado en el hospital y dos centros extrahospitalarios en EE.UU [Limitations of case mix systems in primary care: Comparison of the severity of illness of patients in a hospital clinic and two nonhospital clinics in the U.S.]. *Aten primaria, 12,* 144–147.

Fink MP, Snydman DR, Niederman MS, et al. (1994). Treatment of severe pneumonia in hospitalized patients-results of a multicenter, randomized, double-blind trial comparing intravenous ciprofloxacin with imipenem-cilastatin. *Antimicrob Agents Chemother, 38,* 547–557.

Fisher ES, Whaley FS, Krushat WM, Malenka DJ, Fleming C, Baron JA, & Hsia DC. (1992). The accuracy of Medicare's hospital claims data: Progress has been made, but problems remain. *Am J Public Health, 82,* 243–248.

Gonnella JS, Hornbrook MC, & Louis DZ. (1984). Staging of disease: A case-mix measurement. *JAMA, 251,* 637–644.

*Greenfield S, Apolone G, McNeil BJ, & Cleary PD. (1993). The importance of co-existent disease in the occurrence of postoperative complications and 1-year recovery in patients undergoing total hip replacement: Comorbidity and outcomes after hip replacement. *Med Care, 31,* 141–154.

*Greenfield S, Aronow HU, Elashoff RM, & Watanabe D. (1988). Flaws in mortality data: The hazards of ignoring comorbid disease. *JAMA, 260,* 2253–2255.

Greenfield S, Blanco DM, Elashoff RM, & Aronow HU. (1987). Development and testing of a new index of comorbidity. *Clin Res, 35,* 346A.

*Greenfield S, Blanco DM, Elashoff RM, & Ganz PA. (1987). Patterns of care related to age of breast cancer patients. *JAMA, 257,* 2766–2770.

Guadagnoli E, Ayanian JZ, & Cleary PD. (1992). Comparison of patient-reported outcomes after elective coronary artery bypass grafting in patients aged ≥ and < 65 years. *Am J Cardiol, 70,* 60–64.

*Hartz AJ, Kuhn EM, Kayser KL, Pryor DP, Green R, & Rimm AA. (1992). Assessing providers of coronary revascularization: A method for peer review organizations. *Am J Public Health, 82,* 1631–1640.

Hayward RA, Bernard AM, Rosevear JS, Anderson JE, & McMahon LF. (1993). An evaluation of generic screens for poor quality of hospital care on a general medicine service. *Med Care, 31*, 394–402.

Health Systems International, Inc. (HSI), Horn SD. (1987). *Computerized severity index (CSI) ICD-9-CM severity modification: Adult criteria.* New Haven, CT: HSI, Inc.

Holt AW, Bury LK, Bersten AD, Skowronski GA, & Vedig AE. (1992). Prospective evaluation of residents and nurses as severity score collectors. *Crit Care Med, 20*, 1688–1691.

*Holtzman J, Pheley AM, & Lurie N. (1994). Changes in orders limiting care and the use of less aggressive care in a nursing home population. *J Am Geriatr Soc, 42*, 275–279.

Horn SD, Buckle JM, & Carver CM. (1988). Ambulatory severity index: Development of an ambulatory case mix system. *J Ambul Care Manage, 11*, 53–62.

Horn SD, Bulkley G, Sharkey PD, Chambers AF, Horn RA, & Schramm CJ. (1985). Inter-hospital differences in patient severity: Problems for prospective payments based on diagnosis related groups (DRGs). *N Engl J Med, 313*, 20–24.

Horn SJ. (1986). Measuring severity: How sick is sick? How well is well? *Health Care Finan Manage, 40*, 21–32.

Horn SJ, & Horn RA. (1986). The Computerized Severity Index: A new tool for case-mix management. *J Med Syst, 10*, 73–78.

Iezzoni L. (Ed.). (1994). *Risk adjustment for measuring health care outcomes.* Ann Arbor, MI: Health Administration Press.

Iezzoni LI, Ash AS, Schwartz M, Daly J, Hughes JS, & Mackiernan YD. (1996). Judging hospitals by severity-adjusted mortality rates: The influence of severity-adjustment method. *Am J Public Health, 86*, 1379–1387.

Iezzoni LI, Foley SM, Daley J, Hughes J, Fisher ES, & Heeren T. (1992). Comorbidities, complications, and coding bias: Does the number of diagnosis codes matter in predicting in-hospital mortality? *JAMA, 267*, 2197–2203.

Iezzoni LI, & Moskowitz MA. (1988). A clinical assessment of MedisGroups. *JAMA, 260*, 3159–3163.

Iezzoni LI, Restuccia JD, Shwartz M, Schaumburg D, Coffman GA, Kreger BE, Butterly JR, & Selker HP. (1992). The utility of severity of illness information in assessing the quality of hospital care The role of the clinical trajectory. *Med Care, 30*, 428–444.

Iezzoni LI, Shwartz M, Moskowitz MA, Ash AS, Sawitz E, & Burnside S. (1990). Illness severity and costs of admissions at teaching and nonteaching hospitals. *JAMA, 264*, 1426–1431.

Jencks SF, Williams DK, & Kay TL. (1988). Assessing hospital-associated deaths from discharge data: The role of length of stay and comorbidities. *JAMA, 260*, 2240–2246.

Jollis JG, Ancukiewicz M, DeLong ER, Pryor DB, Muhlbaier LH, & Mark DB. (1993). Discordance of databases designed for claims payment versus clinical information systems: Implications for outcomes research. *Ann Intern Med, 119*, 844–850.

Katz JN, Wright EA, Guadagnoli E, Liang MH, Karlson EW, & Cleary PD. (1994). Differences between men and women undergoing major orthopedic surgery for degenerative arthritis. *Arthritis Rheum, 37*, 687–694.

Kieft H, Hoepelman AIM, Rozenbergarska M, Branger JM, Voskuil JH, Geers ABM, Kluyver M, Hart HC, Poestclement E, Vanbeugen L, Struyvenberg A, & Verhoef J.

(1994). Cefepime compared with ceftazimime as initial therapy for serious bacterial infections and sepsis syndrome. *Antimicrob Agents Chemother, 38,* 415–421.

*Knaus WA, Draper EA, Wagner DP, & Zimmerman JE. (1985). APACHE II: A severity of disease classification system. *Crit Care Med, 10,* 818–828.

*Knaus WA, Wagner DP, Draper EA, Zimmerman JE, Bergner M, Bastos P, Sirio C, Murphy DJ, Lotring T, Damiano A, & Harrell FE. (1991). The APACHE III prognostic system: Risk prediction of hospital mortality for critically ill hospitalized adults. *Chest, 100,* 1619–1636.

Knaus WA, Zimmerman JE, Wagner DP, Draper EA, & Lawrence DE. (1981). APACHE—Acute Physiology and Chronic Health Evaluation: A physiologically based classification system. *Crit Care Med, 9,* 591–597.

Kollef MH. (1993). Do age and gender influence outcome from mechanical ventilation? *Heart Lung, 22,* 442–449.

*Krousel-Wood MA, Re RN, & Abdoh A. (1994). The use of three comorbidity indices in predicting mortality from TURP versus open prostatectomy. *Clin Res, 42,* 248A.

Lahad A, & Yodfat Y. (1993). Impact of comorbidity on well-being in hypertension: Case control study. *J Hum Hypertens, 7,* 611–614.

Le Gall JR, Lemeshow S, Leleu G, Klar J, Huillard J, Rue M, Teres D, & Artigas A. (1995). Customized probability models for early severe sepsis in adult intensive care patients: Intensive Care Unit Scoring Group. *JAMA, 273,* 644–650.

*Le Gall JR, Lemeshow S, & Saulnier F. (1993). A new simplified acute physiology score (SAPS II) based on a European/North American Multicenter study. *JAMA, 270,* 2957–2963.

Lemeshow S, & Le Gall JR. (1994). Modeling the severity of illness of ICU patients A systems update. *JAMA, 272,* 1049–1055.

*Lemeshow S, Teres D, Kalr J, Avrunin JS, Gehlbach SH, & Rapoport J. (1993). Mortality probability models (MPM II) based on an international cohort of intensive care unit patients. *JAMA, 270,* 2478–2486.

Martin LF, Atnip RG, Holmes PA, Lynch JC, & Thiele BL. (1994). Prediction of postoperative complications after elective aortic surgery using stepwise logistic regression analysis. *Am Surg, 60,* 163–168.

*McMahon LF, Hayward RA, Bernard AM, Rosevear JS, & Weissfeld LA. (1992). APACHE-L: A new severity of illness adjuster for inpatient medical care. *Med Care, 30,* 445–452.

Meenan RF, Gertman PM, & Mason JH. (1980). Measuring health status in arthritis: The AIMS. *Arthritis Rheum, 23,* 146–152.

Moscovitz H, Shofer F, Mignott H, Behrman A, & Kilpatrick L. (1994). Plasma cytokine determinations in emergency department patients as a predictor of bacteremia and infectious disease severity. *Crit Care Med, 22,* 1102–1107.

National Committee for the Evaluation of Centoxin. (1994). The French national registry of HA-1A (Centoxin) in septic shock a cohort study of 600 patients. *Arch Intern Med, 154,* 2484–2491.

*O'Connor GT, Plume SK, Olmstead EM, Coffin LH, Morton, JR, Maloney CT, Nowicki ER, Tryzelaar JF, Hernandex F, Adrian L, Casey KJ, Soule DN, Marris CAS, Nugent WC, Charlesworth DC, Clough R, Katz S, Leavitt BJ, Wennberg JE, and the Northern New England Cardiovascular Disease Study Group. (1991). A regional prospective study of in-hospital mortality associated with coronary artery bypass grafting. *JAMA, 266,* 803–809.

*Papadakis MA, Lee KK, Browner WS, Kent DL, Matchar DB, Kagawa MK, Hallenbeck J, Lee D, Onishi R, & Charles G. (1993). Prognosis of mechanically ventilated patients. *West J Med, 159,* 659–664.

Parkerson GR Jr, Broadhead WE, & Tse C-K J. (1992). Quality of life and functional health of primary care patients. *J Clin Epidemiol, 45,* 1303–1313.

Parkerson GR Jr, Broadhead WE, & Tse C-K J. (1993). The Duke Severity of Illness Checklist (DUSOI) for measurement of severity and comorbidity. *J Clin Epidemiol, 46,* 379–393.

Parkerson GR Jr, Broadhead WE, & Tse C-K J. (1995). Health status and severity of illness as predictors of outcomes in primary care. *Med Care, 33,* 53–66.

Parkerson GR Jr, Michener JL, Wu LR, Finch JN, Muhlbaier LH, Magruder-Habib K, Kertesz JW, Clapp-Channing N, Morrow DS, Chen A L-T, & Jokerst E. (1989). Associations among family support, family stress, and personal functional health status. *J Clin Epidemiol, 42,* 217–229.

Perkins NAK. (1991). *Case-mix adjustment of physician practice profiles using claims data.* Unpublished doctoral dissertation, University of Rochester, Rochester, NY.

Romano PS, & Mark DH. (1994). Bias in the coding of hospital discharge data and its implications for quality assessment. *Med Care, 32,* 81–90.

*Romano PS, Roos LL, & Jollis JG. (1993a). Adapting a clinical comorbidity index for use with ICD-9-CM administrative data: Differing perspectives. *J Clin Epidemiol, 46,* 1075–1079.

*Romano PS, Roos LL, & Jollis JG. (1993b). Further evidence concerning the use of a clinical comorbidity index with ICD-9-CM administrative data. *J Clin Epidemiol, 46,* 1085–1090.

Romano PS, Roos LL, Luft HS, Jollis JG, Doliszny K, and the Ischemic Heart Disease Patient Outcomes Research Team. (1994). A comparison of administrative versus clinical data: Coronary artery bypass surgery as an example. *J Clin Epidemiol, 47,* 249–260.

Roos LL, Sharp SM, & Cohen MM. (1991). Comparing clinical information with claims data: Some similarities and differences. *J Clin Epidemiol, 44,* 881–888.

Schneeweiss R, Cherkin DC, Hart LG, Revicki DA, Wollstadt LJ, Stephenson MJ, Froom J, Dunn EV, Tindall HL, & Rosenblatt RA. (1986). Diagnosis clusters adapted for ICD-9-CM and ICHPPC-2. *J Fam Pract, 22,* 69–72.

Schneeweiss R, Rosenblatt RA, Cherkin DC, Kirkwood CR, & Hart G. (1983). Diagnosis clusters: A new tool for analyzing the content of ambulatory medical care. *Med Care, 21,* 105–122.

Starfield B, Weiner J, Mumford L, & Steinwachs D. (1991). Ambulatory care groups: A categorization of diagnoses for research and management. *Health Serv Res, 26,* 53–74.

Tenan PM, Fillmore HH, Caress B, Kelly WP, Nelson H, Graziano D, & Johnson SC. (1988). PACs: Classifying ambulatory care patients and services for clinical and financial management. *J Ambulatory Care Manage, 11,* 36–53.

Thomas JW, & Ashcraft MLF. (1989). Measuring severity of illness: A comparison of interrater reliability among severity methodologies. *Inquiry, 26,* 483–492.

Thomas JW, & Ashcraft MLF. (1991). Measuring severity of illness: Six severity systems and their ability to explain cost variations. *Inquiry, 28,* 39–55.

Weiner JP. (1991). Ambulatory case-mix methodologies: Application to primary care research. In H Hibbard, PA Nutting, & ML Grady (Eds.), *Conference proceedings: Primary care research: Theory and methods.* Rockville, MD: Agency for Health Care Policy and Research, Public Health Service, U.S. Department of Health and Human Services.

Weiner JP, Starfield BH, Steinwachs DM, & Mumford LM. (1991). Development and application of a population-oriented measure of ambulatory care case-mix. *Med Care, 29,* 452–472.

*Wu AW, Rubin HR, & Rosen MJ. (1990). Are elderly people less responsive to intensive care? *J Am Geriatr Soc, 38,* 621–627.

*Ziegler EJ, Fisher CJ, Sprung CL, Straube RC, Sadoff JC, Foulke GE, Wortel CH, Fink MP, Lellinger P, Teng NNH, Allen IE, Berger HJ, Knatterud GL, LoBuglio AF, Smith CR, and the HA-1A Sepsis Study Group. (1991). Treatment of gram-negative bacteremia and septic shock with HA-1A human monoclonal antibody against endotoxin. *N Engl J Med, 324,* 429–436.

4

Cognitive Screening

**Jurgis Karuza, Paul R. Katz,
Robin Henderson**

INTRODUCTION

The focus of this chapter is on cognitive screening for dementia in research and clinical settings. The chapter does not specifically deal with cognitive tests used in the detailed diagnosis of types of dementia. The chapter first reviews some background on the need for and development of cognitive screening instruments, the present ''state of the science,'' and qualities needed in an instrument. Then, the chapter reviews several of the more widely used brief cognitive screening instruments, focusing on the Mini-Mental State Examination (MMSE) because of its stature. The discussion of the MMSE includes some concerns and limits that also apply to cognitive screening in general. Some brief recommendations are given following the sections on the MMSE. Finally, the chapter provides an annotated bibliography on several current representative works on cognitive screening, focusing on the MMSE. The annotated bibliography focuses on empirical studies published since 1990 relevant to currently emerging issues on the use and revision of the MMSE as a screening test. For an overview of the development of ''classic'' screening instruments, the reader is referred to the review below. In addition, the annotated bibliography offers a selected review of current articles detailing the use of alternative dementia screening tools that hold some promise, including cross-cultural screening tests. In keeping with the chapter's focus on screening tests, abstracts on more comprehensive assessment tools were excluded.

For added discussion, readers are alerted to the detailed published review of the MMSE by Tombaugh and McIntyre (1992), the review by Butters, Delis, and Lucas (1995), and a review chapter on brief assessments of cognitive function by Albert (1994). Assessment of behavioral disturbance is beyond the scope of this chapter, but readers are referred to the review by Teri and Logsdon (1994).

HISTORY AND BACKGROUND

Organic mental disorders, with dementia of the Alzheimer's type being the most prevalent, affect 10% of the noninstitutionalized older adult population (e.g., Evans et al., 1989). Among institutionalized people, the prevalence has been estimated at over 50% (Goldman & Lazarus, 1988; Rovner et al., 1986). Epidemiological studies (e.g., Bachman et al., 1993; Schoenberg, Kokman, & Okazaki, 1987) indicate that the incidence of dementia increases with age. In a recent study using the Framingham study cohort, Bachman et al. (1993) determined the 5-year incidence of dementia to be 7 per 1,000 individuals aged 65–69. This increased to an incidence of 118 per 1,000 for individuals aged 85–89. Interestingly, a recently published meta-analysis of nine epidemiological studies found that the prevalence of Alzheimer's disease falls between the ages of 80 and 84 and levels off to 40% (i.e., 400 per 1,000) at age 95, suggesting that Alzheimer's disease should not be considered a natural concomitant of the aging process (Richie & Kildea, 1995).

Despite the high incidence and prevalence of dementias, underdiagnosis remains a problem independent of the discipline of the professions performing the assessment, whether nursing, medicine, social work, or psychology. For example, a recent study of older adults admitted into a university hospital revealed that among those with cognitive deficits, nearly 80% were not diagnosed (McCartney & Palmateer, 1985). It is true that cure of the degenerative dementias remains elusive; still, accurate diagnosis is critical to effective management of patients and support of caregivers.

STATE OF THE SCIENCE

Over the past 20 years considerable work has gone into developing specialized measures of cognitive and functional impairment that characterize dementias and chart the progression of disease. At this point, it is useful to reinforce the distinction between more thorough and involved measurement instruments, which are used in diagnosis and research, and brief screening tests, which are designed to identify individuals for whom a more detailed assessment is warranted.

Several scales have been developed to assess comprehensively the characteristics of dementia, including, for example, the Sandoz Clinical Assessment Geriatric Scale (Lomeo, 1992) and the Alzheimer Disease Assessment Scale (Zec et al., 1992). Typically, these scales cover several domains, such as intellectual functioning, affect, and motor functioning. They are especially useful in assessing outcomes in clinical trials or in performing a comprehensive diagnostic workup of a patient who is suspected of having a dementia. However, such scales are lengthy, take a considerable amount of time and effort to complete, and require specialized training to administer. This makes their use as initial screening tools problematic.

Another assessment approach is based on measuring the patient's functional status. Several studies indicate high correlations between patients' functional and behavioral levels and their cognitive scores (Lomeo, 1992; *Weiler, Chiriboga, & Black, 1994). Scales that are based specifically on measures of patients' functional status include the Blessed Dementia Scale (Blessed, Tomlinson, & Roth, 1968), Functional Assessment Staging (Reisberg, 1988), and the Cognitive Performance Test (Burns, Mortimer, & Merchak, 1994). Function-based assessments of cognitive impairment can be especially useful in assessing patients with severe cognitive impairment because they do not rely on patients' verbal capacity.

Still other approaches focus on supplementary characteristics of dementia in older adults, such as measures of psychiatric symptoms—e.g., the Brief Psychiatric Rating Scale (Overall & Gorham, 1988; Sultzer, Levin, Mahler, High, & Cummings, 1992)—and behavioral symptoms (Cohen-Mansfield, 1986). An interesting new screening strategy is found in the Information Questionnaire of Cognitive Decline (IQCODE) developed by Jorm and Jacomb (1989). The IQ-CODE consists of 26 questions that ask an informant who has known the patient for 10 years to rate the patient in a variety of functional domains. Specifically, the informant is asked to rate, as compared with 10 years ago, whether the subject's function is better or worse on a five-point Likert scale. Functional domains that are sampled include following a story line on a television show and remembering the family's street address. Preliminary data indicate a solid correlation with the MMSE ($r = -0.74$) and good internal consistency ($\alpha > 0.95$). The structure of the test, and its use of informants, makes this test attractive for epidemiological research, especially research using telephone formats. The stipulation of a 10-year time frame in answering the questions, however, raises the issue of the IQCODE's feasibility for longitudinal studies as an outcome measure.

Recent advances in genetic research may lead to the identification of genetic markers for some dementias such as Alzheimer's disease. Also promising is the development of simple noninvasive neurobiological tests for Alzheimer's disease, such as the pupil dilation test (Scinto et al., 1994). However, it is much too early to determine the reliability, validity, and practicality of these new diagnostic tools. Assessments focusing on clinical, neurological, and behavioral criteria are still the primary diagnostic tools.

In contrast to the comprehensive specialized tests enumerated above, there remains an important need for effective screening tools that identify individuals for whom further diagnostic workup is warranted and for epidemiologic and clinical research. Pressures to limit unnecessary diagnostic testing and to identify individuals at risk of functional losses will increase as concerns about cost containment increase and the move to managed care accelerates. In the past 25 years, a parallel effort has gone into developing and validating brief, objective measures of cognitive function. The use of these tests in research and clinical practice has, not surprisingly, increased dramatically.

DESIRABLE QUALITIES OF THE TEST

From a practical perspective, several qualities are desirable in a screening test. They include being nonthreatening, appealing, and easily administered (*Albert & Cohen, 1992). From this perspective, subjecting patients and families to a comprehensive battery of cognitive tests can be emotionally draining and stressful for both patient and family. Also, many of the instruments described above are too long and cumbersome to be used as screening tools. From a psychometric perspective, the screening tests need to be reliable and valid. Especially important is that screening tests be sensitive and specific. A useful cognitive screening test should "screen in" those with dementia; ideally, all individuals who truly have a dementia would test positive. A useful cognitive screening test also should "screen out" those without dementia; ideally, all individuals truly not demented would test negative. The proportion of individuals with dementia who test positive is referred to as the test's *sensitivity*. The proportion of individuals without dementia who test negative is referred to as the test's *specificity*.

SELECTED SCREENING TESTS

Historically, screening tools were keyed to deficits of cognitive functioning, such as loss of attention, concentration, memory, language, and visuospatial skills, that reflect the progression of dementia. Since the development of tests like the Mental Status Questionnaire (Kahn, Goldfarb, Pollack, & Peck, 1960) and the Blessed Information Memory and Concentration Test (Blessed et al., 1968), a variety of cognitively based tests have been reported in the literature. As with much of the neuropsychological research on dementia, these screening tests focus on losses in episodic memory, such as recalling personal experiences of specific events; or on changes in semantic memory, such as recall of learned facts. Losses in visuospatial skills, which may be especially relevant in screening for early stages of Alzheimer's disease, are captured to a lesser degree. Some recent tests (e.g., clock-drawing tests) have begun to emphasize measurement of visuospatial function (Schulman, Shedletsky, & Silver, 1986). A summary of selected tests follows.

Blessed Dementia Scale

One of the earliest mental status tests was the Blessed Dementia Scale (BDS), which was developed in England by Blessed et al. (1968). Its original version consists of two parts. The first part has items that focus on activities of daily living and personality. Scores range from 0 to 28, with higher scores indicating more dementia. A second part has items that focus on memory, concentration, and orientation. The scoring system for the second part counts the number of errors made, with scores ranging from 0 (best) to 37 (worst). A six-item version of the BDS, the Blessed Orientation Memory Concentration Test (BOMC), was developed by Katzman et al. (1983). This version consists of the BDS items on orientation (year, month, and time within the hour), memory (delayed recall of a memory phrase), and concentration (counting backwards and reciting months backwards). The BOMC correlates highly with the MMSE (Fillenbaum, Heyman, Wilkinson, & Haynes, 1987; Thal, Grundman, & Golden, 1986) and with plaque in the temporal, parietal, and frontal cortexes of autopsy patients (Katzman et al., 1983), suggesting good validity. The six-item format makes the test especially attractive in epidemiological studies. Factor analysis (*Zillmer, Fowler, Gutnick, & Becker, 1990) indicates that the factor structure of the BOMC is unidimensional, whereas the MMSE structure reflects two factors: memory attention and verbal comprehension. For that reason, the MMSE, arguably, may be a better tool for screening older adults for dementia.

Short Portable Mental Status Questionnaire (SPMSQ)

The SPMSQ, developed by Eric Pfeiffer (1975), is a 10-item test designed to provide a quick assessment of organic brain deficit in both community-dwelling and institutionalized older adults. The items, most of which were used previously in modified form in the Wechsler Memory Scale and the Mental Status Questionnaire (Kahn et al., 1960), address the patient's orientation and long-term memory. A four-level scoring system was developed to map four levels of intellectual functioning. In addition, the scoring system formally takes into account education and racial influences on test performance. For whites with some high school education, the following criteria were established: 0–2 errors, intact functioning; 3–4 errors, mild (or borderline) intellectual impairment; 5–7 errors, moderate (or definite) intellectual impairment; 8–10 errors, severe intellectual impairment. If the patient has only a grade school education, one additional error is allowed. One less error is allowed if the patient has more than a high school education. One more error is allowed for African American patients at each educational level.

Test reliability and validity were found to be mixed. Test-retest reliability was above 0.80 (Pfeiffer, 1975), and interrater reliability on the items was found to be between 0.62 and 0.87 (Fillenbaum & Smyer, 1981). Investigators in several studies have validated the SPMSQ with nonhospitalized older adults and have found that the SPMSQ was related to a clinical interview diagnosis (Fillenbaum, 1980; Haglund & Schuckit, 1976; Pfeiffer, 1975; Smyer, Hofland, & Jonas, 1979). But in the study by Smyer et al. (1979), little support was found for the test's ability to distinguish among the four levels. In particular, the test does not clearly distinguish between those patients who are mildly impaired and those who are intact or moderately impaired. A three-group classification (not impaired–minimally impaired, moderately impaired, severely impaired) was offered as a compromise. In contrast, Dalton, Pederson, Blom, and Holmes (1987) found that the SPMSQ did not significantly relate to clinical or neuropsychological diagnosis in a group of patients hospitalized on Veterans Administration psychiatry or neurology wards.

Cognitive Capacity Screening Examination (CCSE)

The CCSE (Jacobs, Bernhard, Delgado, & Strain, 1977) is a short (30-item), rapid screening tool designed to detect organic brain dysfunction. Items deal with orientation, serial sevens (counting backwards by seven), verbal short-term memory, abstraction, digit recall, and arithmetic. It also contains an interposed task (remembering a list of words). A cutoff score of 20 is used to define diminished cognitive capacity. In their validation studies, the authors acknowledge that a low score alone "does not substantiate a diagnosis of organic mental syndrome" (p. 43). Other factors, such as mental retardation, low level of intelligence, minimal education, impaired English language skills, and poor hearing can affect the scores. The test does not have an extensive literature on its reliability and validity, but in one study (Foreman, 1987) of 66 older adults admitted to a general medical surgical unit, the CCSE was found to have a correlation of 0.88 with the MMSE and 0.63 with the Short Portable Mental Status Examination.

Benton Dementia Screening Measures (BDSM)

The BDSM, based on the work of Benton and his colleagues (Eslinger, Damasio, Benton, & Van Allen, 1985), is a battery of three tests: visual retention, controlled oral word association, and temporal orientation. It takes 15 minutes to complete and is designed to be an easily administered neuropsychological screening instrument to detect abnormal mental decline in older adults. The tests included in the battery were identified empirically as providing the most accurate categorization of probably demented patients and normal control subjects. Using a stepwise linear discriminant function analysis, the three tests were found to classify correctly 85% of the demented and normal patients. Among the rest of the patients, 8.5% could not be classified and 6.5% were misclassified. In a cross-validation study, 4.5% could not be classified and 6.5% were misclassified. Fully 87% of the dementia cases and 91% of the normal subjects were classified correctly. Harper, Chacko, Kotik-Harper, and Kirby (1992) used the following clinically applied cutoff scores: 24 words on the controlled word association task (out of a maximum of 60), less than 4 correct on the visual retention task (the number correct ranged from 0 to 10), and more than 3 errors on the temporal orientation section (perfect score = 0; up to 113 errors possible). They found that the sensitivity of the BDSM in detecting mild and moderate dementia was 88%, and its specificity was 57%. In their sample, the BDSM was more sensitive but less specific than the MMSE.

Tests of Severe Impairment

Several tests that minimize patients' use of language skills have been developed to assess cognitive changes in severely impaired older adults who have lost their verbal capacity. Three of these are the Severe Impairment Battery (Saxton, McGoingle-Gibson, Swihart, Miller, & Boller, 1990), the Modified Ordinal Scales of Psychological Development (Auer, Sclan, Yaffee, & Reisberg, 1994), and the Test of Severe Impairment (TSI; *Albert & Cohen, 1992). This makes these tests, perhaps, most useful in following up on patients in the later stages of dementia. The Test of Severe Impairment (*Albert & Cohen, 1992) takes about 10 minutes to administer and gives scores ranging from 0–24. It consists of six subsections: well-learned motor performance, language comprehension, language production, immediate and delayed memory, general knowledge, and conceptualization. The TSI correlates highly with the MMSE ($r = 0.83, p < 0.001$), providing preliminary evidence for the TSI's construct validity. Test-retest correlations of the TSI's subscales ranged from 0.74 to 0.97 ($p < 0.001$), and the internal consistency of the scale is robust ($\alpha = 0.91$). Factor analysis of the TSI items resulted in three factors with eigenvalues greater than 2.8: factor 1 relates to memory function; factor 2 relates to verbal function; and factor 3 relates to manipulation and identification of body parts.

Syndrome Kurztest (SKT) Neuropsychological Test Battery

Developed in Germany (Erzigkeit, 1989), the Syndrome Kurztest (SKT) is designed to evaluate memory and attention function in older adult patients with mild to moderately severe dementia (*Overall & Schaltenbrand, 1992). The SKT is offered as an instrument that can be used in the evaluation of treatment effects in dementia research. The test takes about 15 minutes to administer and consists of nine subtests. The subtests rely on test materials that consist of stimulus boards, blocks, and cards. Five parallel forms of the test have been developed to facilitate repeated measurements. The subtests are: (1) naming objects (12 pictures presented on a stimulus board); (2) immediate recall (the stimulus board is turned over and the patient is asked to recall the objects from the previous subtest); (3) naming numerals; (4) arranging blocks (numbered blocks are arranged by numerical magnitude); (5) replacing blocks (replacing the numbered blocks into corresponding numbered circles on the stimulus board); (6) counting symbols; (7) reversal naming (cards are presented with two letters, e.g., A B, presented in random sequence and the patient is asked to say B for A and A for B); (8) delayed recall (of the objects in the naming objects subtest presented earlier); and (9) recognition memory (pictures of 36 objects, including the 12 naming objects, are presented and the patient is asked to identify those seen before). Patients are given a maximum of 60 seconds to complete each subtest. The test administrator, rather than following a strict administration protocol, is instructed to interact with the patient, reminding the patient of forgotten instructions, and prompting the patient to respond as quickly as possible. The scores are the number of seconds it took to complete the task or, in the case of memory items, the number of stimuli *not* recalled or recognized. Factor analysis indicates a two-factor solution, with the three memory tasks projecting on one factor and the timed tests projecting on the second factor. Standardized informative scores have been defined for heterogeneous dementia populations (see *Overall & Schaltenbrand, 1992). The test awaits additional validation work using the English language version.

Clock Test

The clock test was originally used by neurologists to examine temporoparietal function (Critchley, 1953). Variants of the clock test have been used recently in screening for cognitive impairment in patients with Alzheimer's disease (e.g., Shulman et al., 1986; Sunderland et al., 1989; *Tuokko, Hadjistavropoulos, Miller, & Beattie, 1992; Wolf-Klein, Silverstone, Levy, & Brod, 1989). In this simple test, patients are given a blank white sheet of paper with instructions to draw a clock and indicate a specific time (e.g., 11:10, 2:45). Judges, using several defined scoring protocols, score the adequacy of the rendition. The task, while requiring the patient to attend to an oral command, remember a clock, and exercise higher order executive functions, hinges more on the visuospatial skills necessary to draw a clock. As such, the clock test can offer information in addition to that provided by purely verbal memory tasks. Correlations reported between scores on the clock test and other measures of dementia, such as the

MMSE or Global Deterioration Scale, while significant, are in the 0.50 range (e.g., Mendez, Ala, & Underwood, 1992; Sunderland et al., 1989). This finding suggests that the clock test is complementary to verbal and memory-based tasks, not redundant. Several scoring systems have been developed, including those based on an overall rating of how well the drawing represents a clock (Sunderland et al., 1989); others require a detailed scoring based on multiple criteria that include these: Is there a totally closed figure without gaps? Are the symbols ordered in a clockwise direction? Are the hands of the clock within the closed figure? (Mendez et al., 1992). To help distinguish deficits on the test due to difficulties in conceptualizing time from constructional apraxia, *Tuokko et al. (1992) suggest adding a clock-setting and a clock-reading task to the clock-drawing test. Both good interrater reliability on the scoring systems and good test-retest reliability for the scores have been reported (e.g., Mendez et al., 1992; Sunderland et al., 1989). Several studies with community-based older adults and institutionalized residents report significant differences in the clock test scores between normal older adults and patients with Alzheimer's disease (Mendez et al., 1992; Sunderland et al., 1989; *Tuokko et al., 1992). The test's sensitivity as a screening tool has been found to be in the 85%–92% range, and its specificity has been found to be in the 86%–93% range (*Tuokko et al., 1992; Wolf-Klein et al., 1989). Even so, these studies caution against using the clock drawing test to replace existing screening tools that are more cognitively based, especially until more validation work has been done.

Cognitive Performance Scale from the Minimum Data Set

A recent approach uses items from the Minimum Data Set (MDS) to develop an MDS Cognitive Performance Scale (CPS) screen for dementia in nursing home residents (*Hartmaier et al., 1995). The MDS is an assessment of nursing home care that requires clinical professionals, such as nurses and social workers, to observe residents directly and assess their performance as well as review medical record data. The resulting MDS assessments are part of the resident's medical record and are performed on admission, every 3 months after admission, and whenever there is any significant change in the resident's status. The MDS has several items that are relevant to cognition and function. The CPS is defined by five MDS cognitive items: comatose status, short-term memory, ability to make decisions, making oneself understood, and eating. These items are combined into a single, hierarchical seven-point rating scale that ranges from 0 (no impairment) to 6 (very severe impairment). The reported correlation between the CPS and the MMSE was −0.863 in a study of 200 nursing home residents from eight facilities (*Hartmaier et al., 1995). Using the MMSE as the ''gold standard,'' the sensitivity and specificity of the CPS were both found to be 0.94.

In a parallel article (Hartmaier, Sloan, Guess, & Koch, 1994), the CPS was validated against the Global Deterioration Scale. The CPS showed poor agreement with the advanced stages of the Global Deterioration Scale. In response, additional items such as long-term memory, recall and orientation, dressing ability, incontinence, and bed mobility were added to develop a new scale, the MDS-COGS. The agreement between the MDS-COGS and Global Deterioration Scale increased to 0.80 (κ). General concerns about the reliability of MDS data collection raise some question about the widespread use of the CPS.

Mini-Mental State Examination (MMSE)

By far the most commonly used and most thoroughly researched screening test is the MMSE. Nearly 90% of primary care physicians who screen for dementia use the MMSE (Somerfeld, Weisman, Ury, Chase, & Folstein, 1991). It is one of the tests recommended by the National Institute of Neurological and Communicative Disorders and Stroke and by the Alzheimer's Disease Centers funded by the National Institute on Aging (Morris, Mohs, Rogers, Fillenbaum, & Heyman, 1988). A testimonial to the respect accorded to MMSE in the field is that in many validation studies, it is the test against which other cognitive assessment tools are compared. The MMSE originally was designed as a short standardized form to separate patients with cognitive disturbance from those without, and to follow the former serially to determine changes in cognitive state. In keeping with its function as a screening tool, the MMSE was not expected to replace a complete diagnostic workup (Folstein, Folstein, & McHugh, 1975) or to provide specific diagnoses.

Since its development, the MMSE not only has gained wide acceptance within clinical circles as a cognitive screening tool but has been adopted as a core measure of cognitive impairment in community-based epidemiological studies, including the National Institute of Mental Health's Epidemiological Catchment Area Program (Robins, Helzer, Croughan, & Ratcliff, 1981). Recent data (*Roccaforte, Burke, Bayer, & Wengel, 1992) suggest the feasibility of a telephone version of the MMSE.

The MMSE Test

The test itself takes 10–15 minutes to administer and consists of 20 separate items, which add up to a maximum score of 30. The questions can be organized heuristically into seven categories: (1) orientation to time, (2) orientation to place, (3) registration of three words, (4) attention and calculation, (5) recall of three words, (6) language, and (7) visual construction. It has been found that, with both nondemented and demented subjects, most errors are made in the recall of three words, calculation (serial sevens—described below—or, alternatively, spelling *world* backwards), visual construction (drawing of two intersecting polygons), and orientation to time (Fillenbaum et al., 1987; Galasko et al., 1990; Magaziner, Bassett, & Hebel, 1987).

Since the test was originally developed, some accepted variations have appeared in the test items. The MMSE was originally developed for use in a hospital setting, and some of the original orientation questions (e.g., What hospital are we in?) are not applicable to community settings. In those cases substitute questions are asked, such as What floor are we on? What is the address (name) of the building we are in? (Robins et al., 1981). The choice of words for tasks on the registration and recall of three words is left to the administrator, but a convention has evolved to use the words *apple*, *penny*, and *table* ever since the MMSE was included in the Diagnostic Interview Schedule used in the Epidemiologic Catchment Area Study. In the original MMSE, a serial sevens task was used that asked the patient to subtract sevens successively from 100 (stopping after five iterations). A substitute task, spelling the word *world* backwards, has emerged. This substitution is frequently reported, but caution should be exercised when using it. Having patients spell *world* backwards has produced higher scores than the serial sevens task in several studies (e.g., Ganguli et al., 1990). Further, Holzer et al. (1984) reported a correlation of only 0.37 between the serial sevens and the score on the spelling backwards task.

Scoring the MMSE

The MMSE score is the total number of correct answers. Since Anthony, LaResche, Niaz, von Korff, and Folstein published their article in 1982, a score of 23 or lower has defined cognitive impairment. This score was chosen because it optimized the sensitivity of the test while still preserving moderate to high specificity. Several studies have tried to change the cutoff scores, but as often happens with diagnostic tests, an increase in sensitivity results in a corresponding decrease in specificity and vice versa (e.g., Anthony et al., 1982; Galasko et al., 1990). Alternative scoring schemes (e.g., George, Landerman, Blazer, & Anthony, 1991) have been developed to distinguish between mild impairment (scores of 18 to 23) and severe impairment (scores of 0 to 17). Recent community-based epidemiological studies have identified population-based norms by age and educational level of the subjects (*Crum, Anthony, Bassett, & Folstein, 1993). No meaningful gender differences in the MMSE have been found (Tombaugh & McIntyre, 1992).

Reliability of the MMSE

Considerable work has been published on the reliability and validity of the MMSE with a variety of populations, including demented and cognitively intact community-based, institutionalized, and hospitalized adults. Test-retest reliability coefficients (see table 1 in Tombaugh & McIntyre, 1992) typically range from 0.80 to 0.90, with a few studies reporting coefficients in the 0.70s. Although this is impressive, the test-retest reliability needs to be interpreted with caution, given the variable delay between administrations, ranging from the same day to 64 days, and the possibility of practice effects. Some studies report on the internal consistency of the MMSE, but the appropriateness of these statistics is open to question, given that the MMSE items appear to be multidimensional (i.e., different items measure different aspects of cognition).

Interrater reliability is found to be above 0.80 (e.g., Anthony, LaResche, Niaz, von Korff, & Folstein, 1982). One area of concern is the visual construction task, in which subjects must draw two intersecting polygons. Several studies (e.g., O'Connor et al., 1989; Olin & Zelinski, 1991) indicate that the lack of explicit scoring criteria for the drawing item may introduce unreliability into the judge's score for that item.

Validity of the MMSE

Review of the literature indicates considerable evidence that the MMSE has convergent validity both with other cognitive tests and with functional measures. The correlations between the MMSE and other screening tests typically fall into the 0.7–0.9 range (Tombaugh & McIntyre, 1992). Comparisons have been made with other major instruments, including the SPMSQ (Foreman, 1987), the Blessed Information Memory Concentration Test (Fillenbaum et al., 1987; Lomeo, 1992; Salmon, Thal, Butters, & Heindel, 1990; Thal et al., 1986), and the CCSE (Lomeo, 1992).

In addition to being highly correlated with cognitive screening tests, the MMSE correlates with other measures of cognitive performance, such as the Wechsler Adult Intelligence Verbal and Performance Scales (Farber, Schmidt, & Logue, 1988; Folstein et al., 1975; Mitrushina & Satz, 1991) and the Wechsler Memory Scale (Giordani et al., 1990). The MMSE also correlates with a number of other cognitive assessment instruments such as the Alzheimer's Disease Assessment Scale Cognitive Score (Zec et al., 1992), the Sandoz Clinical Assessment (Lomeo, 1992), and the Dementia Rating Scale (Bobholz & Brandt, 1993; Salmon et al., 1990).

Several studies show a relationship between the MMSE score and functional measures. Correlations in the moderate to strong range ($r = 0.4$ to 0.7) have been reported between the MMSE and measures of activities of daily living (ADLs), instrumental activities of daily living (IADLs), and the Blessed Dementia Rating Scale in a series of studies (Tombaugh & McIntyre, 1992). In community-based samples, a pattern emerges showing that the MMSE is more highly correlated with measures of IADLs than measures of ADLs (Bassett & Folstein, 1991;

Mahurin, DeBettignies, & Pirozzolo, 1991). This seems reasonable, since it would be expected that instrumental activities of daily living are more dependent on cognitive function than activities of daily living, which measure motor health and mobility more than cognition. Alternatively, the variability of IADL scores may be much greater than ADL scores in the community samples and so less likely to lead to an attenuated correlation coefficient due to a restriction in the range of scores.

Additional evidence for convergent construct validity can be found in the significant relationship between MMSE scores and urinary incontinence (Ouslander, Zarit, Orr, & Muira, 1990), mortality (Uhlmann, Larson, & Buchner, 1987), and abnormal behavior (Cooper, Mungas, & Wieler, 1990). The MMSE has been found to be related to several physiological measures, such as abnormalities detected by CT scans (Colohan, O'Callaghan, Larkin, & Waddington, 1989), cerebral ventricular size (Pearlson & Tune, 1986), and perfusion deficits detected by SPECT scans (DeKosky, Shih, Schmitt, Coupal, & Kirkpatrick, 1990).

This is impressive, but a limitation of this literature is the relative absence of studies that report discriminant validity for the MMSE measure. Discriminant validity (Campbell & Fiske, 1959) reflects the expectation that a test will be more highly related to other tests measuring the same construct (e.g., the MMSE should be highly related to other tests of cognitive function) than to other tests that measure conceptually different variables (e.g., the MMSE should not be highly related to personality measures).

Sensitivity and Specificity of the MMSE

Clinically, and from the standpoint of research, the validity of the MMSE hinges on its ability to screen those with dementia efficiently. Tombaugh and McIntyre (1992) report 25 studies that have examined the sensitivity and specificity of the MMSE with a variety of patient populations. In approximately three fourths of the studies, a sensitivity of 85% or better was found with demented patients. In nearly all of these studies the "gold standard" used to determine whether, in fact, the patient had a dementia was the criteria set forth by the National Institute of Neurological and Communicative Disorders and Stroke and the Alzheimer's Disease and Related Disorders Association (NINCDS-ADRDA; Morris, Mohs, Fillenbaum, & Heyman, 1988) and the *Diagnostic and Statistical Manual for Mental Disorders (DSM-III;* American Psychiatric Association, 1987).

The sensitivity of the test can be seen to decrease as the level of cognitive impairment decreases. In five studies, when the mean MMSE score in the demented group was greater than 20 the sensitivities dropped to the 21% to 54% range. In other words, the milder the dementia, the less likely the MMSE is to identify the patient as cognitively impaired. Three of those five studies were with neurological and psychiatric patients. The MMSE, because of its reliance on verbal items, may be insensitive to functional losses due to damage to the right hemisphere; such damage is better reflected in items that measure visuospatial or constructional praxis (Nelson, Fogel, & Faust, 1986; Schwamm, Van Dyke, Kierman, Merrin, & Mueller, 1987; *Zillmer et al., 1990). Consequently, the MMSE may not be equally sensitive in detecting cognitive impairment across the range of neurologically compromised patients, thus generating an unacceptable rate of false negatives for this patient population.

The sensitivity of the test also decreases when it is used to screen patients in the community, relative to its screening of patients in hospital or clinic settings. It is unclear whether this reflects a potential confounding of testing sites (*Ward et al., 1990) or whether samples recruited from hospital or clinic settings tend to have higher base levels of cognitive impairment. As summarized in Tombaugh and McIntyre (1992), most reported specificities are in the 85% to 100% range. Of the studies reviewed, only four reported specificities of less than 80%.

Concerns and Caveats Regarding the MMSE

The MMSE has built up a strong track record as a screening tool for dementia. However, several cautions and several limitations of the MMSE need to be noted, which also apply to other cognitive screening tests. It is important to keep in mind what the MMSE, as a screening tool, is designed to do. It should quickly and efficiently identify for further diagnostic workup individuals who are suspected of having dementia. It is not designed to be a diagnostic tool.

Mild Dementia.   The literature suggests that the validity of the MMSE is affected by the severity of the dementia. As reviewed above, using a cutoff point between 23 and 24, the sensitivity of the MMSE does appear to drop off when it is used to screen for mild cognitive impairments. The reported specificities tend to be more robust, so the main problem is falsely screening out people with mild cognitive impairments, rather than falsely screening in normal older adults. This problem is compounded, as discussed below, in testing individuals who are more educated, because of the potential effect education may have in masking early cognitive impairments.

Severe Impairment.   At the other extreme, the MMSE has been criticized as not being able to discriminate cognitive changes in patients with severe cognitive impairment (*Albert & Cohen, 1992; Auer et al., 1994). Scores on tests, such as the MMSE, that rely on the patient's verbal skills "bottom out" in the later stages of dementia when the patient's verbal capacity is lost (i.e., a "floor" effect). Auer et al. (1994) estimate that 500,000 demented patients are untestable with the MMSE because their score is near or at zero. This limitation is not a relevant criticism of the MMSE as a screening tool used to identify patients in earlier stages of cognitive impairment. However, since a second stated purpose of the MMSE was to chart cognitive changes in patients with cognitive impairment (Folstein et al., 1975), this limitation becomes a concern when patients in the later stages of dementia are being tracked (e.g., patients at stages 6 and 7 of the Global Deterioration Scale). A consensus seems to be emerging that more function-based measures of cognitive impairment may be better suited to tracking the progression of dementia in the latter stages (e.g., Auer et al., 1994; Galasko, Corey-Bloom, & Thal, 1991).

Several longitudinal studies indicate that the MMSE is a useful tool in serially documenting changes in patients who do *not* have severe cognitive dysfunction (e.g., Folstein et al., 1975; O'Connor, Pollitt, & Hyde, 1991; Salmon et al., 1990; van Belle, Uhlmann, Hughes, & Larson, 1990). Recent studies (e.g., Corey-Bloom, Galasko, Hofstetter, Jackson, & Thal, 1993; Salmon et al., 1990; Teri, Hughes, & Larson, 1990) indicate that annual drops of 2 to 3 points can be expected in patients newly diagnosed with Alzheimer's disease, and the average rate of decline becoming more rapid as the disease progresses (*Teri, McCurry, Edland, Kukull, & Larson, 1995). The danger that scores will be inflated over time because of practice effects associated with frequent administration should not be discounted.

Differential Age Validity.   Many studies of community-based older adults find that MMSE scores decline as the age of the patient increases (e.g., *Crum et al., 1993; Magaziner et al., 1987). This creates the danger of increased false positive results among nondemented older adults. The items that seem to be most affected by age are repeating "no ifs ands or buts," and the recall of three words (Bleeker, Bolla-Wilson, Kawas, & Agnew, 1988).

Interpreting age as a risk factor for lower MMSE scores is difficult because of cohort differences in educational level and because chronic illness and dementia are more prevalent among older adults (e.g., Bachman et al., 1993; Schoenberg et al., 1987). Age-related declines in MMSE scores do not appear to be solely an artifact of educational level, since the age effect persists after controlling for patients' educational level (Magaziner et al., 1987). Bleeker et al. (1988) found that the MMSE total score, while correlated with age, was not correlated with educational level.

Attributing MMSE declines among older age groups simply to aging is somewhat equivocal. Several studies have specifically focused on subject samples that were not diagnosed as having cognitive impairments (e.g., Bleeker et al., 1988), yet age-related declines remained. Further complicating the picture, more recent studies of the "old old" indicate age-related neurobehavioral changes occurring even in the subgroups that are aging most successfully (Nichols et al., 1994). On the other hand, several recent studies question whether there is a purely chronological age effect on cognitive screening tests, independent of pathology.

*Heeren, Lagaay, von Beck, Rooymans, and Hijman (1990), reporting on a survey of Dutch adults over 85 years of age, found no evidence of a decline in MMSE scores with age; the median score was 28. Further, in a study of older adults with mild Alzheimer's disease and healthy controls (Rubin et al., 1992), age was found to affect performance on psychometric tests (e.g., Trailmaking A, Boston Naming Test) but age per se did not affect performance on brief clinical screening instruments, including the Blessed Dementia Scale and the SPMSQ. In response, separate age-based norms have been proposed for different age groups by several researchers (e.g., Bleeker et al., 1988).

Differential Education Validity.   While some research fails to find a relationship between educational level and MMSE scores (e.g., Bleeker et al., 1988; *Heeren et al., 1990), a preponderance of studies indicate that MMSE scores are positively related to the educational level of demented and cognitively intact older adults. Further evidence indicates that the variability of MMSE scores increases among individuals with lower educational levels (*Crum et al., 1993). Weiss, Reed, Klingman, and Abyad (1995) found that the MMSE score was correlated with the individual's reading level in addition to educational level. Several studies found that educational level predicts MMSE scores independently of other social factors (Uhlmann & Larson, 1991) and age (e.g., *Crum et al., 1993). This creates a bias toward overestimation of cognitive impairment among individuals with an eighth grade education or less. But there is an opposite bias toward underestimating cognitive impairment (i.e., there is an increased rate of false negatives) among highly educated patients. The presence of this bias has led some (Tombaugh & McIntyre, 1992) to recommend not using the MMSE with individuals who have less than an eighth grade education or to interpret the scores using education-based and age-based reference standards. On the basis of their own work, Uhlmann and Larson (1991), for example, propose cutoff scores of 24 for college-educated patients, 23 for patients who attended high school, and 21 for patients who did not attend high school. *Crum et al. (1993) have published reference standards based on age and educational level for MMSE scores collected in the community-based Epidemiologic Catchment Area survey.

There is a temptation to explain education-based differences in MMSE scores as an artifact of poor test-taking skills among individuals with less education. In a study of community-based older adults, Jorm, Scott, Henderson, and Kay (1988) found no evidence that the MMSE was biased against individuals with low educational levels. In addition, the MMSE items did not have a differential reliability among individuals of different educational levels. However, the role of education as an etiologic factor in cognitive impairment should not be ignored (Berkman, 1986). Low educational levels could contribute to dementia because of the association between low educational levels and pathological disease (*Crum et al., 1993; Tombaugh & McIntyre, 1992) or other potential risk factors for dementia such as occupational hazards, inadequate use of health care, and mal-adaptive lifestyles (Farmer, Kittner, Rae, Barko, & Regier, 1995; Friedland, 1993). Older adults with low levels of education may, in fact, have had a lifelong history of mild cognitive impairment.

A high level of education may provide a reserve capacity which shields the emergence of the clinical manifestation of dementia or which acts as a buffer against cognitive impairment. In support of this, Farmer et al. (1995), reporting from the Epidemiological Catchment Area Study, indicate that lower educational level was a significant predictor of a cognitive decline over a 1-year period among older (65+) and younger (18–64) subjects who had an MMSE score higher than 23. In a recent study using the Swedish Adoption/Twin Study of Aging data set, Pedersen, Reynold, and Gatz (1996) argue that the correlation between the MMSE score and educational level is due to the fact that both are related to heritable cognitive ability. It is inherited intelligence, presumably indicating greater cerebral capacity—not education per se—that serves as a protective factor.

Using reference-based standards still leaves open the major issue of what defines normal or impaired performance for each educational level and age group. Currently, there are no universally accepted alternative cutoff scores for different ages or educational levels. In adopting age- or education-based norms for the interpretation of MMSE scores, clinicians need to consider the goals of the screening and the relative costs incurred by false negatives and false positives in the assessment of cognitive impairment. Adjusting MMSE scores for patients' age or educational level may be problematic because it is hard to know whether age and education are determinants of cognitive impairment or proxies for under-lying pathology.

Differential Ethnic Validity.   Data from the Epidemiologic Catchment Area Study indicate that race and ethnicity, like education, also affect the distribution of MMSE scores (George et al., 1991). Interpretation of this pattern is equivocal, given the presence of linguistic artifacts, the confounding of education and socioeconomic factors with race and ethnicity, and the higher prevalence of severe dementia among African Americans compared with Hispanics or whites (George et al., 1991). *Murden, McRae, Kaner, and Buckman (1991), in a study of patients from urban primary care geriatrics clinics, found lower MMSE scores among patients with an eighth grade education or less, compared with better educated patients. No racial differences were found among patients with similar educational levels. Recent work has focused on developing cross culturally sensi-tive assessment instruments, which hold the promise of minimizing ethnic, cul-tural, and educational biases, e.g., the Cross-Cultural Cognitive Examination (*Glosser et al., 1993).

Additional Limitations.   A common finding in the cognitive literature is dimin-ished cognitive performance in depressed individuals, although performance on verbal tasks seems to be more immune to the negative effects of lowered affect (Lyness, Eaton, & Schneider, 1994). Clinically speaking, depression is often considered a complicating factor in cognitive assessment because it mimics functional impairments associated with dementias. Research (e.g., Folstein et al., 1975; Harper, Chacko, Kotik-Harper, & Kirby, 1992) indicates that although MMSE scores are lower in depressed patients, the test does distinguish among depressed patients, demented patients, and demented patients with depression.

Sensory deficits, especially hearing impairments, have also been found to lower MMSE scores and affect the specificity of the MMSE (Fiedler & Klingbeil, 1990). It is unclear whether all of the decline in MMSE scores in hearing-impaired individuals can be attributed solely to the sensory loss (Uhlmann, Teri, Rees, Mozlowski, & Larson, 1989).

The testing site may introduce another bias into the MMSE that affects its validity. *Ward et al. (1990) administered the MMSE to 116 geriatric patients at a clinic and in their residences, counterbalancing the order of administration. Scores were 1.5 points higher when subjects were tested in their residences as compared with the clinic. One quarter of the patients had differences of 5 points or more, and 76% achieved better scores when tested in their residence. Factors such as fatigue or anxiety may be present in a clinical setting and may exert a negative influence on performance.

Identifying other sources of method variance in the test scores, such as the test administrator's skill or previous experience, is an important area for future inquiry.

Differential Diagnosis of Dementia.   Starting with Folstein et al. (1975), the use of the MMSE as a diagnostic tool has been discouraged. Because MMSE scores are sensitive to a variety of pathological conditions, the MMSE cannot support a specific categorical diagnosis. Further, as discussed above, the relative insensitivity of the MMSE to right hemispheric damage and subcortical lesions limits its use as a definitive diagnostic tool.

Current Trends with the MMSE

Shortening the Test.   Several studies have tried to identify, within the MMSE, those items that best discriminate between cognitively impaired and normally functioning patients. Using regression techniques, *Brackhus, Laake, and Engedal (1992) identified a 12-item subscale and *Wells et al. (1992) identified a 9-item subscale from the 20 MMSE items. These subscales were found to correlate highly with the MMSE total score and to have sensitivities and specificities similar to the MMSE. Despite the virtues of parsimony, though, the wisdom of shortening the MMSE—which, as its name indicates, is already "mini" (taking about 10 minutes to complete)—is questionable. A major caution in interpreting these two studies is that the subjects were given the entire MMSE, and then items were extrapolated. Administration of solely the 12-item version may yield different results. At the very least, extensive cross-validation work is necessary to make sure that the items selected are equally powerful in diverse patient groups.

Combining Tests. In response to some of the concerns about the MMSE's lower sensitivity with mild dementias and its failure to distinguish among different types of dementia, some authors have suggested including other instruments along with the MMSE. For example, the Alzheimer's Disease Centers—funded by the National Institute of Aging (NIA)—use the Blessed Information Orientation and Concentration Test along with the MMSE. Ideally, added items can provide a more comprehensive instrument that would sample patients' cognitive functioning more broadly and should result in greater sensitivity and specificity across a wider range of patients, including those with mild dementias. Considerable debate revolves around whether to compute a single summary score from the tests or to derive multidimensional scales that differentially weight the items from the tests (*Weiler et al., 1994).

A variant of this approach is to change the MMSE slightly and include additional items that measure different areas of cognition, such as visuospatial functioning. While at first this seems attractive, considerable problems emerge in scoring the test and in comparing the scores in the absence of any normative information or reference standards.

Since the MMSE is so highly correlated with many other cognitive screening tools and the items of many screening tests overlap (e.g., the orientation questions), the assumption underlying the inclusion of other tests is open to question. In fact, adding a second highly correlated test to the battery may, in effect, increase the test's reliability only by increasing the length of the test. Increasing the length of the screening test, however, puts an added burden on the patient and the test administrator and risks reducing patients' compliance. It is questionable whether the increased length and time of administration are appropriate for a screening test, especially since gains in sensitivity or specificity are marginal. More appropriate rationales for combining the MMSE with other cognitive and functional measures are to develop a more comprehensive research tool and to facilitate long-term tracking of patients.

RECOMMENDATIONS

In the past 25 years there has been considerable work in developing brief screening tools to identify individuals with suspected dementia. As our review indicates, many of these screening tools are respectable and have at least limited documentation of their reliability and validity. The MMSE, however, emerges as the most desirable screening tool, not only because of its robust track record of reliability and validity, but also by virtue of its wide use and acceptance. It is the de facto standard against which the other mental screening tools are validated. It is specifically included in many assessment batteries and recommendations. It is short, easily administered, and easily scored. From a practical standpoint, using the recommended cutoff score of 23–24, the MMSE has acceptable sensitivity and specificity to screen individuals effectively for additional diagnostic cognitive workup without generating excessive false positive results. Caution should be exercised in testing for mild dementias, working with very old adults or individuals with less than a ninth-grade education, testing different ethnic groups, or administering the screen to individuals with sensory impairments. Thought needs to be given to whether adjusting the MMSE for patients' age or educational level using norms is desirable. To expect the MMSE to make a definitive diagnosis, distinguish among different types of cognitive impairment, or chart the progress of dementia across its full range is inappropriate and should be avoided. Above all, clinicians and researchers alike must remember what the MMSE is—a screening test.

ANNOTATED BIBLIOGRAPHY

Mini-Mental State Examination (MMSE)

Development and Methods

Brackhus A, Laake K, & Engedal K. (1992). The Mini-Mental State Examination: Identifying the most efficient variables for detecting cognitive impairment in the elderly. *J Am Geriatr Soc*, 40, 1139–1145.
Design.   A retrospective analysis was done to evaluate the utility of individual items on the MMSE for predicting cognitive impairment. A Norwegian translation of the MMSE was utilized. Modifications included substituting "country" for "state" and "part of the country" for "county" and omitting serial sevens. The median total MMSE score was 22/30. Factor analyses and multiple logistic regression were performed to select the optimal subset of variables for predicting cognitive impairment. A 12-item version was identified which included orientation (year, month, date, day of week, county, postal code), spelling *world* backwards, memory recall, repetition, three-stage command, sentence writing, and copying. Scoring for items that could receive a score of more than one point was changed to a binomial system.
Sample.   Norwegian subjects ($n = 850$) included geriatric inpatients, independent community dwellers, and community dwellers requiring supervision. The sample were predominantly women (74%), with a mean age of 82 years (range: 54–99).
Summary.   The revised 12-item exam yielded a sensitivity of 98% and specificity of 91% when a cutoff point between 9 and 10 was utilized. Comparative analysis of the full

MMSE and the 12-item version with diagnosis by psychogeriatricians yielded similar results. The authors conclude that the shortened version is equally effective.

Discussion.   The utilization of a Norwegian sample and changes in individual items to accommodate this population may affect generalizability to an American population. Caution is also advised, since the entire MMSE was administered and then items were extrapolated. Administration of solely the 12-item version may yield different results. The 12-item version is included in an appendix to the article.

Crum RM, Anthony JC, Bassett SS, & Folstein MF. (1993). Population based norms for the Mini Mental State Examination by age and educational level. *JAMA, 269,* 2386–2391.

Design.   The distribution of the MMSE scores by age and educational level was determined on the basis of an assessment of individuals surveyed in the National Institute of Mental Health's Epidemiologic Catchment Area Program. Two substitutions were made on the MMSE items. First, subjects were asked to do serial sevens and to spell *world* backwards. Also, instead of being asked for their county of residence, subjects were asked for the names of two main streets nearby.

Sample.   The survey was conducted from 1980 to 1984 in five communities: New Haven, CT; Baltimore, MD; St. Louis, MO; Durham, NC; and Los Angeles, CA. It involved adults selected by probability sampling within census tracts and households. The MMSE was included as part of the diagnostic interview schedule administered to an average of 76% of the initially selected subjects ($n = 18,571$).

Summary.   Results indicated a decline in total MMSE score with age and with educational level. Further, the variability of scores increased with age and was greater for lower educational levels compared with higher levels. For individuals with a minimum of 9 years of education, the median MMSE score was 29, compared with 26 for those with 5–8 years of schooling and 22 for those with 0–4 years of schooling.

Discussion.   The authors propose these average scores as normative reference values for clinicians and researchers, but a cautionary note should be sounded. The inability of large epidemiologic surveys such as this to control for a host of comorbidities and other socioeconomic factors that potentially have an impact on cognitive status is a concern. The increased variability in test scores seen in subjects with lower educational levels may in fact reflect the known increased prevalence of disease associated with lower educational level and lower socioeconomic status. The study highlights the need for increasing research aimed at defining more useful clinical cutoff values for the MMSE and on investigating the relationships between MMSE scores and other social and demographic characteristics.

Heeren TJ, Lagaay AM, von Beck WCA, Rooymans HGM, & Hijman W. (1990). Reference values for the Mini Mental State Examination (MMSE) in octo- and nonagenarians. *J Am Geriatr Soc, 38,* 1093–1096.

Design.   A population study of the very old (85+) adult residents of Leiden, Netherlands ($n = 1,258$), which included the MMSE.

Sample.   Of the 1,258 subjects selected, 222 died before the interview took place. Subjects were excluded if they had a neurological disorder as assessed by an internist or a psychiatric disorder as assessed by a psychiatrist. Patients who were illiterate or who had less than a fourth grade education were also excluded. A total of 532 individuals were included in the analysis.

Summary.   While significant differences in the mean MMSE were found among the age groups, the median scores were identical (28), and the lowest quartile cutoff was nearly the same: 26 for the 85–89 age group and 25 for the 90–94 and the 95+ age groups. Significant age differences were found on only one item (copying polygons). Ten percent of the patients used psychoactive medicines; 81%, a benzodiazepine; 15%, a neuroleptic; and 4%, an antidepressant. No differences in the MMSE scores were found between users and nonusers of psychoactive drugs. Individuals reporting vision or hearing defects were older, and their MMSE median score and lowest quartile cutoff were one point lower than those of the other subjects. The majority of the subjects had 6 to 7 years of education, and there was no evidence of lower MMSE scores among individuals who had less education.

Discussion.   The study provides little indication of a "pure" age-based decline in the MMSE scores, apart from pathology, and suggests the potential use of the MMSE with very old patients (95+ years old).

Murden RA, McRae TD, Kaner S, & Buckman ME. (1991). Mini-Mental State Exam scores vary with education in blacks and whites. *J Am Geriatr Soc, 39,* **149–155.**
Design.   The impact of both education and race on MMSE scores was determined by testing African American and white older adult subjects. African American subjects also were followed longitudinally and retested a minimum of 6 months after the initial evaluation. None of the white subjects was retested. A diagnosis of dementia was based on the presence of all of the following criteria: history of decline in memory and cognition, absence of delirium, MMSE score of 23 or less, and presence of dementia in the opinion of the examiner. The examiners consisted of a geriatrician and a geriatrics-trained physician's assistant.

Sample.   Of 358 individuals 60 years and older screened with the MMSE over a 4-year period, 248 nondemented subjects were identified and constituted the sample for the study. African American subjects ($n = 148$) were recruited from Kings County Hospital in New York, and 100 white subjects were recruited from Bellevue Hospital in New York. Most (76%) of the subjects were female.

Summary.   In both African American and white subjects with at least a ninth grade education, there was a slight but significant decline in MMSE scores with age. No such correlation was demonstrated with patients who had an eighth grade education or less, regardless of race. The mean total MMSE scores were significantly better in the more highly educated group among both African Americans and whites.

Discussion.   An analysis of differences on the individual items indicated differences on only three items, and for two of them only among less educated subjects.

Roccaforte W, Burke W, Bayer B, & Wengel S. (1992). Validation of a telephone version of the Mini-Mental State Examination. *J Am Geriatr Soc, 40,* **697–702.**
Design.   Prospective correlative analysis of a 22-item telephone-administered version of the MMSE and the traditional 30-item MMSE. The study objective was to evaluate the efficacy of a telephone version of the MMSE. The telephone version did *not* include the following: floor of building, following a three-stage command, sentence reading and

follow-through, sentence writing, or copying. Naming was limited to identifying "the thing that you are speaking into as you talk to me." Subjects were contacted at home for the telephone version; the in-person version was conducted at an outpatient geriatric assessment clinic.

Sample. The sample were predominantly women (76%) and white, with a mean age of 79 years, and exhibited a wide range of medical and cognitive problems. Out of 175 potential subjects, 100 completed both assessments.

Summary. Total scores on the two versions (clinic mean = 21.4; home mean = 14.6) were highly correlated for the total sample ($r = 0.85$, $p < 0.0001$). Individual item analysis revealed differences between the two versions on orientation (higher scores by telephone, $p < 0.05$), phrase repetition (lower scores by telephone, $p < 0.05$) and registration of "penny" (lower scores by telephone, $p < 0.05$). Subjects who reported problems with their hearing acuity had lower scores on the telephone version. Sensitivity and specificity were similar for both versions relative to a brief neuropsychiatric screening test (67% and 100% by telephone; 68% and 100% in clinic).

Discussion. The 22-item telephone MMSE may serve as a useful screening instrument. Caution is advised, given the significant discrepancies on multiple individual items and the suggestion that diminished hearing or in-home availability of cues may play a role. The modified version is not appropriate for diagnostic purposes, owing to the omission of multiple items from the standard MMSE.

Ward HW, Ramsdell JW, Jackson E, Revall M, Swart JA, & Rockwell E. (1990). Cognitive function testing in comprehensive geriatric assessment: A comparison of cognitive test performance in residential and clinic settings. *J Am Geriatr Soc,* **38, 1088–1092.**

Design. Scores of MMSEs administered in a clinic or at home were compared to determine the impact of testing site on MMSE scores. The MMSE was administered by a psychiatrist in the clinic and by a geriatric nurse specialist in the patient's residence. Whether the test was first administered in the clinic or the residence varied among the subjects. Interrater reliability was determined by comparing the mean scores of eight subjects who were interviewed by both the psychiatrist and the nurse practitioner. A difference of 5 points or more on the MMSE was defined as "clinically relevant."

Sample. The subjects for this study consisted of 116 patients sequentially registered for a comprehensive assessment program at the University of California at San Diego.

Summary. Patients' test scores were significantly higher in their residences than in the clinic (mean difference was 1.5); for 25% of the subjects, the difference was 5 points or more. Interestingly, 76% of these patients scored higher in their residence. The mean time between testing in the clinic and residence was 11 days (range 1–76 days). No association was demonstrated between testing time interval and differences in test scores. Further, the order of test sites had no effect on differences in test scores, nor was there any significant difference between the nurse's and the physician's scores. Of the 29 patients who experienced a clinically significant change in test scores between the test sites, 10 had concurrent changes in medication. Four of these patients scored better on the clinic test. Age, gender, living situation, and education were not associated with differences in scores between the sites. Finally, patients whose scores were higher in their residences had higher scores in the following domains: orientation, attention-calculation, language.

Discussion.   This study suggests a significant effect of screening site on the MMSE scores. Clinic-based MMSE scores may underestimate the patient's ability to perform. A difference of 5 points on the MMSE, as noted by the investigators, has significant implications for treatment and diagnosis. Although these authors do not explicitly define the manner in which the test sites were ordered, and although the impact of changes in medication may be underestimated, this study points to the potential of confounding by environmental and pharmacological factors in the assessment of cognitive status using the MMSE.

Weiler PG, Chiriboga DA, & Black SA. (1994). Comparison of mental status tests: Implications for Alzheimer's patients and their caregivers. *J Gerontol*, *49*, S44–S51.
Design.   This study was designed to compare the utility of the Blessed Information Orientation Memory and Concentration Test (IOMC) summary score, the MMSE summary score, and a combined scale score derived from a factor analysis of a combined instrument in predicting patients' functional independence and caregivers' burden and distress. Measures included the IOMC, MMSE, Activities of Daily Living (ADLs), a rating by a nurse practitioner concerning level of care for which the patient was certified, Assistance with Daily Life scale, Caregiver Burden scale, a 13-item Depression subscale from the Symptoms Checklist 90 (SCL-90), and the Anxiety subscale from the SCL-90.
Sample.   Subjects were older adults with a diagnosis of probable dementia of Alzheimer's type ($n = 201$) and their adult children caregivers ($n = 394$). The first sample consisted of community and institutionalized older adults recruited from six counties in northern California. These subjects' average age was 77 years, and 77% of them were women. Among the men, 66% were married, compared with 31% of the women. Most of the subjects (93.3%) were whites of European decent. The sample of caregivers consisted of 245 primary and 149 secondary caregivers. Caregivers had an average age of 47.7 years old; 68% were daughters and 32% were sons of the patient.
Summary.   Factor analysis was performed on the combined IOMC and MMSE items. Five factors were extracted and named: General Cognitive Function, Orientation, Abstract Memory, Item Recall, and Copy Design. It should be noted the last factor, Copy Design, had an eigenvalue of 0.83, and consisted of only a single item, the polygon copying item on the MMSE. Separate hierarchical regression analyses were performed to predict ADL and ratings of level of care using the cognitive scores as predictors. In each analysis, demographic characteristics, health history, and psychological characteristics (e.g., depression) were entered first. Then one of following alternative cognitive scoring approaches was entered as the predictor: summary score of the IOMC, summary score of the MMSE, summary score of the two tests combined (overlapping items removed), unit-based summary scores from the five factor scales derived from the factor analysis (i.e., the five-scale alternative), or scores from the General Cognitive Function and Orientation subscales (i.e., the two-scale alternative). Each of the alternative cognitive scoring approaches significantly predicted ADLs: Change in R^2 after entering the cognitive predictors ranged from 0.40 to 0.46. A slightly higher proportion of variance was accounted for by the five-scale and two-scale alternatives. A parallel pattern was found for the rating of the required level of care, for which change in R^2 after entering the cognitive predictors ranged from 0.20 to 0.23. Among caregivers, anxiety and depression were poorly explained by the cognitive predictors. Only the five-score cognitive alternative significantly predicted assis-

tance provided and perceived burden (change in $R^2 = 0.02$). Of special note was the observation that parents who scored higher on the general cognitive function items received more assistance from their children.

Discussion. The five-factor derived subscale explained slightly more variance than the summary scores, but, as the authors admit, the differences were small. The authors urge the consideration of the multiple dimensions underlying cognitive tests in guiding new research and in adapting cognitive tests for research purposes. It would be desirable to cross-validate the relationship between the cognitive score on the one hand and patients' function and caregivers' outcomes on the other, on a sample different from the one used to generate the factor scores.

Wells J, Keyl P, Chase G, Aboraya A, Folstein M, & Anthony J. (1992). Discriminant validity of a reduced set of Mini-Mental State Examination items for dementia and Alzheimer's disease. *Acta Psychiatry Scand, 86,* **23–31.**

Design. A series of discriminant function analyses were computed to identify the efficacy of a reduced-item MMSE.

Sample. Subjects were obtained from both a subset of a large epidemiological investigation (65 normal controls; 22 with dementia) and a clinical case series from an Alzheimer's Disease Research Center (ADRC; 55 controls and 181 individuals with Alzheimer's disease, AD). Both samples were predominantly white and composed of women. Age ranged from 50 to over 80 years.

Summary. Discriminant function analyses were performed using the MMSE variables, as well as age, race, gender, and education. The model that best distinguished demented subjects from controls was a nine-item discriminant function that included the MMSE variables (time orientation, recall, calculation, figure copying, sentence writing, three-step command, naming), age, and race. The highest-ranked variables were recall, time orientation, calculation, and copying. Sensitivity and specificity for classification in the epidemiologic sample were 91% and 88%, respectively. The ADRC sample findings for this model were 96% sensitivity and 98% specificity for classification of AD versus controls.

Discussion. These findings highlight the value of a subset of MMSE and demographic variables in screening for dementia. These findings should not be viewed as supporting a shortened version of the MMSE, however, since the entire MMSE was administered. It may best be viewed as highlighting important discriminators of dementia that are present in the MMSE in concert with demographic information.

Zillmer EA, Fowler PC, Gutnick HN, & Becker E. (1990). Comparison of two cognitive bedside screening instruments in nursing home residents: A factor analytic study. *J Gerontol, 45,* **P69–P74.**

Design. To examine the factor structure of MMSE and BOMC items for nursing home residents using factor analytic techniques. Within a 4-week period, the subjects received the MMSE and BOMC. Both instruments were administered by the nursing and social work staffs.

Sample. Subjects were 120 older adults from a skilled nursing home providing intermediate long-term care. Ten subjects were excluded because of cognitive and physical impairment. Of the subjects, 77% were women and 99% were white. Their average age was 84.4 years, and their average level of education was 10.2 years.

Summary. The mean MMSE score was 14.4 (*SD* = 10.8), and the mean BOMC score was 20.4 (*SD* = 8.4). The correlation between the MMSE and BOMC was −0.77, $p <$ 0.001. Factor analysis of the combined items from the MMSE and BOMC yielded a two-factor solution accounting for 57% of the variance. The first factor was defined as Memory-Attention, which was characterized by loadings of items from the MMSE and BOMC measuring orientation, memory, attention concentration, and recall. The second factor was Verbal Comprehension, which was defined by loadings from the MMSE items measuring word-finding reading and language.

Discussion. The MMSE, by sampling language and cognitive praxis, is seen as a conceptually different test from the BOMC, which seems to measure only memory-attention. The results suggest that the somewhat longer MMSE may be preferable, since it measures two factors, compared with the one factor measured by the BOMC. Even so, brief mental status examinations should be recognized as measuring limited dimensions of mental processes. Limits to the study include a relatively small and homogeneous sample.

Applications

Pedersen NL, Reynolds CA, & Gatz M. (1996). Source of covariation among Mini-Mental State Examination scores, education, and cognitive abilities. *J Gerontol*, *51B*, P55–P63.

Design. This adoption–twin study examines the relationship between MMSE performance, cognitive ability, and educational level. General cognitive ability was measured by Dureman-Salde battery tests (synonyms, figure logic, block design, and figure identification), which are based on Thurstone's primary mental abilities. Mean score for general cognitive abilities was 101.32 (*SD* = 15.31) for men and 99.27 (*SD* = 14.17) for women. The MMSE incorporated an elaboration of the three-item recall question. Multivariate model-fitting approaches were used to examine genetic and environmental influences on the variation and covariation of MMSE, general cognitive abilities, and education scores.

Sample. Subjects were drawn from same-sex twins from the Swedish Adoption/Twin Study of Aging data set. The subjects were 44 pairs of monozygotic twins reared apart, 66 pairs of monozygotic twins reared together, 91 dizygotic pairs reared apart, and 86 dizygotic pairs reared together. Educational level (66.7% did not extend their education beyond elementary school) and MMSE score distributions (59.3% had scores above 28) were skewed. Only eight subjects were diagnosed as having dementia. They were retained in the sample. In-person data collection was done by trained registered nurses.

Summary. Heritability for the MMSE was 0.32 for men and 0.19 (not significant) for women. Twenty to thirty percent of the variation in MMSE was associated with level of education and cognitive ability. The correlation between education and MMSE performance (0.21 for men and 0.16 for women) was reduced to nearly zero when general cognitive ability was partialed out; this suggests that the relationship between education and MMSE can be attributed to genetic effects for cognitive abilities.

Discussion. Pedersen, Reynolds, and Gatz argue that lower MMSE scores among less educated individuals are not due to test bias or health-endangering lifestyles. It is inherited intelligence, presumably indicating greater cerebral capacity, not education per se, that serves as a protective factor. Limitations of the study include the fact that measurements of education, cognitive ability, and MMSE were not made at the same point in time and that the distributions on the measures were skewed. Questions remain about the generalizability of the results to demented samples and to other populations.

Teri L, McCurry SM, Edland SD, Kukull WA, & Larson EB. (1995). Cognitive decline in Alzheimer's disease: A longitudinal investigation of risk factors for accelerated decline. *J Gerontol, 50A,* **M49–M55.**

Design. A longitudinal design was employed to investigate the relationship between the rate of cognitive decline and demographic, behavioral, and health factors in a community-based sample. Measures included the Mini-Mental Status Exam, the Mattis Dementia Rating Scale, a 21-item checklist of behavior problems, physician-identified health problems, and demographic variables. Data were analyzed using multivariate regression analysis. To avoid floor or ceiling effects, subjects with MMSE less than 5 or greater than 25 were dropped from the analysis ($n = 13$).

Sample. Subjects were recruited from an Alzheimer's Disease Patient Registry maintained by the University of Washington and the Group Health Cooperative in Seattle, Washington. Criteria for inclusion consisted of (1) subjects' meeting the criteria established by the National Institute of Neurologic and Communicative Diseases and the Alzheimer's Disease and Related Disorders Association for probable Alzheimer's disease and (2) subjects' completing two or more cognitive evaluations. A total of 156 subjects met both criteria. Their mean age was 79 years old, and 67% were women. Thirty percent of the subjects had less than a high school education.

Summary. Average rates of annual decline increased as the level of impairment increased. At about an MMSE level of 10, the decline stabilized at a rate of loss of 5 MMSE points per year. For less-educated patients, the stabilization occurred at MMSE level of 9 with an annual loss of 4 points. Higher levels of education lead to a more rapid rate of decline. Age, gender, duration of illness, number of health problems, and number of behavior problems did not significantly predict a decline in MMSE points. Presence of behavioral problems involving agitation was related to more rapid annual decline. A total of 37% of the decline in MMSE points was explained by level of dementia, education, and agitated behavior.

Discussion. There is a heterogeneity of change among individuals with Alzheimer's disease. Contrary to expectations, rates of decline were greater among more educated patients. Results suggest that more educated individuals can escape early detection by screening instruments. For those individuals, clinically observable dysfunction may appear at a later stage of the disease. Education and severity of dementia should be specifically considered in future analyses of cognitive change in Alzheimer's disease. Additional research on the relationship between agitation and the rate of decline is needed.

Other Current Screening Tests

Syndrome Kurztest (SKT) Neuropsychological Test Battery

Overall JE, & Schaltenbrand R. (1992). The SKT Neuropsychological Test Battery. *J Geriatr Psychiatry Neurol,* **5, 220–227.**

Design. This article introduces the Syndrome Kurztest (SKT) Neuropsychological Test Battery to an American audience and reports validation data from previous studies. The

SKT was developed by Dr. Hellmut Erzigkeit in Germany and is widely used in German-speaking countries as an outcome measure with dementia patients.

Sample.   Results from a previously reported Vinpocetine study were presented (n = 582 patients).

Summary.   Cluster analysis yielded one cluster reflecting a predominant memory deficit and a second cluster reflecting predominant deficits in the attentional domain. Test-retest reliability ranged from 0.51 to 0.91, with most in the 0.7–0.8 range. Analysis of covariance of data obtained from the Vinpocetine study were presented ($n = 582$ patients). Differences of 3.2 units on the attentional factor and 1.5 units on the memory factor between the treatment and control groups were significant, $p < 0.0001$.

Discussion.   Although a full SKT profile sheet with norms for demented populations was presented for all subtests, no sensitivities or specificities of the test are reported. The SKT is offered as an instrument for clinical outcome studies; but it holds promise as a screening tool because of its short but controlled format, its demonstrated reliability, and its derivation of T scores for the subscales for use with cognitively impaired individuals.

Clock Test

Tuokko H, Hadjistavropoulous T, Miller JA, & Beattie BL. (1992). The clock test: A sensitive measure to differentiate normal elderly from those with Alzheimer's disease. *J Am Geriatr Soc*, 40, 579–584.

Design.   This article presents a validation study of an augmented clock test as a screening tool for dementia. Data were reported on the interrater reliability of the scoring and on the percentage of normal and demented patients who were correctly classified. The clock test was augmented with two additional tasks—setting a clock and reading a clock—to help determine whether deficiencies in drawing a clock are related to the individual's ability to conceptualize time or to deficits in constructional skills. A more detailed scoring system was also developed for the clock test that scores specific errors. The clock test was administered by giving the subject a predrawn circle and asking him or her to imagine it was the face of a clock. Subjects were then requested to place the numbers in the appropriate positions and to place the clock hands to indicate "10 past 11." For the clock-setting task, the subject was shown a circle with marks indicating the hour locations (without numbers). On separate circles subjects were asked to draw in the hands to indicate 1 o'clock, 10 past 11, 3 o'clock, 9:15, and 7:30. For the clock-reading test, the subjects were asked to read predrawn clocks that indicated the same times as on the previous task.

Sample.   The subjects in the study were 62 volunteers recruited from senior citizen centers and 58 patients with Alzheimer's disease referred by community physicians to an outpatient diagnostic setting. The average score on the MMSE for the Alzheimer's disease group was 15.5 ($SD = 7.69$).

Summary.   The article presents a table of types of errors that were quantitatively scored for the clock-drawing test (i.e., omissions, preservations, rotations, misplacement, distortions, substitutions, and additions). The clock-setting and clock-reading tests were scored as follows: 1 point for every correct placement or reading of the clock hands and an extra point if both hands were placed or read correctly. The interrater reliability was in the range of 0.90–0.95 for the ratings. A test-retest reliability of 0.70 was reported. Analysis of covariance, with education as the covariate, was performed on the drawing error score.

A significant difference ($p < 0.001$) was found between the group with Alzheimer's disease and the other group. Using a cutoff score of more than two errors resulted in a correct classification of 92% of the subjects without Alzheimer's disease and 86% of the subjects with Alzheimer's disease. Significant differences on the clock-setting task were found ($p < 0.001$) between the two groups. A cutoff score of 13 resulted in the correct classification of 87% of the subjects without Alzheimer's disease and 97% of those with Alzheimer's disease. Significant differences were also found on the clock-reading test ($p < 0.001$). Using the same cutoff score of 13 correctly classified 92% of the subjects without Alzheimer's disease and 85% of those with Alzheimer's disease. Combining the tests and using the criterion of impairment on two or more components of the three tests yielded a correct classification of 94% of the subjects without Alzheimer's disease and 93% of those with Alzheimer's disease.

Discussion.   These authors interpret the results as suggesting that deficits in clock drawing may reflect a disturbance in the conceptualization of time rather than constructional apraxia. The clock-drawing test in combination with the clock-setting and clock-reading tests is offered as a useful research and screening tool. The clock-setting and clock-reading tests added to the clock drawing seem to increase the sensitivity and specificity of the screening tool slightly. Whether physicians will endure the burden of administering two additional tests is a concern.

Cognitive Performance Scale (CPS)

Hartmaier SL, Sloan PD, Guess HA, Koch GG, Mitchell M, & Phillips CD. (1995). Validation of the Minimum Data Set Cognitive Performance Scale: Agreement with the Mini-Mental State Examination. *J Gerontol*, *50A*, M128–M133.

Design.   This study reports on a validation of the Cognitive Performance Scale (CPS). The CPS is defined by five cognitive items: (1) comatose status, (2) short-term memory, (3) ability to make decisions, (4) making oneself understood, and (5) eating. These items were drawn from the Minimum Data Set (MDS) assessment of residents that is made by clinical professionals in nursing homes. A geriatric research nurse was responsible for collecting information on the MDS cognitive items from review of charts and direct observation of subjects. A medical resident assessed the resident using the MMSE. The CPS items are combined into a single, hierarchical seven-point rating scale that ranges from 0 (no impairment) to 6 (very severe impairment).

Sample.   Two hundred subjects were randomly recruited from a convenience sample of eight nursing homes in North Carolina. Subjects were excluded if they did not have good working command of the English language, were seriously ill, or were due to be discharged shortly. To recruit the sample, 526 subjects were approached. The sample were primarily women (72%) and white (86%). The mean age was 80.5 years, and the mean educational level was 10.84 years.

Summary.   The mean MMSE score was 12.7 ($SD = 9.47$), and the mean CPS score was 2.99 ($SD = 1.9$). The reported correlation between the CPS the and MMSE was −0.863. Using the MMSE cut scores as the "gold standard," both the sensitivity and the specificity of the CPS were 0.94 after adjustment for educational level. The positive predictive value was 0.97, and the negative predicative value was 0.80.

Discussion. Using MDA data that have already been collected is an attractive way to do cognitive screening within a nursing home population. A concern with the study is that it permits the MMSE, rather than a comprehensive assessment, to define cognitive impairment. The potential lack of reliability of MDS data collection across facilities raises some question about the widespread use of the CPS. At the very least, using the CPS would require a highly trained staff who would follow the MDS protocols. Additional work is needed, examining the robustness of the CPS as a screening tool in less than optimal nursing home settings.

Test for Severe Impairment (TSI)

Albert M, & Cohen C. (1992). The Test for Severe Impairment: An instrument for the assessment of patients with severe cognitive dysfunction. *J Am Geriatr Soc*, **40, 449–453.**

Design. This article reports on a validation study of the Test for Severe Impairment (TSI). TSI scores were correlated with MMSE scores, and TSI test-retest coefficients were reported. Factor analysis of the results of the TSI was performed to investigate its factor structure. The TSI was developed as a test of cognitive function in patients with severe cognitive impairment. The article contains the full test in an appendix. The guiding principles for the design of the test were to minimize the need for subjects to use language, to cover a broad range of cognitive function by extending the range of measurement downward in some areas of cognitive functioning, and to minimize the administration time. Subjects were first screened through the MMSE and were included in the study only if they had a score less than 10. The TSI was administered after the MMSE. The TSI was also readministered to 19 subjects 2 weeks later.

Sample. Subjects for the validation study were 40 residents of a chronic care facility. Subjects' ages ranged from 72 to 98. Patients suffered from a variety of dementias, including Alzheimer's disease, multi-infarct dementia, and Parkinson's disease with dementia. They also required nursing care to maintain activities of daily living.

Summary. The TSI score was highly correlated with the MMSE ($r = 0.83$, $p < 0.001$), which provides preliminary evidence for the TSI's construct validity. Test-retest correlations of the TSI's subscales ranged from 0.74 to 0.97, $p < 0.001$. The internal consistency of the scale ($\alpha = 0.91$) was higher than the internal consistency of the MMSE for this sample ($\alpha = 0.56$). Factor analysis of the TSI items resulted in three factors with eigenvalues greater than 2.8: factor 1 related to memory function; factor 2 related to verbal function; and factor 3 related to manipulation and identification of body parts. No evidence was found of a relationship between TSI scores and educational level or age.

Discussion. The results indicated that the TSI may be a useful test for following up on severely impaired patients. Its advantages include shorter administration time and the ability to evaluate severely impaired patients. This should assist with management of patients and with the examination of rates of decline among more severely demented patients. Unanswered questions remain about the relationship of the TSI to other tests of cognitive function, and its use with other patient populations, especially patients with different brain diseases and disorders.

Cross-Cultural Cognitive Examination (CCCE)

Glosser G, Wolfe N, Albert M, Lavine L, Steele J, Caine D, & Schoenberg B. (1993). Cross-Cultural Cognitive Examination: Validation of a dementia screening instrument for neuroepidemiological research. *J Am Geriatr Soc*, *41*, 931–939.

Design. This is a validation study of the Cross-Cultural Cognitive Examination (CCCE), which was developed for use in a neuroepidemiologic survey designed to detect dementia associated with amyotrophic lateral sclerosis–Parkinsonism in Guam. This study investigated the utility of the CCCE as a new dementia screening instrument that minimizes the effects of cultural, age, and educational factors. Designed to assess a range of cognitive functions (attention, language, visuospatial, verbal memory, visual memory, recent memory, abstraction, and psychomotor speed), it includes both a screening section and a more in-depth mental status evaluation. It is designed so that the in-depth evaluation is administered only if the screen is failed. The initial screening section can be completed in 5 minutes; the extended evaluation reportedly takes 20 minutes. There are 13 tasks and 3 behavioral ratings in the total exam. All subjects in the study on the American mainland were given the complete CCCE, as well as the MMSE and the Blessed-Roth Information Memory Concentration Test (Katzman, Brown, Fuld, Peck, Schecter, & Schimmel, 1983), and correlations among the tests were reported. Sensitivities and specificities of the three tests in detecting dementia were also provided.

Sample. The exam was initially validated on a random sample of 115 community-dwelling subjects, aged 40–87 (39% men), on the island of Guam. Subsequent evaluation was performed on samples in the mainland United States, including healthy volunteers (*n* = 64; mean age = 60.5; 45% men), individuals with probable Alzheimer's disease (*n* = 18; mean age = 80; 44% men), and individuals with idiopathic Parkinson's disease (*n* = 14; mean age = 61.3; 57% men).

Summary. CCCE screening was 100% sensitive and 92% specific (healthy versus clinically demented). The complete exam was found to have 100% sensitivity and 99% specificity. The correlation of both the CCCE screen and the complete CCCE with the MMSE were high ($r = 0.79$ and 0.83, respectively). Correlations between both the CCCE screen and the complete CCCE and the Blessed-Roth were $r = 0.55$ and 0.64, respectively. The ability of these three instruments to detect dementia was as follows: MMSE had sensitivity = 79% and specificity = 100%; Blessed-Roth had sensitivity = 79% and specificity = 96%; and the CCCE had sensitivity = 100% and specificity = 99%. Language, education, and social factors did not compromise sensitivity or specificity of the CCCE in the study samples.

Discussion. This is a potentially important new screening instrument that correlates well with the MMSE, exhibits excellent sensitivity and specificity, and addresses some of the purported weaknesses of the MMSE, namely, susceptibility to cultural and educational influences and relative insensitivity to subcortical dementias.

REFERENCES

Albert, M. (1994). Brief assessments of cognitive function in the elderly. In MP Lawton & JA Teresi (Eds.), *Annual review of gerontology and geriatrics* (pp. 93–106). New York: Springer.

*Albert M, & Cohen C. (1992). The Test for Severe Impairment: An instrument for the assessment of patients with severe cognitive dysfunction. *J Am Geriatr Soc*, *40*, 449–453.

American Psychiatric Association. (1987). *Diagnostic and statistical manual of mental disorders* (Rev. 3rd ed.). Washington, DC: Author.

Anthony JC, LaResche L, Niaz U, von Korff MR, & Folstein MF. (1982). Limits of the "Mini-Mental State" as a screening test for dementia and delirium among hospital patients. *Psychol Med*, *12*, 397–408.

Auer SR, Sclan GS, Yaffee RA, & Reisberg B. (1994). The neglected half of Alzheimer disease: Cognitive and functional concomitants of severe dementia. *J Am Geriatr Soc*, *42*, 1266–1272.

Bachman DL, Wolf PA, Linn RT, Knoefel JE, Cobb JL, Belanger AJ, White LR, & D'Agostino RB. (1993). Incidence of dementia and probable Alzheimer's disease in a general population: The Framingham Study. *Neurology*, *43*, 515–519.

Bassett SS, & Folstein MF. (1991). Cognitive impairment and functional disability in the absence of psychiatric diagnosis. *Psychol Med*, *21*, 77–84.

Berkman LF. (1986). The association between educational attainment and the mental status examinations: Of etiologic significance or not? *J Chronic Dis*, *29*, 1771–1774.

Bleeker ML, Bolla-Wilson K, Kawas C, & Agnew J. (1988). Age-specific norms for the Mini-Mental State Exam. *Neurology*, *33*, 1565–1568.

Blessed G, Tomlinson BE, & Roth M. (1968). The association between quantitative measures of dementia and senile change in the cerebral gray matter of older adult subjects. *Br J Psychiatry*, *114*, 797–811.

Bobholz JH, & Brandt J. (1993). Assessment of cognitive impairment: Relationship of the Dementia Rating Scale to the Mini-Mental State Examination. *J Geriatr Psychiatry Neurol*, *6*, 210–213.

*Brackhus A, Laake K, & Engedal K. (1992). The Mini-Mental State Examination: Identifying the most efficient variables for detecting cognitive impairment in the elderly. *J Am Geriatr Soc*, *40*, 1139–1145.

Burns T, Mortimer JA, & Merchak P. (1994). Cognitive performance test: A new approach to functional assessment in Alzheimer's disease. *J Geriatr Psychiatry Neurol*, *7*, 46–54.

Butters N, Delis DC, & Lucas JA. (1995). Clinical assessment of memory disorders in amnesia and dementia. *Ann Rev Psychol*, *46*, 493–523.

Campbell DT, & Fiske DW. (1959). Convergent and discriminant validation by the multitrait-multimethod matrix. *Psychol Bul*, *56*, 81–105.

Cohen-Mansfield J. (1986). Agitated behaviors in the elderly: II. Preliminary results in the cognitively deteriorated. *J Am Geriatr Soc*, *34*, 722–727.

Colohan H, O'Callaghan E, Larkin C, & Waddington JL. (1989). An evaluation of cranial CT scanning in clinical psychiatry. *Ir J Med Sci*, *158*, 178–181.

Cooper JK, Mungas D, & Wieler PG. (1990). Relation of cognitive status and abnormal behaviors in Alzheimer's disease. *J Am Geriatr Soc*, *38*, 867–870.

Corey-Bloom J, Galasko D, Hofstetter R, Jackson JE, & Thal LJ. (1993). Clinical features distinguishing large cohorts with possible AD, probable AD and mixed dementia. *J Am Geriatr Soc*, *41*, 31–37.

Critchley M. (1953). *The parietal lobes*. London: Hafner.

*Crum RM, Anthony JC, Bassett SS, & Folstein MF. (1993). Population based norms for the Mini Mental State Examination by age and educational level. *JAMA, 269,* 2386–2391.

Dalton JE, Pederson SL, Blom BE, & Holmes NR. (1987). Diagnostic errors using the Short Portable Mental Status Questionnaire with a mixed clinical population. *J Gerontol, 42,* 512–514.

DeKosky ST, Shih WJ, Schmitt FA, Coupal J, & Kirkpatrick C. (1990). Assessing utility of single photon emission computed tomography (SPECT) scan in Alzheimer disease: Correlation with cognitive severity. *Alzheimer Dis Assoc Disord, 4,* 14–23.

Dufouil C, Fufrer R, Dartigues JF, & Alperovitch A. (1996). Longitudinal analysis of the association between depressive symptomatology and cognitive deterioration. *Am J Epidemiol, 144,* 634–641.

Erzigkeit H. (1989). SKT: A short cognitive performance test as an instrument for the assessment of clinical efficacy of cognitive enhancers. In W Bergner & B Reisberg (Eds.), *Diagnosis and treatment of senile dementia.* Heidelberg: Springer Verlag.

Eslinger PJ, Damasio AR, Benton AL, & Van Allen M. (1985). Neuropsychological detection of abnormal mental decline in older persons. *JAMA, 253,* 670–674.

Evans DA, Funkenstein HH, Albert MS, Scherr PA, Cook NR, Chown MJ, Herbert LE, Hennekens CH, & Taylor JO. (1989). Prevalence of Alzheimer's disease in a community population: Higher than previously reported. *JAMA, 262,* 2251.

Farber JF, Schmitt FA, & Logue PE. (1988). Predicting intellectual level from the Mini-Mental State Examination. *J Am Geriatr Soc, 36,* 509–510.

Farmer ME, Kittner SJ, Rae DS, Barko JJ, & Regier DA. (1995). Education and change in cognitive function: The Epidemiologic Catchment Area study. *Ann Epidemiol, 5,* 1–7.

Fiedler IG, & Klingbeil G. (1990). Cognitive-screening instruments for the elderly. *Top Geriatr Rehab, 5,* 10–17.

Fillenbaum GG. (1980). Comparison of two brief tests of organic brain impairment, the MSQ and the Short Portable MSQ. *J Am Geriatr Soc, 28,* 381–384.

Fillenbaum GC, Heyman A, Wilkinson WE, & Haynes CS. (1987). Comparison of two screening tests in Alzheimer's disease: The correlation and reliability of the Mini Mental State Examination and the Modified Blessed Test. *Arch Neurol, 44,* 924–927.

Fillenbaum GC, & Smyer M. (1981). The development, validity and reliability of the ORS multidimensional functional assessment questionnaire. *J Gerontol, 36,* 428–434.

Folstein MF, Folstein SE, & McHugh PR. (1975). "Mini-Mental State:" A practical method for grading the cognitive state of patients for the clinician. *J Psychiatr Res, 12,* 189–198.

Foreman MD. (1987). Reliability and validity of mental status questionnaires in elderly hospitalized patients. *Nurs Res, 36,* 216–220.

Friedland RP. (1993). Epidemiology, education, and the ecology of Alzheimer's disease. *Neurology, 43,* 246–249.

Galasko D, Corey-Bloom J, & Thal LJ. (1991). Monitoring progression in Alzheimer's disease. *J Am Geriatr Soc, 39,* 932–942.

Galasko D, Klauber MR, Hofstetter CR, Salmon DP, Lasker B, & Thal LJ. (1990). The Mini-Mental State Examination in the early diagnosis of Alzheimer's dementia. *Ann Neurol, 47,* 49–52.

Ganguli M, Ratcliff G, Huff FJ, Belle S, Kancel MJ, Fischer L, & Kuller LH. (1990). Serial sevens versus word backwards: A comparison of the two measures of attention from the MMSE. *J Geriatr Psychiatry Neurol*, *3*, 246–252.

George LK, Landerman R, Blazer DG, & Anthony JC. (1991). Cognitive impairment. In LN Robbins & DA Regier (Eds.), *Psychiatric disorders in America* (pp. 291–337). New York: Free Press.

Giordani B, Boivin MJ, Hall AL, Foster NL, Lehtinen SJ, Bluemlein LA, & Berent S. (1990). The utility and generality of Mini-Mental State Examination scores in Alzheimer's disease. *Neurology*, *40*, 1884–1886.

*Glosser G, Wolfe N, Albert M, Lavine L, Steele J, Caine D, & Schoenberg B. (1993). Cross-Cultural Cognitive Examination: Validation of a dementia screening instrument for neuroepidemiological research. *J Am Geriatr Soc*, *41*, 931–939.

Goldman LS, & Lazarus LW. (1988). Assessment and management of dementia in the nursing home. *Clin Geriatr Med*, *4*, 589–600.

Haglund R, & Schuckit MA. (1976). A clinical comparison of test of organicity in elderly patients. *J Gerontol*, *31*, 645–659.

Harper RG, Chacko RC, Kotik-Harper D, & Kirby HB. (1992). Comparison of two cognitive screening measures for efficacy in differentiating dementia from depression in a geriatric inpatient population. *J Neuropsychiatry Clin Neurosci*, *4*, 179–184.

Hartmaier SL, Sloane PD, Guess HA, & Koch GG. (1994). The MDS Cognition Scale: A valid instrument for identifying and staging nursing home residents with dementia using the Minimum Data Set. *J Am Geriatr Soc*, *42*, 1173–1179.

*Hartmaier SL, Sloan PD, Guess HA, Koch GG, Mitchell M, & Phillips CD. (1995). Validation of the Minimum Data Set Cognitive Performance Scale: Agreement with the Mini-Mental State Examination. *J Gerontol*, *50A*, M128–M133.

*Heeren TJ, Lagaay AM, von Beck WCA, Rooymans HGM, & Hijman W. (1990). Reference values for the Mini Mental State Examination (MMSE) in octo- and nonagenarians. *J Am Geriatr Soc*, *38*, 1093–1096.

Holzer CE, Tischler GL, & Leaf PJ, et al. (1984). An epidemiologic assessment of cognitive impairment in a community population. In JR Greenley (Ed.), *Research in community mental health* (pp. 3–32). London: JAI.

Jacobs JW, Bernhard MR, Delgado A, & Strain JJ. (1977). Screening for organic mental syndromes in the medically ill. *Ann Int Med*, *86*, 40–46.

Jorm AF, & Jacomb P (1989). The Informant Questionnaire on Cognitive Decline in the Elderly (IQCODE): Sociodemographic correlates, reliability, validity and some norms. *Psychol Med*, *19*, 1015–1022.

Jorm AF, Scott R, Henderson AA, & Kay DW. (1988). Educational level differences on the Mini-Mental State: The role of test bias. *Psychol Med*, *18*, 727–731.

Kahn RL, Goldfarb AI, Pollack M, & Peck A. (1960). Brief objective measures for the determination of mental status in the aged. *Am J Psychiatry*, *117*, 326–328.

Katzman R, Brown T, Fuld P, Peck A, Schechter R, & Schimmel H. (1983). Validation of a short orientation-memory-concentration test of cognitive impairment. *Am J Psychiatry*, *140*, 734–739.

Lomeo VC. (1992). Alzheimer's disease: Correlational analysis of three screening tests and three behavioral scales. *Acta Neurol Scand*, *86*, 603–608.

Lyness SA, Eaton EM, & Schneider LS. (1994). Cognitive performance in older and middle aged depressed outpatients and controls. *J Gerontol, 49*, P129–P136.

Magaziner J, Bassett SS, & Hebel JR. (1987). Predicting performance on the Mini-Mental State Examination: Use of age- and education-specific equations. *J Am Geriatr Soc, 35*, 996–1000.

Mahurin RK, DeBettignies BH, & Pirozzolo FJ. (1991). Structured assessment of independent living skills: Preliminary report of a performance measure of functional abilities in dementia. *J Gerontol, 46*, 58–66.

McCartney JR, & Palmateer LM. (1985). Assessment of cognitive deficit in geriatric patients: Study of physician behavior. *J Am Geriatr Soc, 33*, 467–471.

Mendez MF, Ala T, & Underwood KL. (1992). Development of scoring criteria for the clock drawing task in Alzheimer's disease. *J Am Geriatr Soc, 40*, 1095–1099.

Mitrushina M, & Satz P. (1991). Reliability and validity of the Mini-Mental State Exam in neurologically intact elderly. *J Clin Psychol, 47*, 537–543.

Morris JC, Mohs RC, Rogers H, Fillenbaum G, & Heyman A. (1988). Consortium to Establish a Registry for Alzheimer's Disease (CERAD): Clinical and neurological assessment of Alzheimer's disease. *Psychopharmacol Bull, 24*, 641–652.

*Murden RA, McRae TD, Kaner S, & Buckman ME. (1991). Mini-Mental State Exam scores vary with education in blacks and whites. *J Am Geriatr Soc, 39*, 149–155.

Nelson A, Fogel BS, & Faust D. (1986). Bedside cognitive screening instruments: A critical assessment. *J Nerv Ment Dis, 174*, 73–82.

Nichols ME, Meador KJ, Loring DW, Poon LW, Clayton GM, & Martin P. (1994). Age-related changes in the neurologic examination of healthy sexagenarians, octogenarians, and centarians. *J Geriatr Psychiatry Neurol, 7*, 1–7.

O'Connor DW, Pollitt PA, & Hyde JB. (1991). The progression of mild idiopathic dementia in a community population. *J Am Geriatr Soc, 39*, 246–251.

O'Connor DW, Pollitt PA, Hyde JB, Fellows JL, Miller ND, Brock CP, & Reiss BB. (1989). The reliability and validity of the Mini-Mental State in a British community survey. *J Psychiatr Res, 23*, 87–96.

Olin JT, & Zelinski M. (1991). The 12-month reliability of the Mini-Mental State Examination. *Psycholog Assess, 3*, 427–432.

Ouslander JG, Zarit SH, Orr NK, & Muira SA. (1990). Incontinence among elderly community-dwelling dementia patients: Characteristics, management and impact on caregiver. *J Am Geriatr Soc, 38*, 440–445.

Overall JE, & Gorham DR. (1988). Introduction—The Brief Psychiatric Rating Scale (BPRS): Recent developments in ascertainment and scaling. *Psychopharmacol Bull, 24*, 97–99.

*Overall JE, & Schaltenbrand R. (1992). The SKT Neuropsychological Test Battery. *J Geriatr Psychiatry Neurol, 5*, 220–227.

Pearlson GE, & Tune LE. (1986). Cerebral ventricular size and cerebrospinal fluid acetylcholinesterase levels in senile dementia of the Alzheimer type. *Psychiatry Res, 17*, 23–29.

*Pedersen NL, Reynold CA, & Gatz M. (1996). Sources of covariation among Mini-Mental State Examination scores, education and cognitive abilities. *J Gerontol, 51B*, P55–P63.

Pfeiffer E. (1975). A Short Portable Mental Status Questionnaire for the assessment of organic brain deficit in elderly patients. *J Am Geriatr Soc, 23,* 433–441.

Reisberg B. (1988). Functional assessment staging (FAST). *Psychopharmacol Bull, 24,* 633–639.

Richie K, & Kildea D. (1995). Is senile dementia "age-related" or "aging-related"? Evidence from meta-analysis of dementia prevalence in the oldest old. *Lancet, 346,* 931–934.

Robins LN, Helzer JE, Croughan J, & Ratcliff KS. (1981). The National Institute of Mental Health Diagnostic Interview Schedule: Its history, characteristics and validity. *Arch Gen Psychiatry, 38,* 381–389.

*Roccaforte W, Burke W, Bayer B, & Wengel S. (1992). Validation of a telephone version of the Mini-Mental State Examination. *J Am Geriatr Soc, 40,* 697–702.

Rovner B, Kafonek W, Filipp S, Lucas L, Folstein MJ, & Marshall F. (1986). Prevalence of mental illness in a community nursing home. *Am J Psychiatry, 143,* 1446–1449.

Rubin E, Storandt M, Miller P, Grant E, Kinscherf D, Morris J, & Berg L. (1992). Influence of age on clinical and psychometric assessment of subjects with very mild or mild dementia of the Alzheimer type. *Arch Neurol, 50,* 380–383.

Salmon DP, Thal LJ, Butters N, & Heindel WC. (1990). Longitudinal evaluation of dementia of the Alzheimer's type: A comparison of three standardized mental status examinations. *Neurology, 40,* 1225–1230.

Saxton J, McGoingle-Gibson K, Swihart A, Miller V, & Boller F. (1990). Assessment of the severely impaired patient: Description and validation of a new neuropsychological test battery. *Psychol Assess, 12,* 298–303.

Schoenberg BS, Kokmen E, & Okazaki H. (1987). Alzheimer's disease and other dementing illnesses in a defined United States population: Incidence rates and clinical features. *Ann Neurol, 22,* 724–729.

Schwamm LH, Van Dyke C, Kierman RJ, Merrin EL, & Mueller J. (1987). The Neurobehavioral Cognitive Status Examination: Comparison with the Cognitive Capacity Screening Examination and the Mini-Mental State Examination in a neurosurgical population. *Ann Int Med, 107,* 486–491.

Scinto LF, Daffner KR, Dressler D, Ransil BI, Renth D, Weintraub S, Mesulam M, & Potter H. (1994). A potential noninvasive neurobiological test for Alzheimer's disease. *Science, 266,* 1051–1054.

Shulman K, Shedletsky R, & Silver IL. (1986). The challenge of time: Clock drawing and cognitive function in the elderly. *Int J Geriatr Psychiatry, 1,* 135–140.

Smyer SM, Hofland BF, & Jonas EA. (1979). Validity study of the Short Portable Mental Status Questionnaire for the elderly. *J Am Geriatr Soc, 27,* 263–269.

Somerfeld MR, Weisman CS, Ury W, Chase GA, & Folstein MF. (1991). Physician practices in the diagnosis of dementing disorders. *J Am Geriatr Soc, 39,* 172–175.

Sultzer DL, Levin HS, Mahler ME, High WM, & Cummings JL. (1992). Assessment of cognitive, psychiatric and behavioral disturbances in patients with dementia: The Neurobehavioral Rating Scale. *J Am Geriatr Soc, 40,* 549–555.

Sunderland T, Hill JL, Mellow AM, Lawlor BA, Gundersheimer J, Newhouse PA, & Grafman JH. (1989). Clock drawing in Alzheimer's disease: A novel measure of dementia severity. *J Am Geriatr Soc, 37,* 725–729.

Teri L, Hughes JP, & Larson EB. (1990). Cognitive deterioration in Alzheimer's disease: Behavioral and health factors. *J Gerontol, 45*, 58–63.

Teri L, & Logsdon RG. (1994). Assessment of behavioral disturbance in older adults. In MP Lawton & JA Teresi (Eds.), *Annual review of gerontology and geriatrics* (pp. 107–124). New York: Springer.

*Teri L, McCurry SM, Edland SD, Kukull WA, & Larson EB. (1995). Cognitive decline in Alzheimer's disease: A longitudinal investigation of risk factors for accelerated decline. *J Gerontol, 45*, 58–63.

Thal LJ, Grundman M, & Golden R. (1986). Alzheimer's disease: A correlational analysis of the Blessed Information-Memory-Concentration test and the Mini-Mental State Exam. *Neurology, 36*, 262–264.

Tombaugh TN, & McIntyre NJ. (1992). The Mini-Mental State Examination: A comprehensive review. *J Am Geriatr Soc, 40*, 922–935.

*Tuokko H, Hadjistavropoulos T, Miller JA, & Beattie BL. (1992). The clock test: A sensitive measure to differentiate normal elderly from those with Alzheimer disease. *J Am Geriatr Soc, 40*, 579–584.

Uhlmann RF, & Larson EB. (1991). Effect of education on the Mini-Mental State Examination as a screening test for dementia. *J Am Geriatr Soc, 39*, 876–880.

Uhlmann RF, Larson EB, & Buchner DM. (1987). Correlations of Mini-Mental State and Modified Dementia Rating Scale to measures of transitional health status in dementia. *J Gerontol, 50A*, M49–M55.

Uhlmann RF, Teri L, Rees TL, Mozlowski KJ, & Larson EB. (1989). Impact of mild to moderate hearing loss on mental status testing: Comparability of standard and written Mini-Mental Status Examinations. *J Am Geriatr Soc, 37*, 223–228.

van Belle G, Uhlmann RF, Hughes JP, & Larson EB. (1990). Reliability of estimates of changes in mental status test performance in senile dementia of the Alzheimer type. *J Clin Epidemiol, 43*, 589–595.

*Ward HW, Ramsdell JW, Jackson E, Revall M, Swart JA, & Rockwell E. (1990). Cognitive function testing in comprehensive geriatric assessment: A comparison of cognitive test performance in residential and clinic settings. *J Am Geriatr Soc, 38*, 1088–1092.

*Weiler PG, Chiriboga DA, & Black SA. (1994). Comparison of mental status tests: Implications for Alzheimer's patients and their caregivers. *J Gerontol, 49*, S44–S51.

Weiss BD, Reed R, Klingman EW, & Abyad A. (1995). Literacy performance on the Mini-Mental State Examination. *J Am Geriatr Soc, 43*, 807–810.

*Wells J, Keyl P, Chase G, Aboraya A, Folstein M, & Anthony J. (1992). Discriminant validity of a reduced set of Mini-Mental State Examination items for dementia and Alzheimer's disease. *Acta Psychiatry Scand, 86*, 23–31.

Wolf-Klein GP, Silverstone FA, Levy AP, & Brod MS. (1989). Screening for Alzheimer's disease by clock drawing. *J Am Geriatr Soc, 37*, 730–734.

Zec RF, Landreth ES, Vicari SK, Feldman E, Belman J, Andrise A, Robbs R, Kumar V, & Becker R. (1992). Alzheimer disease assessment scale: Useful for both early detection and staging of dementia of the Alzheimer type. *Alzheimer Dis Assoc Disord, 6*, 89–102.

*Zillmer EA, Fowler PC, Gutnick HN, & Becker E. (1990). Comparison of two cognitive bedside screening instruments in nursing home residents: A factor analytic study. *J Gerontol, 45*, P69–P74.

5

Screening for Depression

**Deborah Ossip-Klein, Barbara M. Rothenberg,
Elena M. Andresen**

OVERVIEW: DEPRESSION IN LATER LIFE

Depression is the psychological disturbance most frequently encountered in older adults (Kaszniak, 1990). Depression among the elderly has been reported in terms of both *clinically diagnosed* depression and prevalence of reported depressive *symptoms*. The prevalence of clinically diagnosed major depression in community-dwelling older adults has been estimated at 2%–5% (Blazer & Williams, 1980; Myers et al., 1984). Depressive symptomatology is more frequently found in this population, with a prevalence of 15% consistently reported across studies of community-dwelling older adults (e.g., Blazer, 1994).

Prevalence of depression also varies across types of older populations, with differing levels found for older adults in different settings: primary care, acute care, and institutional care. For example, Callahan, Hui, Nienaber, Musick, and Tierney (1994) and Barsa, Toner, Gurland, and Lantigua (1986) reported that nearly one third of patients seen in primary care exhibit significant symptoms of depression. Koenig and Blazer (1992) found significant depressive symptoms in 40% of older inpatients in acute care settings. Similarly, a prevalence of 11.5% for major depression and 23% for depressive symptomatology has been found for men aged 70 and older on an acute care Veterans Affairs Medical Service (Koenig, Meador, Cohen, & Blazer, 1988a, 1988b). Higher prevalence has been found among adults in institutional long-term-care settings, with up to 50%

showing significant symptoms of depression (Abrams, Teresi, & Butin, 1992; Koenig & Blazer, 1992).

In contrast to clinical lore—according to which depression occurs more frequently in later life—research has demonstrated that the frequency of both current and lifetime major depression tends to be higher in youth and middle age, as compared with later life (Blazer, 1994; Myers et al., 1984), although recent research suggests a modest increase in depressive symptoms after age 75 (*Kessler, Foster, Webster, & House, 1992). However, despite overall lower rates of depression in older groups as compared with younger groups, suicide rates are higher among persons 65 and older than among any other age group in the United States (Cohen, 1990).

As reflected in the relatively low prevalence of depression and depressive symptoms for older populations, the norm is for stable mental health in later years (Cohen, 1990). Thus, deviations from psychological health are significant and are not consistent with normal aging. There is a clinical need to detect and treat depressive symptoms and depression in older adults, particularly given the relationship of these conditions to increased morbidity and mortality. Both major depression and depressive symptoms have been related to increased mortality (Gurland, 1992) and to decline in functional health status (Gurland, 1992; Wells et al., 1989).

The vast majority of older adults with depressive symptoms do not seek mental health services but, rather, rely on their primary care providers (Koenig & Blazer, 1992). Unfortunately, recognition and appropriate treatment of depression by primary care physicians is inadequate (Abrams et al., 1992; Perez-Stable, Miranda, Munoz, & Ying, 1990; Rapp, Parisi, Walsh, & Wallace, 1988).

ISSUES IN SCREENING FOR DEPRESSION

Depression screening scales are standardized instruments designed to assess the presence, the severity, or both of self-reported depressive symptoms in a given population. This approach offers several advantages. For epidemiologic research, it provides an efficient means of tracking the incidence and prevalence of depressive symptoms in communities. Depression screening instruments can typically be administered using either interview or paper-and-pencil formats; they usually do not require extensive training of raters (with the exception of the Hamilton Rating Scale for Depression—Hamilton, 1967); and they provide consistent measurement criteria across samples and time. For clinical use, these scales can be administered routinely and will provide brief indicators of patients who are most likely to be depressed and for whom more complete assessment might be indicated.

It is important to note that depression screening scales are not diagnostic instruments. The clinical diagnosis of depression requires more intensive assessment, using diagnostic criteria such as those provided by the *Diagnostic and Statistical Manual* (*DSM-IV*; American Psychiatric Association, 1994), the Schedule for Affective Disorders and Schizophrenia/Research Diagnostic Criteria (Endicott & Spitzer, 1978; Spitzer, Endicott, & Robins, 1978), and the recently released Agency for Health Care Policy and Research (AHCPR) Clinical Practice Guideline for detection, diagnosis, and treatment of depression (Depression Guideline Panel, 1993). The degree to which self-reported symptoms of depression correspond with the diagnosis of major or minor depression varies across screening instruments. In general, the prevalence of depressive symptoms is higher than the prevalence of depressive disorder based on diagnostic criteria, although at least some depression screening scales may actually underestimate the prevalence of minor depression (e.g., Harper, Kotik-Harper, & Kirby, 1990).

The value of the screening instruments lies in the wide-reaching ability, which is due to their relative ease of administration, to measure and track populations most likely to become clinically depressed. In addition, as noted above, depressive symptoms are themselves related to increased morbidity and mortality. They thus may be viewed as valid variables themselves, although they are, at best, imperfect indicators of clinical depression.

Screening for depression in older adults poses several challenges. First, a number of depression scales contain both affective items (e.g., feeling sad or blue) and somatic items (e.g., changes in appetite or sleep patterns). There is some controversy regarding the appropriateness of including somatic items in depression screening instruments for older adults. To the extent that somatic items may be influenced by other changes in health or medications that are more typical of older populations, inclusion of such items may inflate estimates of depressive symptoms among older adults (e.g., *Kessler et al., 1992). Thus, there currently appears to be a preference for scales such as the Geriatric Depression Scale (GDS) that do not include somatic content. On the other hand, depression may manifest itself in physical or vegetative symptoms in older adults (Koenig, Cohen, Blazer, Krishnan, & Sibert, 1993). In fact, some studies have found that older adults are less likely than younger groups to report dysphoria and are more likely to report such symptoms as emptiness, worry, insomnia and a pattern of multiple somatic complaints (e.g., Koenig, Cohen, et al., 1993; Weiss, Nagel, & Aronson, 1986). However, the ability of these symptoms to discriminate between depressed and nondepressed elderly people is less clear. It is notable that at least some studies have found good correlations between the GDS (which does not include somatic items) and the Beck Depression Inventory (BDI, which does include somatic items), and between both of these scales and clinical diagnoses of depression (e.g., *Norris, Gallagher, Wilson, & Winograd, 1987). The Center for Epidemiologic Studies Depression Scale (CES-D) also contains somatic items, and some studies report that this does not bias the results for older adults (e.g., *Foelker & Shewchuk, 1992).

A second and related challenge is that older adults are more likely than younger groups to have comorbid conditions and to be using multiple medications that may adversely affect mood and cognitive function. These conditions place older adults at increased risk of secondary depressions (Cohen, 1990) and underscore the importance of screening for depression. However, symptoms related to other illness or medications may also confound the diagnosis of depression. For example, symptoms of depression and dementia may overlap. Both depressed and demented people may report memory difficulties, decrements in concentration, slower performance, lack of personal grooming, etc. (Kaszniak, 1990).

A final issue in screening for depression is a lack of data on the reliability and validity of depression screening scales among the "old old," typically defined as persons older than 75 years (Weiss et al., 1986).

DEPRESSION SCREENING SCALES

A number of depression screening scales have been used with older adults. These include the Beck Depression Inventory (*Beck, Ward, Mendelson, Mock, & Erbaugh, 1961), the Center for Epidemiologic Studies Depression Scale (*Radloff, 1977), the CORE-CARE (Golden, Teresi, & Gurland, 1984), the SHORT-CARE (Gurland, Golden, Teresi, & Challop, 1984), the Cornell Scale for Depression in Dementia (Alexopoulos, Abrams, Young, & Shamoian, 1988), the Dementia Mood Assessment Scale (Sunderland et al., 1988), the D scale of the Minnesota Multiphasic Personality Inventory (Kaszniak & Allender, 1985), the Depression Adjective Check List and Multiple Affect Adjective Check List (Lubin & Rinck, 1986), the Geriatric Depression Scale (*Yesavage et al., 1983), the Hamilton Rating Scale for Depression (Hamilton, 1967), the Medical Outcomes Study Short Form or SF-36 (Ware & Sherbourne, 1992), and the Zung Self-Rating Depression Scale (Zung & Zung, 1986). Scales vary in administration format; some require interviews and observation, and others provide self-report or options for self-report or interview formats. It appears that an interviewer-administered format is most appropriate for frail and cognitively impaired older adults (e.g., Toner, Gurland, & Teresi, 1988). Readers are referred to a recent chapter by Pachana and colleagues (1994) for a more complete discussion of the scales noted above. All these scales were developed and tested before *DSM-IV* (1994). Thus some may now need to be tested further.

Currently and overall, the most widely used screening measures for depression in older populations appear to be the Center for Epidemiologic Studies Depression Scale (CES-D), the Geriatric Depression Scale (GDS), and the Beck Depression Inventory (BDI). The GDS was designed specifically for older populations and may be considered the most sensitive and widely accepted scale, although data on its appropriateness with cognitively impaired older adults are mixed (Pachana, Gallagher-Thompson, & Thompson, 1994). The BDI and CES-D both have extensive literatures demonstrating their reliability and validity with older populations, and they have the added advantage of allowing for comparisons with other age groups. However, the BDI and most versions of the CES-D have a more complex response format than the GDS and may be most appropriate for older adults who are more highly educated and cognitively intact. Although the BDI is widely used, there is also concern about its inclusion of somatic items. The CORE-CARE and SHORT-CARE assess both depression and dementia, and the Cornell Scale for Depression in Dementia and the Dementia Mood Assessment Scale were designed specifically for use with demented patients. The Hamilton Rating Scale for Depression has a considerable literature, but the reliability and validity of this instrument among older adults are less clear. The depression items of the MOS SF-36 are coming into wider use with the increasing application of this instrument as a measure of general health status; for more information on this measure, the reader is referred to Chapter 2. A substantial literature is also available on the Zung Self-Rating Depression Scale. However, because of its heavy somatic content, this scale is currently considered less appropriate for older populations.

Three depression screening measures—the CES-D, Geriatric Depression Scale, and Beck Depression Inventory—have been selected for more detailed review here because they are among those most commonly used with older adults, have well-documented reliability and validity, and represent a variety of approaches (e.g., multi-item response versus yes-no format, and a varying number of somatic items). For specific screening in cognitively impaired populations, however, scales such as the Cornell Scale for Depression in Dementia might be considered. Brief overviews of the CES-D, Geriatric Depression Scale, and Beck Depression Inventory are provided below. These overviews are followed by summary recommendations, and then by annotated bibliographies and a reference list of a sampling of other articles for each scale.

Center for Epidemiologic Studies Depression Scale (CES-D)

Introduction

The Center for Epidemiologic Studies Depression (CES-D) Scale was first introduced to the research community in 1977 (*Radloff, 1977). This scale was intended to meet the need for a screening tool for depressive symptoms applicable to a broad population. The 20 items of the CES-D scale were derived from a pool of items from other instruments used for the diagnosis and screening of depression. Radloff used factor analysis to look for "grouped" items and compared these with components of depressive symptoms from the literature to identify the most important items. The final version of the CES-D consists of 20 items that describe feelings. For each item, the respondents are asked how often they have felt this way in the past week, from never or rarely (0 points) to most or all of the time (3 points). Four of the 20 items are worded positively, to break up any tendency toward a response set as well as to assess a "positive affect" factor. The four positive items are scored by reversing the order of responses so that a higher score represents increased depressive symptoms. The CES-D is then scored as a sum of points across all items. Total scores range, in theory, from 0 to 60 points. Four factors were identified among the 20 items: (1) depressive affect, (2) positive affect, (3) somatic symptoms, and (4) interpersonal (subsequent publications sometimes rename these factors, but the terms are similar). The CES-D factors are not independently scored as subscales.

The early developmental work with the CES-D found that subjects who scored at least 16 points on the scale could be categorized as having "depressive symptoms." For example, in a depressed patient group the mean score was 39 points, with no patient scoring below the diagnostic cutoff of 16 (*Radloff, 1977). However, persons who score at or above 16 points are not necessarily suffering from major clinical depression. Radloff (*1977) and others (Boyd, Weissman, Thompson, & Myers, 1982) emphasize that the CES-D was originally designed as a population research tool, not as a clinical diagnostic tool. The CES-D is, however, an appropriate screening tool for identifying individuals who need further workup for clinically significant levels of depression.

Radloff and Teri (1986) later reviewed the use of the CES-D among older adults. They note that administration problems, including nonresponse and missing items, may increase with age. Missing items can be scored by substituting the average response from items that were completed. A more conservative approach, allowing fewer missing values, is suggested in some publications (*Andresen, Malmgren, Carter, & Patrick, 1994; *Callahan & Wolinsky, 1994). Generally the CES-D scale should be considered invalid if more than five items are unanswered or if all of the items are answered with either high or low extreme values. Because it includes reversed items, consistently high or low extreme values indicate that a person has completed the survey in a response "set."

Generally, Radloff and Teri (1986) report that the CES-D yields consistent results across varied age ranges and is not overly affected by negative health. It has been especially well tested among community-dwelling older adults. Perhaps the best examples of use of the CES-D (including two brief versions) come from publications of the sites of the Established Populations for Epidemiological Studies of the Elderly (EPESE) (Berkman et al., 1986; *Blazer, Burchett, Service, & George, 1991; *Colantonio, Kasl, & Ostfeld, 1992; Mendes de Leon, Rapp, & Kasl, 1994; O'Hara, Hinrichs, Kohout, Wallace, & Lemke, 1986; O'Hara, Kohout, & Wallace, 1985; *Oxman, Berkman, Kasl, Freeman, & Barrett,

1992; *Salive & Blazer, 1993; *Wallace & O'Hara, 1992). Other uses of the CES-D or its shorter derivatives with older adults include population-based studies in Alabama (*Foelker & Shewchuk, 1992), studies with members of a health maintenance organization in California (*Goldstein & Hurwicz, 1989), national studies (DiPietro, Anda, Williamson, & Stunkard, 1992; Eaton & Kessler, 1981; *Kessler, Foster, Webster, & House, 1992; *Stallones, Marx, & Garrity, 1990), and studies in the Epidemiologic Catchment Area Program (e.g., Kennedy et al., 1989). The four-factor structure of the CES-D has been explicitly tested among older adults and has usually been found to be supported (*Davidson, Feldman, & Crawford, 1994; *Kohout, Berkman, Evans, Cornoni-Huntley, 1993), although Callahan and Wolinsky (*1994) did not confirm a positive affect factor.

Most investigators agree that the CES-D works relatively well with older adults. Somatic symptoms included in the CES-D might be present for reasons other than depression and may be reported. For example, a person who responds that, frequently in the last week, "My sleep was restless" may be reporting common sleep disturbances that are related to increasing age. A number of publications have concentrated on interpreting the measurement bias of the CES-D among older adults, members of ethnic groups, and persons with health problems that are common at older ages.

Stommel and colleagues (*1993) suggest that gender bias in the CES-D explains part of the higher prevalence of depressive symptoms reported among women. Callahan and Wolinsky (*1994) suggest removing five items that account for much of the differences in measurements by gender and race. Cho and colleagues (1993) found that the CES-D might overreport depressive symptoms for Cuban Americans and Puerto Ricans. They recommended a CES-D cutoff point: a score of 18 for Cuban Americans and a score of 20 to 21 for Puerto Ricans. Garcia and Marks (1989) examined the results of the CES-D among Mexican American adults who responded to the Hispanic Health and Nutrition Examination Survey (H-HANES) conducted from 1982 to 1984 and reported that the factor structure was generally similar to prior studies. Mahard (1988) also confirmed the measurement properties of the CES-D among older Puerto Ricans. Liang, Van Tran, Krause, and Markides (1989), however, suggested that the CES-D has a three-factor rather than a four-factor structure among Mexican Americans. Frerichs, Aneshenel, and Clark (1981) found that social factors and age were significant predictors of depressive symptoms and that including social variables in a predictive model yielded lower association with race and ethnicity and higher CES-D scores. Other tests of the CES-D among ethnic groups have had generally favorable results (Rankin, Galbraith, & Johnson, 1993; Somervell et al., 1993).

Authors disagree as to the ability of the CES-D to measure depression without error among general older adult or patient groups. Blalock, DeVellis, Brown, and Wallston (*1989) found that four CES-D items seem to explain much of the measurement bias of the CES-D among patients with arthritis, although

Himmelfarb and Murrell (1983) reported that the CES-D was valid with a higher cutoff point (20) among these patients. Foelker and Shewchuk (*1992) concluded that the CES-D did not inappropriately measure somatic symptoms as depressive symptoms among a population-based sample of older adults. The CES-D has tested well among stroke patients (Parikh, Eden, Price, & Robinson, 1988; Shinar et al., 1986). The conclusions of all authors as to the bias of the CES-D among subgroups are based on the expectation that some, but not all, differences among groups are due to measurement bias and not to actual differences in depressive symptoms.

The CES-D has also been used in studies of older adults with specific diseases, conditions, or social circumstances, including, for example, the following: stroke (*Colantonio ct al., 1992), arthritis (Hurwicz & Berkanovic, 1993; Nicassio & Wallston, 1992), frailty and depression among public housing residents (Bojrab et al., 1988; *Davidson et al., 1994), the effect of social support (*Oxman et al., 1992), poverty (Mendes de Leon et al., 1994), bereavement (Jacobs, Hansen, Berkman, Kasl, & Ostfeld, 1989), depression among chronic obstructive pulmonary disease patients and their caretakers (Keele-Card, Foxall, & Barron, 1993), hip fracture (Marottoli, Berkman, & Cooney, 1992; *Mossey, Knott, & Craik, 1990), obesity (DiPietro et al., 1992), smoking (Colsher et al., 1990; *Salive & Blazer, 1993), and the cross-sectional nature of depression and decreased cognitive function (Dufouil et al., 1996). Variation in the use of health services by those with depressive symptoms has also been studied using the CES-D (Colantonio, Kasl, Ostfeld, & Berkman, 1993).

Versions of CES-D

Most publications use the traditional 20-item version of CES-D and categorize individuals as "positive" for depressive symptoms if they score 16 or more points. As with many good scales, the CES-D has been revised, and there are now versions with fewer items and different scoring techniques.

Some studies suggest using higher cutoff scores to categorize subjects as having depressive symptoms (Himmelfarb & Murrell, 1983; Murrell, Himmelfarb, & Wright, 1983; Shinar et al., 1986). The use of higher cutoff scores is recommended because many individuals categorized as having depressive symptoms are judged to be "false positives" when compared with a strict clinical diagnosis of depression. Using different cutoff scores makes it difficult to compare results among research publications. If one chooses to use a higher CES-D score to classify individuals with depressive symptoms, it seems advisable to compare results against the traditional cutoff score of 16 points.

There are a number of brief versions of CES-D in the research literature (*Andresen et al., 1994; *Blalock et al., 1989; *Callahan & Wolinsky, 1994; *Kessler et al., 1992; *Kohout et al., 1993; Nicassio & Wallston, 1992; O'Hara et al., 1985; Shrout & Yager, 1989; *Stommel et al., 1993). There is also a composite screening tool with six CES-D items and two Diagnostic Interview Schedule (DIS) items (Burnam, Wells, Leake, & Landsverk, 1988). Alternative scoring methods for the full scale (*Blazer et al., 1991; Colsher et al., 1990) are available. The versions of CES-D developed and used primarily among older adults are as follows: those used in two sites of the EPESE project described by Kohout et al. (*1993), a 10-item version proposed by Andresen and colleagues (*Andresen et al., 1994), a 15-item version (*Callahan & Wolinsky, 1994), and a 20-item version recommended by Blazer et al. (*1991) that collapses the response categories to "yes" or "no" (see also *Salive & Blazer, 1993). Kessler et al. (*1992) describes two versions of the CES-D used in national surveys: a 13-item version with three response categories, and a 12-item version with eight response categories (representing number of days, from 0 to 7, in the past week when a subject has experienced each symptom).

Several versions with fewer items are the result of testing the CES-D among specific patient groups (or ethnic populations, as described above). Nicassio and Wallston (1992) took the precaution of removing the CES-D item on sleep and using a 19-item version when examining the relationships among sleep, pain, and depressive symptoms for patients with rheumatoid arthritis. Blalock and colleagues (*1989) also suggest dropping items to correct for overestimating depression among patients with arthritis.

There may be practical advantages to using a shorter version of the CES-D with older adults in some settings. If the CES-D is part of a long questionnaire, then the overall length of the survey can become taxing, and a brief version may be preferable, especially with self-administered forms. Simplified response categories, especially when reduced to "yes" and "no" (*Blazer et al., 1991), may be easier for subjects to handle than the four "frequency" categories of the original version. However, any version that offers simplification also reduces the point spread of either individual items or the overall points of the CES-D and may reduce the sensitivity of the instrument to real differences among individuals. It may be important to compare the results of any brief version in a specific study group or population with the full CES-D; if so, formal statistical guidance for transforming scores is offered by some authors (e.g., *Kohout et al., 1993).

There is, however, no universal agreement that an abbreviated or simplified version of the CES-D ought to be used among older adults. The argument for a brief form is especially weak when the CES-D is administered in an interview. A well-trained and experienced interviewer can overcome communication barriers due to vision, hearing, lack of education, and poor health. Furthermore, a well-designed self-administered format should pose few problems for respondents. Self-administered forms used with older adults should adhere to time-honored formatting rules whenever space and money allow. Professionally printed forms with a large, easy-to-read typeface will reduce problems with missing responses.

Using response categories that are arranged vertically beneath each CES-D item, rather than horizontally, may seem repetitive, but it clearly reminds the respondent of the answers for each CES-D statement. It can reduce errors that arise with a horizontal format when subjects answer two items on a single line (a potential problem as items change from negative to positive responses). Careful survey formatting and pilot testing of the CES-D in each proposed setting will help to determine if the 20-item version is inappropriate.

Geriatric Depression Scale (GDS)

Introduction

The Geriatric Depression Scale (GDS) was developed in the early 1980s by Yesavage, Brink, and colleagues (*Brink et al., 1982; *Yesavage et al., 1983) specifically for use with older adults. Items were selected from an initial pool of 100 questions identified by geriatric specialists as potentially distinguishing between depressed and nondepressed elderly people. The 30 items that correlated most highly with the total score were selected. It is interesting that none of the 12 original somatic items correlated sufficiently with the total score, and they were not included in the final scale. The final 30-item scale consists of 20 items that indicate depression when answered positively and 10 that indicate depression when answered negatively. A yes-no response format is used to simplify responding and to avoid the confusion of multiple response choices that may occur in scales such as the Zung (Zung & Zung, 1986) and the CES-D. Items tap affective and behavioral components of depression. The GDS can be answered in either a self-administered or an interviewer-administered format; some researchers recommend the interview format particularly for cognitively impaired older adults (e.g., Parmelee & Katz, 1990). The scale takes approximately 8 to 10 minutes to administer, and individuals are typically asked to respond to each item on the basis of how they have felt in the past week.

Cutoff scores have varied across studies. The original report recommended using a score of 11+ to provide the best sensitivity and specificity for detecting possible depression (*Brink et al., 1982). Scores of 11–20 and 21–30 have been used to indicate mild depression and moderate to severe depression, respectively (e.g., *Alden, Austin, & Sturgeon, 1989), although other groupings have also been reported in the literature. Although the variety of cutoff scores may be confusing to the reader, a generally accepted rule of thumb is to use the cutoff scores that have been reported for samples that will serve as comparison groups for the population being examined.

The reliability and validity of the GDS have been demonstrated for community-dwelling older adults, for both outpatient and hospitalized older adults, and for geriatric stroke patients (e.g., *Agrell & Dehlin, 1989; *Brink et al., 1982; *Burke,

Nitcher, Roccaforte, & Wengel, 1992; Koenig, Meador, Cohen, & Blazer, 1988a, 1988b; Rapp et al., 1988; *Yesavage et al., 1983). The sensitivity and specificity of the GDS have generally been in the 0.55–0.86 and 0.75–0.95 range, respectively (*Brink et al., 1982; *Koenig, Ford, & Blazer, 1993; *Koenig, Meador, Cohen, & Blazer, 1992). Mixed results have been found for use of the GDS in cognitively impaired populations. Some studies have found that the scale was unable or less able to detect depression in patients with dementia (*Burke, Houston, Boust, & Roccaforte, 1989; Burke, Roccaforte, & Wengel 1991; *Kafonek et al., 1989), but others suggest no differences in performance for cognitively impaired versus intact populations (*Burke, Roccaforte, & Wengel, 1991; O'Riordan et al., 1990; *Parmelee, Lawton, & Katz, 1989). At least one study has suggested that the GDS may be less appropriate for older African Americans relative to whites (Koenig et al., 1992). There is also some evidence that the GDS is more effective in identifying moderate or severe depression than minor depression, which it may underestimate (Harper et al., 1990; *Lesher & Berryhill, 1994; *Parmelee et al., 1989).

The GDS has been used in a range of clinical research applications that have examined depression in relation to attitudes toward life-sustaining therapy (Gerety, Chiodo, Kanten, Tuley, & Cornell, 1993; Lee & Ganzini, *1992, 1994; Schonwetter, Teasdale, Taffet, Robinson, & Luchi, 1991), functional dependency (Harris, Mion, Patterson, & Frengley, 1988), use of religion for coping (*Koenig, Cohen, Blazer, Pieper, et al., 1992), pain (*Parmelee, Katz, & Lawton, 1991), caregivers' burden (Printz-Feddersen, 1990), psychopharmacologic treatment (Altamura et al., 1988; Ambrosio, Marchese, Filippo, Romano, & Musacchio, 1993; Thapa, Meador, Gideon, Fought, & Ray, 1994; Vida, Gauthier, & Gauthier, 1989), memory (Cipolli, Neri, Andermarcher, Pinelli, & Lalla, 1990; Hanninen et al., 1994), and other topics.

Versions of GDS

The 30-item GDS is the most widely used version of the GDS in the literature. A 15-item short form of the GDS was developed by Sheikh and Yesavage (1986), using the 15 items having the highest correlation with depressive symptoms. The following cutoff scores for the short form have been recommended: 0–4 (nondepressed), 5–9 (mild depression), and 10–15 (moderate to severe depression). Relatively fewer data are available on this form, compared with the original 30-item GDS. High correlations between the short and long forms of the GDS have been reported by at least two sets of researchers ($r = 0.84$–0.89; *Lesher & Berryhill, 1994; Sheikh & Yesavage, 1986). However, a lower correlation between the two forms ($r = 0.66$) was reported by Alden and colleagues (*1989), who suggested that the short form is not an acceptable alternative to the 30-item GDS. The GDS has been translated into a 15-item Chinese version, with an optimum cutoff score of ≥ 8 and a sensitivity and specificity of 0.96 and 0.88, respectively (*Woo et al., 1994). The GDS has also been translated into Dutch, French, German, Hebrew, Italian, Japanese, Portuguese, Romanian, Spanish, and Yiddish (Pachana et al., 1994), and thus may be useful for cross-cultural comparisons of depressive symptomatology.

At least two other depression scales have been developed from the GDS (the Geriatric Depression Rating Scale by Jamison & Scogin, 1992, and an 11-item scale for the medically ill by Koenig, Cohen, Blazer, Meador, & Westlund, 1992); and several scales, for depression as well as other symptoms, have been validated using the GDS as a criterion measure (e.g., Gerety et al., 1994; Mahoney et al., 1994).

Beck Depression Inventory (BDI)

The Beck Depression Inventory (BDI) was developed in the early 1960s by a psychiatrist and his colleagues at the University of Pennsylvania (*Beck et al., 1961) and is based on clinically observed behaviors associated with depression. It has been used widely in a variety of populations, including older adults. It consists of a graded series of statements regarding 21 of categories of symptoms and attitudes (e.g., sense of failure, indecisiveness, and social withdrawal). The original version had four or five self-evaluative statements for each item; it was later modified so that all items have four statements ranging from "least severe" to "most severe." Respondents are asked to select the statement that best describes them in the past week. A number of cutoff scores have been used. One possible categorization is the following (Gallagher, 1986): 0–9, no depression; 10–15, mild depression; 16–19, mild to moderate depression; 20–29, moderate to severe depression; 30–63, severe depression. A short version of the BDI was developed in the mid-1970s. It contains only 13 items, with the order of the statements reversed so that the most severe responses are listed first. One range of scores for the short form is 0–4, none or minimal depression; 4–7, mild depression; 8–15, moderate depression; and 16 or greater, severe depression. The BDI has also been translated into several other languages, including German, Spanish, and French. (For a good overview of use of the BDI among older adults as of 1986, including its utility as an index of change and in clinical practice, see Gallagher, 1986.)

The original and the shortened instruments have been tested extensively and have been to be found reasonably reliable and valid among older adults (see, for example, *Gallagher, Breckenridge, Steinmetz, & Thompson, 1983; *Gallagher, Nies, & Thompson, 1982; *Scogin, Beutler, Corbishley, & Hamblin, 1988). The short form has also been shown to have a factor structure among older adults similar to that in a more general adult population (*Foelker, Shewchuk, & Niederehe, 1987).

There have been two primary criticisms of the BDI. The first is that it is more difficult to complete than some alternatives, such as the Geriatric Depression Scale, because of the need to respond to a series of ordered statements. The second is that it includes a number of items regarding somatic symptoms and may therefore overestimate the prevalence of depression among older adults. The short form of the BDI is less subject to this criticism, since many of the somatic items have been omitted from it (*Foelker et al., 1987). It is also interesting that in at least one study (*Norris et al., 1987), the BDI correctly identified more cases of depression based on *DSM-III* or Research Diagnostic Criteria (Spitzer et al., 1978) than the GDS. Another recent study (Lyness et al., 1995) among psychiatric inpatients showed that age is negatively correlated with overall BDI score and with the psychologic-affective items on the BDI, but there was no association between age and scores on the somatic items on the BDI. These results held up even after controlling for other variables such as education, gender, and a measure of overall medical burden (the Cumulative Illness Rating Scale). A final concern that has been expressed regarding the BDI is that it may contain a social desirability response set; that is, individuals' responses may be biased by whether the individual who completes the instrument views the statements as reflecting socially desirable or undesirable sentiments. However, this potential weakness is not limited to the BDI (Gallagher, 1986).

Despite the criticisms of the BDI, it has been used widely among older adults for a long time and continues to be used. Recent examples of the types of topics or conditions assessed using the BDI among older adults include the following: the relationship between age and depression in individuals with chronic back pain (Herr, Mobily, & Smith, 1993), the use of surrogate respondents to detect depression in individuals with Alzheimer's disease (in a study that also compares the performance of the BDI to the GDS and CES-D, Logsdon & Teri, 1995), sex differences in detection of depression (Allen-Burge, Storandt, Kinscherf, & Rubin, 1994), mood disorder following stroke (*House et al., 1991), the association between depression and type 2 diabetes (Palinkas, Barrett-Connor, & Wingard, 1991), age differences in recovery after coronary artery bypass graft surgery (*Artinian, Duggan, & Miller, 1993), and the effects of bereavement (Tudiver, Hilditch, & Permaul, 1991).

RECOMMENDATIONS

There are supportive data for the use of each of the three scales reviewed (CES-D, GDS, and BDI). Overall, the CES-D and the BDI have been validated across a range of ages and thus are particularly appropriate for studies comparing older and younger groups and for research on the aging of cohorts beginning at younger ages. Drawbacks of these two instruments include the multiple-choice format, which may be difficult for cognitively impaired older adults, and the heavy inclusion of somatic items in the BDI, which may misrepresent depressive symptoms in older adults. The CES-D has been reviewed somewhat more favorably, despite its somatic content. Generally favorable results have been found for both scales across several ethnic groups.

The GDS has the advantages of a simplified response format, which may enhance its appropriateness in mildly cognitively impaired older adults (although mixed results have been found for this group), and the inclusion of nonsomatic items specifically targeted to an older population. However, because this instrument was developed for older adults, it is not appropriate for studies comparing older and younger populations. The sensitivity of this scale to depressive symptoms in African Americans has been questioned by at least one study.

No clear empirical guidelines were identified for selecting one instrument over the other. In general, epidemiologic studies tended to use the CES-D, studies published in geriatric journals tended to use the GDS, and the BDI tended to be used for psychological publications. However, considerable overlap was found in these areas. Therefore, readers are encouraged to select the instrument most often used by the body of research most salient to their research or clinical interests, in order to maximize the ability to compare results across studies or clinical practices.

ANNOTATED BIBLIOGRAPHY

Center for Epidemiologic Studies Depression Scale (CES-D)

Development and Methods—Original and Revised CES-D Versions

Radloff LS. (1977). The CES-D Scale: A self-report depression scale for research in the general population. *Appl Psychol Meas*, *1*, 385–401.

Design. The CES-D scale was derived from a pool of over 300 items from other instruments. After initial item reduction, field tests were conducted which compared the CES-D with other scales of depression and well-being (Bradburn, Lubin, Cantril, others) for content, criterion, and construct validity. Test-retest reliability was assessed by comparing interviews and a mail-back of retests from the same community subjects. Households were sampled in two communities (Kansas City, MO; Washington County, MD), and an individual was randomly selected from each household. Trained interviewers administered a 1-hour interview, usually within 1 week of the sample selection, between 1971 and 1973. Reinterviews and mailed retests were administered for reliability and change analysis. A clinical validation sample was also selected and interviewed.

Sample. Subjects were all 18 years or older. A total of 1,173 interviews were completed in Kansas City (75% response) and 1,673 in Washington County (80% response). A shorter survey was tested in Washington County in 1973–1974 with 1,089 completed. Mailed retests to these last subjects received about 56% response ($n = 419$). Reinterviews in both sites were attempted for a sample; 343 (78% response) were repeated in Kansas City and 1,209 (79% response) were repeated in Washington County. Repeated interviews took place 3, 6, and 12 months after the first interview. Two clinically depressed samples were also interviewed (inpatients and outpatients), for a total of 105 patients.

Summary.   The CES-D was judged acceptable to clinical and population samples; the items most commonly missed (skipped) by respondents were: "I felt hopeful about the future" (2.2%) and "I felt I was just as good as other people" (1.6%). Nonparametric tests of the CES-D were required because of the skewness of results: The scale has potential scores of 0 to 60 points, but most respondents score below the "diagnostic" cutoff of 16 points. The variability of scores among interviewers and populations suggested some problems with the CES-D scale, but it was considered to be of no practical importance by the authors. Measures of internal consistency were high (about 0.85 for the general population and 0.90 in patient samples). Test-retest correlations were between 0.45 and 0.70 and were higher for shorter intervals (2 weeks versus 12 months). Correlations between the CES-D scale and nurse-clinician ratings were 0.56. In a group of depressed patients, the mean score was 39 points; no patient scored below the diagnostic cutoff of 16. Correlations between the Hamilton and Raskin scale and the CES-D were 0.44 to 0.54 at the time of admission for patients who were depressed and increased to 0.69 and 0.75 after 4 weeks of treatment.

Discussion.   This article introduces the CES-D to the scientific literature and is the standard reference for its development. The author cautions that the CES-D was designed specifically for use in general population studies of depressive symptoms, not as a clinical or diagnostic scale. The article also suggests problems in measurement for bilingual respondents, and the potential for interviewers to bias responses.

Andresen EM, Malmgren JA, Carter WB, & Patrick DL. (1994). Screening for depression in well older adults: Evaluation of a short form of the CES-D. *Am J Prev Med, 10,* 77–84.

Design.   The study used subjects from a randomized trial of health-promotion interventions among older adults. A lengthy mailed baseline survey included a 10-item shortened version of the CES-D, as well as 11-point Likert stress and pain scales and a 10-item Positive Affect Scale. Correlations among measures were computed, as were retest correlations. The items of the short CES-D (CESD-10) were tested by linear regression for their ability to predict the full 20-item version score. The CESD-10 results were also compared with the full version for agreement on categorizing subjects as having depressive symptoms using κ statistics. The CESD-10 scale scores range from 0 to 30 points.

Sample.   From a total of 4,250 randomly sampled members of a health maintenance organization (HMO) in Seattle aged 65 and older, 1,206 completed mailed surveys and were available for analysis after exclusions, refusals, and incomplete CESD-10 surveys (28.4%). Those who completed this baseline survey were sampled, and 102 were sent retested items after 4 weeks; 99 (97%) completed the retest. The larger study group was 61.2% female and 83% white; and these subjects were 72.8 years old, on average, at the time of the baseline survey. They were somewhat younger and healthier than all potential older adult members of the HMO.

Summary. Two cutoff points for the CESD-10 were tested: scores of 8 points (the arithmetic equivalent of the full CES-D scores of 16) and 10. For subjects tested with both versions of CES-D, the cutoff point of 8 resulted in many who would be classified as having depressive symptoms on the CESD-10 but not on the full 20-item version. Overall prevalence of depressive symptoms was 19.3% with a cutoff point of 8 and 11.7% with a cutoff of 10. The prevalence was higher among women and increased with age for women but not for men. The authors conclude that a cutoff point of 10 might be useful in some settings to avoid false positive results. The mean CESD-10 score was 4.7 for all subjects and 5.7 for retest subjects. Scores were predictably (although in some cases not too strongly) correlated with stress ($r = 0.43$) and pain ($r = 0.30$), and negatively correlated with Positive Affect ($r = -0.63$). Decreasing self-assessed health was also positively correlated with increasing depressive symptoms ($r = 0.37$). The CESD-10 test-retest over 4 weeks was high ($r = 0.71$). Of the original 1,206 subjects, 1,006 also completed the CES-D after 12 months, and the scores were strongly correlated at $r = 0.59$.
Discussion. The study reports a high prevalence of depressive symptoms in a large sample of healthy community-dwelling older adults. The study results are biased toward healthier individuals because of low response to the mailed survey, and one would assume that the prevalence would be higher in a broader population. The shorter CES-D is shown to be reliable in test-retest studies and strongly predicts depressive symptoms measured with the longer version. This 10-item depression screening survey may be used when the full CES-D survey is considered too long.

Callahan CM, & Wolinksky FD. (1994). The effect of gender and race on the measurement properties of the CES-D in older adults. *Med Care, 32*, 341–356.
Design. The authors had observed a marked difference in the prevalence of depression among four patient groups defined by race (African American versus white) and by gender. They conducted psychometric testing of the CES-D to determine whether measurement properties of the screening instrument could explain the differences. A large, older adult, primary care patient population was interviewed using the CES-D, the Short Portable Mental Status Questionnaire (SPMSQ), and the CAGE alcohol screening questions. (Interviewers used direct data entry to laptop computers during interviews with patients.) The data obtained were merged with computerized medical information about the subjects' active diagnoses. If subjects did not answer one to four CES-D items, their mean item score was substituted for the missing item or items. Those who answered fewer than 16 items were excluded. Differences among groups were tested for (1) missing information, (2) differences between mean item and mean summary scores by one-way ANOVA, (3) internal consistency by Cronbach's α for those answering all 20 items, (4) CES-D categories using principal components analyses, and (5) questionnaire scores and demographic information.
Sample. All outpatients aged 60 and older from an urban, university-affiliated primary care practice of 35 faculty general internists and 118 internal medicine residents were selected for the survey. Some patients were excluded (e.g., prisoners, nursing home patients, non–English-speaking individuals, hearing-impaired patients). Over a 16-month period, 3,319 patients were contacted: 185 were ineligible, 77 refused, and 3,057 were interviewed (an impressive 97.5% of those eligible). There were 1,392 African American women, 741 white women, 597 African American men, and 317 white men. The mean

age of the study group was 68.8 years (range, 60–102); age was significantly different among races by gender; African American men and women were older than their white counterparts. Among those willing to give income data (about two thirds), 80% had a monthly income under $800.

Summary. The study included a formal test of interviewer interrater reliability on 30 patients, and Pearson correlation coefficients (rather than the preferred intraclass correlation coefficients) were very high, from 0.97 to 0.99. The mean administration time for the CES-D was about 8 minutes and did not differ by study group. Overall, 5.1% were unable to complete the CES-D. This percentage was similar across groups, as was the internal consistency for those who answered all 20 items (Cronbach's α overall = 0.85). However, the proportion of subjects with imputed data (up to four missing items) differed among groups. It was greater for both white women and men compared with African American women (40% versus 33%) and men (43% versus 39%), respectively. There were also marked differences among groups in not answering specific items of the CES-D. Imputed data were most common for items in the positive affect construct. Imputed data were not considered responsible for the differences in the prevalence of depressive symptoms among groups. Factor analysis among subjects with all 20 items of the CES-D answered yielded constructs similar to the original CES-D for women, but not for either African American or white men, who also had different results from each other. For the large number of subjects with imputed values (37%), the factor analysis was quite different from that of the original CES-D. There were differences among groups, but the positive affect dimension disappeared for all groups. Elimination of seven items from the CES-D resolved the race and gender differences. The authors conclude that an abbreviated scale of 15 items might be adequate for a diverse population. This scale of 15 items would use a score cutoff of 14 points (compared with 16 on the CES-D). However, even this abbreviated CES-D yielded striking differences in the prevalence of depression among the four groups similar to the full scale. The prevalence of depressive symptoms among the four groups was as follows: white women, 25.4%; African American women, 12.8%; white men, 15.5%; and African American men, 9.0%.

Discussion. The study is important and unique in exploring both practical and psychometric issues of using CES-D in a heterogeneous population. The results suggest that the measurement properties, including the underlying factor structure of the CES-D, are not the same for all population subgroups. It is intriguing that the positive affect construct items were most often missing; these items all require reversing answer categories as compared with other CES-D items. In other words, a "frequent" response to these items is associated with *fewer* depressive symptoms. The abbreviated CES-D suggested by these authors may resolve the problem in factor structure, but it does not resolve or explain the continued differences in depressive symptoms across race and gender.

Kessler RC, Foster C, Webster PS, & House JS. (1992). The relationship between age and depressive symptoms in two national surveys. *Psychol Aging, 7,* **119–126.**
Design. This is a secondary analysis of two large national surveys, both of which used the CES-D as a component of the interviews. However, the two surveys did not use the same version of the CES-D. The Americans Changing Lives (ACL) survey used a 13-item version with three rather than four response categories, and the National Survey of Families and Households (NSFH) used a 12-item short form with eight response categories

(representing number of days, from 0 to 7, in the past week that a subject had experienced each symptom). To analyze the data, each scale was configured to use the items that were part of the original "somatic" dimension (4) and the "depressive affect" dimension (3 in the ACL and 4 in the NSFH). Summary scores were transformed to a continuous scale of 0 to 1, and also a dichotomous category comparing the 20% of subjects with highest scores on each version (categorized as having depressive symptoms) and the remainder. These authors subjected each scale to psychometric tests, including factor analysis and internal consistency (Cronbach's α). They also explored the relationship between age and depressive symptoms using simple and polynomial regression modeling.

Sample.   Respondents to two national surveys are used for the report; 3,617 subjects from the ACL and 13,017 individuals from the NSFH.

Summary.   Factor analysis confirmed that the two factors were present for each study population in both men and women, although somewhat less clearly in the NSFH study. The authors suggest that the three-category response used on the ACL version of the CES-D discriminated better than the expanded response categories of the NSFH version. The relationship between increasing age and depressive symptoms was weak, but there was evidence for a nonlinear relationship where symptoms declined with age in the middle years, then rose somewhat with older age. The lowest scores were for ages 50 and 63. The relationship with age was similar for both the depressive affect and the somatic symptoms subscales for both men and women.

Discussion.   This article provides an excellent review of the evidence for the nonlinear association between age and depressive symptoms and the common methodological mistakes of other studies. Simply, depression is low in the middle years, and high for younger and older subjects. For older adults, the association grows only after about age 75, so that simple linear models with smaller data sets will not pick up the association. In addition, the authors provide two very large and representative samples to demonstrate the associations. The results also show a relationship between age and both somatic and nonsomatic depressive symptoms, suggesting that age-related changes in health are not the only explanation for the increase in measured depressive symptoms. Unfortunately, the unique scoring schemes used here make comparisons with data from other studies difficult.

Kohout FJ, Berkman LF, Evans DA, & Cornoni-Huntley J. (1993). Two shorter forms of the CES-D depression index. *J Aging Health*, **5,** 179–193.

Design.   Three sites of the Established Populations for Epidemiological Studies of the Elderly (EPESE) each used a different version of the CES-D with in-home interviews of older adults. The Yale project used the original 20-item version; the East Boston site used 10 items with dichotomous responses comparing those who responded that they had experienced a symptom "much of the time" versus those who gave no response; and the Iowa site added one additional item (appetite) for an 11-item form with three rather than the traditional four response categories. Both abbreviated forms were tested for internal consistency (Cronbach's α) and factor analysis validity, then tested by simulating the scales among the Yale sample CES-D results.

Sample.   The three sites of the EPESE yielded samples of adults aged 65 and older of 2,811 (Yale), 3,673 (Iowa), and 3,812 (East Boston). Other publications from each site give details about the methods and study samples (e.g., *Colantonio, Kasl, & Ostfeld, 1992; Oxman, Berkman, Kasl, Freeman, & Barrett, 1992; *Wallace & O'Hara, 1992).

Summary. The Yale sample confirmed the original factor loading of the CES-D. The brief forms yielded similar results and suggested that the brief forms tapped all four of the original factors. Internal consistency was good for the Yale 20-item CES-D ($r = 0.86$) and for simulations with the two brief forms (Iowa form, 0.86; East Boston form, 0.73). Comparing the results with a national survey from the National Center for Health Statistics, the Iowa short form appeared to correspond more closely to the scale cutoff of the CES-D 20-item form. The authors also report the results of regression equations, suggesting that the brief forms can be transformed for comparison with results from studies using the original 20-item form. However, the cutoff values for these forms may have to be adjusted from the arithmetic equivalence of the traditional 16 points.

Discussion. The article confirms the good psychometric properties of the CES-D for older adults even when fewer items are included. The problem of multi-item forced-choice responses was eliminated in the East Boston form and reduced in the Iowa form. When one is considering a shorter form, the Iowa 11-item version of the CES-D may be a good choice. This form still requires respondents to choose among three frequency options for each statement; this is less complicated than the original CES-D (with four choices) but more difficult than the East Boston form (response versus no response).

Stommel M, Given BA, Given CW, Kalaian HA, Schulz R, & McCorkle R. (1993). Gender bias in the measurement properties of the Center for Epidemiologic Studies Depression Scale (CES-D). *Psychiatry Res, 49,* 239–250.

Design. This is a cross-sectional, multicenter study of a single administration of the CES-D among cancer patients and their caregivers. The original four-factor model of the CES-D was tested against exploratory models among the cancer patients. The factor model from patients was then tested among caregivers.

Sample. Subjects for the exploratory analyses were 708 diverse cancer patients from three home-care studies. Among the three sites, patients' mean ages were 59, 62, and 63 years (range, 19–89). Patient groups were 70% to 96% white and about 50% women. Confirmatory analyses were conducted on 504 caregivers. Caregivers were mostly white (92.5%) and ranged from 18 to 88 years of age (mean, 63.4).

Summary. These authors found that a three-factor model (excluding the original interpersonal factor) yielded similar properties in both men and women. Fifteen of the original 20 items appeared to yield a relatively better gender-free measurement of depression. The reduced scale correlated very highly with the 20-item scale ($r = 0.98$), and Cronbach's α (alpha) for internal consistency was virtually the same (0.88 versus 0.89 for the full version). The prevalence of depression was still significantly higher for both patient and nonpatient groups of women, but the mean absolute difference between men and women was reduced.

Discussion. These authors' argument for gender bias in the CES-D is largely based on the compelling evidence of a gender-biased factor structure. However, their reduced scale does not remove the traditional interpretation that there is a greater prevalence of depressive symptoms among women. Either women do have a greater propensity for depressive symptoms or there is still a gender bias in the CES-D and other screening tools. Although the study populations represented a wide range of ages, the results are likely to represent older ages because of the older mean ages of the samples.

Applications

Blalock SJ, DeVellis RF, Brown GK, & Wallston KA. (1989). Validity of the Center for Epidemiological Studies Depression Scale in arthritis populations. *Arthritis Rheum*, 32, 991–997.

Design. Arthritis may affect the measurement properties of depression screening scales because of somatic symptoms or other aspects of the disease. These authors report secondary analysis of the CES-D among three study populations of patients with arthritis. Data were analyzed by study rather than aggregated. The CES-D was administered by interviewers in two studies and mailed to subjects in the third. Among the studies, various other measures of psychological distress and health status were also used. The authors examined correlations between the CES-D and pain and lower extremity function. The primary analysis was conducted using a "depression-corrected" measure of health status and the CES-D items to suggest which items were biased for arthritis patients.

Sample. Study 1 was of 67 women whose mean age was 56.6 years; study 2 was of 59 patients, 64% women, whose mean age was 53.2 years; study 3 was of 369 patients, 75% women, whose mean age was 52.7 years.

Summary. Depressive symptoms were significantly correlated with pain in the two studies that included pain measures ($r = 0.63, 0.53$). When regressions of the corrected measures were used, some CES-D items were still strongly correlated. The same was found when measures of lower extremity function were examined. These four items were item 7, "I felt that everything I did was an effort"; item 8, "I felt hopeful about the future"; item 11, "My sleep was restless"; and item 20, "I could not get going." The study groups were then analyzed with a modified CES-D from which these four items were dropped. Not surprisingly, the mean CES-D scores were lower, and the percentage of subjects scoring above the cutoff score of 16 was lower, although not significantly lower. Correlations among other measures of psychological distress and the two versions were nearly identical.

Discussion. Specific items of the CES-D may overestimate depressive symptoms among arthritis patients, but these authors still find that the scale works relatively well. In addition, the authors make a strong argument that such patients have real increases in depressive symptoms.

Blazer D, Burchett B, Service C, & George LK. (1991). The association of age and depression among the elderly: An epidemiologic exploration. *J Gerontol*, 46, M210–M215.

Design. These authors sought to disentangle the various causes of depression from the effect of age. A community-based cross-sectional survey of older adults assessed depressive symptoms using a modified version of the CES-D, physical disability measured by the Nagi Scale and the Rosow and Breslau Scale, chronic illness, cognitive impairment measured by the Short Portable Mental Status Questionnaire (SPMSQ), social support, and economic status. The modified CES-D used all 20 items but collapsed the answers to a yes-no format. This version was considered successful in retaining the original factor structure of the CES-D; when it was tested for potential scoring cutoffs with the original version, a cutoff of 9 points (out of 0 to 20 points) was found to represent the diagnosis of depressive symptoms of the usual CES-D cutoff score of 16 points (out of 0 to 60 points).

Sample.   The CES-D and other study variables were complete for 3,998 of 5,223 selected (76.5%) community-dwelling adults aged 65 and older in the Established Populations for Epidemiologic Studies of the Elderly (EPESE; this sample included only the five communities in the north-central Piedmont of North Carolina). The study sample was selected to balance information by race and rural and urban residence. The group was 62.4% women and 34.9% African American. Subjects' ages were distributed as follows: 63.9% ages 65 to 74, 30.1% ages 75 to 84, and 6.0% ages 85 and older.

Summary.   Chronic conditions were reported for 8.0% of the sample, 22.0% had no functional disability on either the Nagi or the Rosow-Breslau scale, and 8.3% were classified as having cognitive impairment. Nine percent were categorized as having depressive symptoms. The CES-D scores increased with age, as expected in univariate analysis. When regression analysis controlled for the factors of functional disability, cognitive impairment, chronic illness, social support, marital status, and income, the trend was reversed. In this multivariate analysis, depressive symptoms decreased significantly with increasing age.

Discussion.   The study presents data from a large, heterogeneous sample. Despite some bias from nonresponse, the ability to analyze over three quarters of the selected sample is impressive. The authors' use of a modified CES-D with simplified response categories will benefit from use among other populations. The yes-no format may prove particularly useful for telephone interviews, where the usual four-category response can be confusing, as it is not visible to the respondent. The important finding of the study is that increasing prevalence of depressive symptoms with increasing age can be explained by other experiences common to aging (e.g., decreased physical, social, and cognitive function and income, and being unmarried). A prospective cohort study (rather than the cross-sectional data presented here) is needed to explore the causal nature of the factors found to be associated with depressive symptoms among older adults.

Colantonio A, Kasl SV, & Ostfeld AM. (1992). Depressive symptoms and other psychosocial factors as predictors of stroke in the elderly. *Am J Epidemiol*, 136, 884–894.

Design.   This was a prospective cohort study of the effect of psychosocial factors on incidence of stroke. From a population-based sample of older adults, incidence was ascertained using multiple overlapping methods, including vital statistics, hospital admissions, self-reports, and Health Care Financing Administration data. Baseline data were obtained by interviews in 1982 and included physical measures, self-reported medical history, the Pfeiffer scale for cognitive impairment, the Katz Activities of Daily Living Scale, the Rosow and Breslau scale for gross mobility, the Berkman and Syme social network index, a measure of religiousness, and the CES-D. The CES-D was considered positive at a cutoff of 16 points. A Cox proportional hazards model was used to analyze the relative risks of stroke for the primary measure of depressive symptoms and other measures. Correlations among measures were also analyzed with Kendall's τ-β.

Sample.   This is a study derived from the longitudinal Yale Health and Aging Project (YHAP), part of the program Established Populations for Epidemiologic Studies of the Elderly. The current study used the probability sample of 2,812 noninstitutionalized adults aged 65 and older from New Haven, CT. Of individuals sampled, response was 89% for men and women living in public housing and 82% for men and 84% for women living in private housing. Only 24 subjects dropped out of the study. There were 2,604 stroke-free individuals at the baseline interview in 1982 who were followed for incidence of stroke through 1988 ($n = 167$, for an incidence of 0.01 per person-year). These adults were on average 74 years old at baseline, 59% were women, 70% were white, and 40% had annual incomes below $5,000.

Summary. The authors do not report general descriptive results of the psychosocial measures. In univariate analysis, the incidence of stroke increased with increasing quartiles of CES-D scores. Correlations were statistically significant, but only moderate, for a number of combinations of demographic and medical variables and the CES-D. The CES-D score increased the risk of stroke slightly in a univariate Cox model but demonstrated no relationship with stroke in multivariate modeling (i.e., after controlling for other medical and demographic variables).

Discussion. The study found that the usual biomedical and demographic variables were associated with stroke, for example, increasing age and hypertension. None of the psychosocial measures were independently associated with incidence of stroke. The prospective cohort design strengthens this conclusion.

Davidson H, Feldman PH, & Crawford S. (1994). Measuring depressive symptoms in the frail elderly. *J Gerontol, 49,* **P159–P164.**

Design. The deterioration of health among some older adults has been suspected to cause false-positive results with screening for depression because such persons may have high scores on scale items that measure somatic symptoms. The authors report on a study of frail older adults who were the subjects of an evaluation of a cluster care program. In-person interviews in either Spanish or English included the Katz Activity of Daily Living (ADL) scale and the CES-D. The CES-D was considered positive for depressive symptoms at a cutoff score of 16 points. Interviews were repeated after 18 months. The CES-D factor structure (*Radloff, 1977) was retested. The authors also tested for a single, second-order factor structure that would confirm that the CES-D scale could yield a single unified score for depressive symptoms. The somatic factor of the CES-D was further tested against the other factors using Pearson pairwise correlations. Finally, regression analyses were conducted to determine the relationship of demographic and ADL variables to each of the four subscales.

Sample. Subjects were 303 (of 347; 87.3%) frail residents of federally subsidized housing in New York City, aged 65 and older (mean, 79.8 years; range, 65–102). They were also receiving home care services. Eighty-five percent of the group were women, 47% were white, and 26% were Hispanic.

Summary. Mean scores for the CES-D were as follows: 16.7 for men, 18.9 for women, 18.7 for those ages 65 to 84, and 18.2 for those 85 or older. The prevalence of depressive symptoms was among the highest ever reported for a community-dwelling sample: 46.7% of men and 53.9% of women had scores of 16 points or higher. CES-D scores were reported for other demographic and health categories. Only white race and decreased health status, as measured using the Katz ADLs, were associated with a statistically significant increased prevalence of depressive symptoms.

The internal consistency of the CES-D was as high as in other samples (Cronbach's α, alpha = 0.86). The original four-factor model was statistically confirmed, as well as the second-order model confirming a single scale structure. The somatic factor was found to have high correlation with other CES-D factors; this suggests that it measures increasing depressive symptoms in tandem with, and not independently of, other factors. In multivariate regression models, ADL limitations had strong correlations not only with the somatic factor but also with other factors of the CES-D.

Discussion.　While decreasing health was confirmed to be associated with greater depressive symptoms in this study, it was not independently associated with the somatic factor of the CES-D. This finding suggests that the CES-D does not overreport depressive symptoms for the elderly because of a higher prevalence of somatic symptoms. However, the extremely high prevalence of depressive symptoms in this study as measured by the CES-D suggests either that this population is, indeed, at high risk of depressive symptoms, or that the CES-D measures in part some other negative aspect of the study population of poor and frail older adults.

Foelker GA, & Shewchuk RM. (1992). Somatic complaints and the CES-D. *J Am Geriatr Soc*, *40*, 259–262.

Design.　Because of the increasing somatic complaints that accompany the changes in health of older age, these authors tested whether the CES-D tended to yield false positive results in that population. They compared cross-sectional results from the CES-D (especially the somatic subscale) with the Philadelphia Geriatric Center's Multi-Level Assessment Instrument (MAI); specifically, the Physical Health Domain Index (PHDI) composite score and its three component indices were examined. Surveys were administered by interviewers as part of the 1987 Statewide Survey of Alabama Elderly. A score of 16 was considered positive for the CES-D.

Sample.　Participants were 1,060 community-dwelling persons aged 55 and older from 13 rural and urban counties in Alabama. No response figure is given. The group's mean age was 69.1 years. It was 72.9% white and 26.8% African American, and 67.5% women. About one-third reported an annual income under $6,000.

Summary.　The CES-D total score and the somatic scale were not related to age increases in the sample, nor to the PHDI composite score or to the three index scores. Among those screened as depressed, the PHDI and the three indices were not related to the CES-D total score or to three of the four subscales. The CES-D somatic factor was positively related to high total PHDI somatic complaints. However, among the depressed group there were more persons with extreme (high) scores on the CES-D depressive affect scale than on the somatic scale. The authors conclude that the CES-D and its somatic factor are relatively unbiased by the respondent's somatic complaints and that the CES-D can continue to be considered valid under the circumstances of poor health and increasing age.

Discussion.　The study is important in providing evidence that the CES-D is not measuring somatic complaints of aging as depressive symptoms.

Goldstein MS, & Hurwicz ML. (1989). Psychosocial distress and perceived health status among elderly users of a health maintenance organization. *J Gerontol*, *44*, P154–P156.

Design.　This is a cross-sectional survey of older adults enrolling in a Medicare HMO plan in southern California. Telephone interviews consisted of the CES-D, recent life events, a measure of social strain, the Lubben Social Network Scale, and a three-item health status index. The CES-D was considered positive at the usual cutoff score of 16 points. The authors used hierarchial regression modeling to examine the relationships between these measures and health status.

Sample.   Of 1,145 new Medicare enrollees who gave informed consent, 1,034 completed interviews. The authors do not report the number of new enrollees who were eligible. The authors report that about 60% of the sample were women, 38% had education beyond high school, 38% were non-Hispanic whites, and 25% had annual incomes under $25,000. About two thirds were between 65 and 74 years old. The subjects were better educated and healthier and more likely to be white than others in the HMO.

Summary.   Sixty-one percent of subjects were classified as having excellent or good health. During the 6 months prior to the interviews, 44% had not experienced one of 11 life events common to older adults and 22% had experienced 2 or more such events. Only 11.4% scored 16 points or higher on the CES-D. Social support was measured as at least moderately high for 88% of the group. Regression modeling showed that CES-D scores consistently yielded the largest regression coefficients and the largest explained variance in heath status.

Discussion.   This very brief paper does a nice job of looking at interrelationships among measures of psychosocial distress and a very simple measure of health status, but the relationships are cross-sectional in nature, so no inferences about causation can be drawn from the results. The sample was not completely representative of all older adults, but it was typical of HMO enrollees. Depressive symptoms in this group were relatively uncommon, compared with other populations.

Mossey JM, Knott K, & Craik R. (1990). The effects of persistent depressive symptoms on hip fracture recovery. *J Gerontol, 45,* M163–M168.

Design.   This is a secondary analysis of a prospective study of the determinants of recovery from hip fracture. Patients were interviewed after surgery (median lag, 14 days) and at 2, 6, and 12 months postoperatively. Interviews were in person except for a telephone interview at 12 months. Preoperative function was determined by interview and from medical charts. The Short Portable Mental Status Questionnaire (SPMSQ) and the CES-D (cutoff score of 16 points) were administered in interviews. History of prior depression was assessed from five questions of the Eysenck Personality Inventory (EPI). Activities of daily living (ADL) were determined during follow-up interviews. Analyses concentrated first on the general determinants of recovery; then a logistic model was built controlling for strong predictors and examining the effect of persistent depressive symptoms.

Sample.   The patients were recruited from 17 hospitals in the Philadelphia area, and 219 (about 60%) were enrolled in the study between 1984 and 1986. A total of 196 patients had complete data and survived to 12 months for the analyses reported in this paper.

Summary.   Those with consistently low depressive symptoms had the most positive recovery; those with both initially high symptoms and persistently high symptoms were at increased risk of poorer recovery. As expected, older age and poor health preoperatively also were related to poorer outcomes.

Discussion.   The study does not report on those with the poorest outcome (death); such a report might make the findings of the effect of depression on recovery even more dramatic. As expected, age and prior function were strongly related to recovery, but even with these variables in a multivariate model, persistent depressive symptoms had an independent association with poor outcomes. It is possible that the measured variables did not adequately control for the severity of the hip fracture and that the relationship with increased depressive symptoms might be partly confounded. Given the magnitude of the association, however, residual confounding is unlikely to be the only explanation for the association.

Oxman TE, Berkman LF, Kasl S, Freeman DH, & Barrett J. (1992). Social support and depressive symptoms in the elderly. *Am J Epidemiol, 135,* 356–368.

Design.   The results are part of the New Haven Established Populations for Epidemiologic Study of the Elderly. The investigators sought to examine prospectively the impact of social networks and social support on depressive symptoms in the elderly. Individuals were interviewed using a 75-page, 1-hour structured form, including the CES-D (using a cutoff of 16 points), in 1982 and 1985. Other questions included items regarding social network and social support and a 15-item functional disability index (FDI). Change scores were computed by subtraction (CES-D 1985 score minus CES-D 1972 score). In addition to univariate analyses, regression analyses were conducted to seek a model that would explain 1985 CES-D scores.

Sample.   In 1982, 2,806 older adults were interviewed, and 2,487 were alive and interviewed in 1985 (88.6%). The CES-D could be scored (at least 17 items were answered) for 1,962 (79% of those interviewed).

Summary.   The mean CES-D score in 1985 was 8.1, and it was higher for women, compared with men; and higher for those living in public housing, compared with private or community housing. The baseline CES-D, functional status (the FDI), and education explained nearly a quarter of the variance in 1985 CES-D scores. Of the 13 social support and social network variables, four remained significantly associated with the 1985 CES-D in adjusted, multivariate modeling; lower depressive symptoms were associated with contacts with children, other relatives, and friends, and with loss of spouse prior to 1982. The social support variables were also associated with CES-D scores. Decreases in social support from 1982 to 1985 were associated with increased CES-D scores, although changes in social network were not (except for changes involving offspring). The statistical relationship was maintained even when the regression model was adjusted for relevant demographic and health measures. In addition, when older adults lost close relationships (confidants), depression increased. The authors also note that acquiring close relationships did not buffer the effect of loss in older adults as it does in younger persons.

Discussion.   The authors provide concise and well-analyzed prospective data on the relationships among depressive symptoms, social support, and social networks. The number of adults who did not have complete CES-D scales, even though this was a study using trained interviewers, suggests problems in measuring depressive symptoms with this population and may bias the results somewhat.

Salive ME, & Blazer DG. (1993). Depression and smoking cessation in older adults: A longitudinal study. *J Am Geriatr Soc, 41,* 1313–1316.

Design.   This is a prospective cohort study of older adults with self-reported smoking status (including prospective changes in smoking) and an in-person, interviewer-administered CES-D. At baseline, subjects were categorized as current, former, or never smokers. The CES-D scoring was modified to use a yes-no format rather than the traditional symptom frequency scoring (scale scores range from 0 to 20) and using a cutoff score of 9 points or higher to classify individuals as having depressive symptoms. Gender-specific logistic regression models were tested for the relationship between cessation of smoking (outcome) and depressive symptoms and other measured variables. These results are reported for the North Carolina stratified cluster sample of the Established Populations for the Epidemiologic Studies of the Elderly (EPESE).

Sample. At baseline, there were 3,936 subjects with complete data (95% of those who were interviewed). Women were 65.1% of the sample, and 54.2% of the subjects were African American.

Summary. More current smokers had high CES-D scores (11.2%) than either lifelong nonsmokers (9.5%) or former smokers (7.1%). The prevalence of depression for subcategories of subjects by gender, age, and smoking status is also presented in the paper. At the 3-year follow-up, there were too few "relapsed" smokers ($n = 32$) to determine whether depressive symptoms were a risk factor. Women with depressive symptoms were much more likely than other women to stop smoking during the 3 years of follow-up (55% versus 25%). This pattern was not apparent among men. In logistic regression models (controlled by confounding characteristics), depression at baseline was significantly associated with cessation of smoking among women (odds ratio = 3.7) but not among men (odds ratio = 0.6).

Discussion. The results suggest that for both men and women, successful cessation of smoking may not follow the same pattern among older smokers. The paradoxical relationship of depression to successful cessation among older women needs more study.

Stallones L, Marx MB, & Garrity TF. (1990). Prevalence and correlates of depressive symptoms among older U.S. adults. *Am J Prev Med, 6,* 295–303.

Design. These investigators analyze telephone interviews with older adults conducted in 1985 which included the CES-D (cutoff score of 16 points); Holmes and Rahe's Schedule of Recent Events; and other measures of health, health behavior, and social networks. Correlations between depressive symptoms and the other measures were tested in stepwise logistic regression models.

Sample. The subjects were a random sample of 1,232 community-dwelling adults age 65 chosen from across the United States. Of the randomly called telephone numbers, 1,794 were appropriate households for the 1985 survey, and 68.7% of the selected households agreed to participate. Analyses in this report are on 990 individuals with complete data. The group closely resembled the characteristics of adults ages 65 and older from the 1980 Census. The subjects were 60.4% women and 89.7% white, and 20.1% reported annual incomes under $5,000.

Summary. Tables display the proportion of subjects with CES-D scores of 16 points or above separately for the two genders, broken down by categories of the various demographic and health variables. Overall, 9.9% of those sampled scored 16 or above. For both men and women, the prevalence of depressive symptoms increased with increasing age in univariate analyses. These prevalence estimates might be considered as basic comparative data for other studies of older adults. In addition, depressive symptoms increased with decreasing health, lower income, and a number of other tested variables. In the final multivariate model, age was not a factor and the global health rating had the strongest association with depressive symptoms. In addition, subjects' "illness behavior" and the number of clubs and organizations they reported belonging to showed significant associations with depressive symptoms. Interestingly, it appears from the logistic regression analyses that marital status and gender interact so that only among men was being unmarried associated with depression. Recent life events were not correlated with depressive symptoms.

Discussion.   This national probability sample yields lower estimates of the prevalence of depressive symptoms than many studies using the CES-D. The analytic technique of allowing stepwise regression to select the best predictive variables from many should be considered preliminary, and the results should be followed up with more hypothesis-driven research with other populations. However, these exploratory analyses confirm other research findings that poor health and some negative demographic and social factors are associated with depressive symptoms.

Wallace J, & O'Hara MW. (1992). Increases in depressive symptomatology in the rural elderly: Results from a cross-sectional and longitudinal study. *J Abnormal Psychol, 101,* **398–404.**

Design.   These are data from the Iowa component of the Established Populations for Epidemiologic Studies of the Elderly (EPESE). A cross-sectional baseline in-home survey of all residents aged 65 and older in two counties in 1981 and 1982 was followed up 3 and 6 years later. A modified CES-D was used with 11 items and three, rather than four, response categories. The scoring scheme transformed points to represent the standard 20-item scores; and a cutoff score of 16 was used for categorizing a person as having depressive symptoms. In addition, a health history was obtained and questions were asked about instrumental activities of daily living (IADL). Responses to social support items were also collected. Mean CES-D scores were analyzed for differences among groups by baseline characteristics. Multivariate relationships among interview times and other factors were examined with ANOVA, and regression analysis explored baseline predictors of subsequent depressive symptoms.

Sample.   At baseline, 3,159 persons had complete data (of 4,601 residents aged 65 and older in two counties; 68.6%), of whom 2,896 were interviewed at 3 years and 2,259 at 6 years. The baseline characteristics of the sample were as follows: 63% were women (this rose to 66% at 6 years), 23% were ages 80 and older, 38% had an elementary school education, and 21% reported annual incomes under $5,000.

Summary.   At baseline, 9% of subjects were classified as having depressive symptoms, and this rose to 12.2% after 6 years. The proportion rose with age group, was higher for women, and decreased with increasing education and income. Results of the ANOVA suggested that age, gender, and interview were significantly associated with greater CES-D scores, and the scores of the older age groups were more likely to increase than the scores of the younger groups. There were different predictive regression models for the 3- and 6-year follow-up interviews. Baseline CES-D score, education, and social support were predictive of depressive symptoms for both follow-up interviews. Gender was predictive at 3 years, and age was predictive of the 6-year scores. Mean chronic illnesses at baseline predicted depressive symptoms at 6 years only. Depressive symptoms were predicted by IADLs at both times despite the fact that the group overall had very high functioning.

Discussion.   These findings are hard to interpret: Different baseline measures had different effects on future depression depending on the length of follow-up. Perhaps the variables that remained predictive through both time periods should be emphasized if no other cohort analyses show similar patterns. Unfortunately, characteristics found here to predict depression—age, gender, and, to a lesser degree, education—are not amenable to intervention. Physical health, measured by function and chronic illness, showed a strong relationship with depressive symptoms (especially at 6 years). It would be of interest to demonstrate that interventions that improve health status in older adults might decrease depressive symptoms.

Geriatric Depression Scale (GDS)
Development and Methods: Long and Short Forms

Yesavage JA, Brink TL, Rose TL, Lum O, Huang V, Adey M, & Leirer VO. (1983). Development and validation of a geriatric depression screening scale: A preliminary report. *J Psychiat Res, 17*, 37–49.

Design. Results of two studies on the construction as well as reliability and validity of the Geriatric Depression Scale (GDS) were reported. In study 1, an initial item pool of 100 questions believed to distinguish older depressives from normals were generated by a team of geriatric psychiatry clinicians and researchers. Questions covered somatic symptoms, cognitive complaints, motivation, future-past orientation, self-image, losses, agitation, obsessive traits, and mood. A yes-no format was selected for ease of administration. The questionnaire was administered to 47 subjects in paper-and-pencil format to determine the correlation of individual items with the total score. In study 2, the revised 30-item scale was administered to three groups of subjects, along with the Hamilton Rating Scale for Depression (HRS-D; interviewer rating) and the Zung Self-Rating Depression Scale (SDS; self-administered) for determination of reliability and validity of the scale. Order of presentation of questionnaires was randomized across subjects, and interviewers assisted subjects who were unable to complete self-rating forms independently.

Sample. Study 1 had 47 subjects aged 55+ who either were normal older adults living in the community with no reports of depression or history of mental illness, or were hospitalized for depression in several hospitals in California. Study 2 had two groups of subjects: normal older adults recruited at local senior centers and housing projects who had no history of mental illness and were functioning well in the community ($n = 40$), and subjects in treatment for depression in inpatient or outpatient settings at Veterans Administration, county, or private facilities ($n = 60$). This second group was subdivided into subjects with "mild" depression ($n = 26$) or "severe" depression ($n = 34$), using Research Diagnostic Criteria (RDC) and on the basis of a clinical interview.

Summary. In study 1, the 30 items chosen were those that correlated significantly and most highly with the total score (median correlation = 0.675, range = 0.47–0.83). Interestingly, the 12 original somatic items did not correlate highly with total score (median correlation = 0.33, range = 0.02–0.45) and were not included in the final scale. Of the final 30 questions comprising the GDS, 20 indicated depression when answered positively and 10 indicated depression when answered negatively. In study 2, four measures of internal consistency were calculated for each of the three measures of depression: (1) median correlations of items with corrected-item total score (0.56, 0.44, 0.56 for GDS, SDS, and HRS-D, respectively); (2) mean interitem correlations (0.36, 0.25, 0.34 for

GDS, SDS, and HSR-D); (3) Cronbach's α (0.94, 0.87, and 0.90 for GDS, SDS, and HSR-D); and (4) split-half reliability (0.94, 0.81, and 0.82 for GDS, SDS, and HRS-D). Discriminant validity was determined by the ability of the GDS (and the SDS and HRS-D) to classify subjects as normal, mildly depressed, and severely depressed, using separate ANOVAs for depression scores across types of subject. All scales significantly discriminated across groups of subjects, and the scales were significantly correlated with each other (0.80–0.84). Finally, both the GDS and the HSR-D showed a significantly greater relationship with RDC diagnoses than did the SDS.

Discussion.   This article is the most often cited reference to the GDS. Overall, results showed the GDS to be a valid and reliable screening instrument for depression in older adults. Drawbacks to this study include the relatively small sample and the fact that the ''normal'' control group was defined subjectively (i.e., these subjects could also have had depressive symptomatology that would bias comparisons). In addition, the generalizability of this scale to the oldest adults, or to older adults with multiple physical or cognitive challenges, cannot be determined. Some of these issues are addressed in later studies.

Brink TL, Yesavage JA, Lum O, Heersema PH, Adey M, & Rose TL. (1982). Screening tests for geriatric depression. *Clin Gerontol*, *1*, 37–43.

Design.   The development of the Geriatric Depression Scale was described as in *Yesavage et al. (1983), reviewed above. In addition, the 30-item GDS was administered to a separate group of older adults in paper-and-pencil format, along with the Zung SDS (self-administered) and the HRS-D (interviewer ratings) to determine sensitivity and specificity of the GDS in relation to the other two scales.

Sample.   Subjects were 20 normal older adults and 51 geriatric patients receiving treatment for depression (age and recruitment sources not specified).

Summary.   These authors conclude that the GDS offers the best trade-off for sensitivity and specificity relative to the other two scales. At the suggested normal range for older adults (0–10 GDS, 20–45 SDS, 0–10 HRS-D), sensitivity was 84%, 80%, and 86% for the GDS, SDS, and HRS-D, respectively; and specificity was 95%, 85%, and 80% for these three scales, respectively. Sensitivity and specificity are also reported for other possible cutoff scores.

Discussion.   The GDS appears to have the best trade-off between sensitivity and specificity for the population tested. Because data on age, other demographics, recruitment, and diagnosis were not provided for subjects (e.g., whether any subjects in the normal group could be classified as depressed), the comparability of these results with other studies is reduced.

Alden D, Austin C, & Sturgeon R. (1989). A correlation between the Geriatric Depression Scale Long and Short Forms. *J Gerontol Psychol Sci*, *44*, P124–P125.

Design.   The original 30-item GDS Long Form and a 15-item Short Form (Sheikh & Yesavage, 1986) were administered to older adults. Order of administration of the two forms was randomized across subjects, and the forms were administered at a 2-week interval.

Sample.   Subjects were 81 older adults (mean age = 76, range = 58–94 years) in Texas who volunteered to participate. The gender of participants was not reported. The group consisted of 34 residents of a continuing care center, and 47 helpers employed in a program to provide foster grandparents for the mentally retarded.

Summary. Mean scores were significantly lower for the foster grandparents group, as compared with the continuing care group, on both the long and the short forms. (Long Form: mean = 5.66, SD = 4.68 and mean = 11.0, SD = 6.29, respectively, t (80) = 4.33, $p < 0.05$; Short Form: mean = 2.11, SD = 1.84 and mean = 4.71, SD = 3.06, respectively, t (80) = 4.70, $p < 0.05$). The overall correlation between scores on the two forms was significant, though moderate (r = 0.66, $p < 0.01$), with no differences between the two subject groups in the magnitude of the correlation.

Discussion. Although the correlation between the long and short forms was significant, these authors state that it was not sufficiently high to recommend using the GDS Short Form as a substitute for the Long Form. It is possible that the lower correlation obtained in this study, as compared with other studies, is due to the restricted range of GDS scores obtained in this essentially nondepressed sample.

Burke WJ, Roccaforte WH, & Wengel SP. (1991). The Short Form of the Geriatric Depression Scale: A comparison with the 30-item form. *J Geriatr Psychiatry Neurol*, **4,** 173–178.

Design. Two groups of patients were given the GDS Long Form. Patients unable to self-administer the form were assisted by an interviewer. The 15 items of the GDS Short Form were extracted from the Long Form for comparison of the two forms. Results of the GDS were compared with *DSM-III* diagnoses of depression that had been established on the basis of chart review.

Sample. Subjects were 141 patients seen at the University of Nebraska Geriatric Assessment Center over a 2-year period. Two groups of patients were included: 69 cognitively intact patients and 72 patients who had mild dementia of the Alzheimer's type (DAT). Determination of cognitive status was established through a clinical dementia rating (CDR) of patients' charts, in which patients were rated on memory, orientation, judgment, and problem solving, involvement in community affairs, involvement at home and in hobbies, and personal care. This resulting sample included 19% men in the intact group and 29% men in the mild DAT group. Mean age was 77.6 (SD = 7.2) for the intact group and 78.3 (SD = 8.1) for the mild DAT group.

Summary. Data were analyzed using receiver operating characteristic (ROC) curves to examine the ability of the GDS long and short forms to discriminate between depressed and nondepressed patients. Overall, depression was diagnosed in 22% of cognitively intact patients and 14% of patients with mild DAT using *DSM-III* criteria. The GDS Short Form produced an area under the curve (AUC) of 0.86, or 86% of the total area under the curve for intact subjects (Wilcoxon z = 3.55; $p < 0.001$), and an AUC of 0.65 for subjects with mild DAT (Wilcoxon z = 0.54; NS). Similar results were found when subjects were divided into two groups based on scores on the Mini-Mental State Examination. For purposes of screening for depression, the best trade-off of sensitivity and specificity was found for a cutoff of $\geq$ 5, with sensitivity and specificity of 0.93 and 0.48, respectively, for cognitively intact patients; 0.60 and 0.63 for mild DAT; and 0.80 and 0.56 for the total group.

Discussion. Data on the Long Form and on the diagnostic rating procedures are presented elsewhere (*Burke et al., 1989). Overall, results suggested that the GDS Short Form, like the Long Form, is an appropriate screening tool for cognitively intact older adults but loses its validity in patients with mild DAT.

Lesher EL, & Berryhill JS. (1994). Validation of the Geriatric Depression Scale-Short Form among inpatients. *J Clin Psychol, 50,* 256–260.

Design. A battery of tests including the GDS Long Form (GDS-LF) were administered orally to newly admitted psychiatric patients. The 15-item GDS Short Form (GDS-SF) was evaluated using this subset of items from the Long Form. Results were compared with patients' discharge diagnoses assigned by the geropsychiatric treatment staff.

Sample. Subjects were 46 patients with a diagnosis of major depression, 13 patients with a diagnosis of dementia, and 13 patients with a diagnosis of some type of thought disorder. Confirmation of the diagnoses of major depression was conducted by independent chart reviews of patients postdischarge to ensure that the required 5/9 *DSM-III-R* symptoms of major depression were present.

Summary. One-way ANOVAs across patient groups were used to compare scores on the GDS-LF and GDS-SF. Significant overall differences were found for both measures. (GDS-LF: depressed patients, mean = 19.90, SD = 8.11; demented patients, mean = 20.67, SD = 6.39; thought-disordered patients, mean = 10.08, SD = 4.75. GDS-SF: depressed patients, mean = 8.04, SD = 4.62; demented patients, mean = 2.69, SD = 3.77; thought-disordered patients, mean = 5.31, SD = 2.67.) For the GDS-SF, a comparison of group means showed each patient group to be significantly different from both of the others in GDS-SF scores. For the GDS-LF, all groups were different from each other, except for the patients with dementia and the patients with thought disorders, whose scores were not significantly different. The GDS-LF and GDS-SF were highly correlated for the total sample (r = 0.89, p < 0.001) and for each group; the lowest correlation was for dementia patients (r = 0.60, p < 0.001). Sensitivity ranged from 0.72 to 0.91 for GDS-SF cutoff scores ranging from 5–10 for the total sample; specificity ranged from 0.54 to 0.92. For the GDS-LF, similar sensitivity (ranging from 0.70 to 0.91) and specificity (ranging from 0.42 to 0.85) were found. For the demented and thought-disordered patients, sensitivity ranged from 0.77 to 0.92 and 0.31 to 0.85, respectively, across cutoff scores for the GDS-SF; and from 0.38 to 0.85 and 0.46 to 0.85, respectively, for the GDS-LF.

Discussion. The GDS-SF is a reasonable substitute for the GDS-LF, with a cutoff of ≥ 7 recommended as optimal. Both scales have similar and adequate sensitivity but may overdiagnose depression in demented and thought-disordered groups.

Baker FM, & Miller CL. (1991). Screening a skilled nursing home population for depression. *J Geriatr Psychiatry Neurol, 4,* 218–221.

Design. All patients in a skilled nursing facility serving the Audie L. Murphy Memorial Veterans Hospital were screened for the presence of depression. Patients were interviewed using the MMSE, Hamilton Depression Scale, and 15-item GDS Short Form in a single session (unless additional sessions were required to complete the forms). Patients scoring ≥ 6 on the GDS or ≥ 18 on the Hamilton were evaluated by senior psychiatry residents for depression using *DSM-III-R* criteria. Order of presentation of forms was not specified.

Sample. Of 80 patients approached, 74% (n = 59) were able to complete most of the battery. The final sample consisted of 57 men and 2 women, of whom 73% were white,

7% were African American, and 20% were Mexican American. Subjects had a mean age of 70 and an average of seven medical problems and five medications per patient.

Summary. A total of 33 patients (56%) were referred to the psychiatry residents for evaluation; 20 (61%) were classified as depressed, with a *DSM-III-R* diagnosis of major depressive disorder or adjustment disorder with depressed mood. When either the Hamilton alone or GDS alone was positive, 1 of 7 patients (14%) and 6 of 11 (54%) patients, respectively, were diagnosed as depressed. When elevated GDS score was combined with increasing Hamilton scores, the concordance with diagnosis of depression increased. For example, for patients with a GDS score of 6–10 and a Hamilton score of 30–45, 100% had a diagnosis of depression.

Discussion. The Hamilton Depression Scale was less effective than the GDS in identifying depression in the older medical sample, unless patients were quite symptomatic (i.e., scored above 24). In addition, the scale was difficult for patients to answer. The GDS yes-no format was easier for patients and relatively effective at identifying depression in frail elderly veterans in a skilled nursing home. Several methodological problems were present. The reliability of diagnoses of depression was not provided. In addition, only patients who scored above a certain score on the GDS or Hamilton were referred for diagnosis of depression; this made it impossible to assess the false negative rate of either of the two screening instruments. Finally, because only subjects with depressive symptoms were referred for diagnosis, psychiatry residents were not blinded to mood status of patients and thus may have been biased in their ratings.

Burke WJ, Houston MJ, Boust SJ, & Roccaforte W. (1989). Use of the Geriatric Depression Scale in dementia of the Alzheimer type. *J Am Geriatr Soc, 37*, 856–860.

Design. The validity of the GDS as a screen for depression in elderly adults with dementia of the Alzheimer type (DAT) was evaluated. All patients seen at the University of Nebraska Geriatric Assessment Center over a 2-year period were targeted. Patients were assessed on a number of variables; those relevant to the present chapter were measures of cognitive status (e.g., MMSE), functional status (IADL), and mood (GDS). The GDS was self-administered, with assistance as needed. Patients were seen on an "as needed" basis by a psychiatrist or psychologist in year 1, and routinely by one of two geropsychiatrists (the authors) in year 2, independently of subjects' scores on the GDS. To establish consistent diagnoses, the geropsychiatrists reviewed patients' records from year 1 and assigned a *DSM-III* diagnosis and clinical dementia rating (CDR). Interrater reliability for the CDR was adequate for a subsample of 50 patients ($\kappa = 0.83$).

Sample. Of 283 patients evaluated, 184 were selected, including patients who either were cognitively intact ($n = 70$) or had DAT ($n = 72$; CDR ratings of 0 or 1). The final sample included 81% and 71% women for the intact and DAT groups, respectively, with a mean age of 77.7 years ($SD = 7.1$) and 78.3 years ($SD = 8.1$), respectively. Diagnoses of major depression were given to 21% of intact patients and 14% of DAT patients.

Summary. ROC curves were used to assess the ability of the GDS to discriminate between the two subject groups regardless of cutoff score. For the total sample, the area under the curve (AUC) was 0.77 ($z = 5.33$, $p < 0.0001$). For cognitively intact subjects, the GDS produced an AUC of 0.85 ($z = 6.35$, $p < 0.0001$). For DAT subjects, the AUC was 0.66 ($z = 1.92$, NS). For intact subjects, sensitivity and specificity were maximized with cutoffs in the range of 14–16 (sensitivity and specificity were 80% and 78% to 73%

and 88%, respectively). For DAT subjects, no cutoff could be identified at which sensitivity and specificity both exceeded 65%.

Discussion. This study supported the use of the GDS in cognitively intact older adults but found that it was no better than chance in identifying depression in patients with mild dementia of the Alzheimer type. Note that the sample of depressed subjects in the DAT group was quite small ($n = 7$). The reader is also referred to comments by Christensen and Dysken (1990) and the response by Burke, Roccaforte, and Boust (1990).

Burke WJ, Nitcher RL, Roccaforte WH, & Wengel SP. (1992). A prospective evaluation of the Geriatric Depression Scale in an outpatient geriatric assessment center. *J Am Geriatr Soc, 40*, 1227–1230.

Design. This study evaluated the GDS in cognitively intact versus impaired outpatients at a geriatric assessment clinic, in comparison with prospective clinical diagnoses by geriatric psychiatrists. All patients evaluated at the clinic over a 1-year period underwent a comprehensive medical examination, cognitive evaluation including the MMSE, and measures of physical status (Illness Rating Scale) and functional status (ADL and IADL). Patients self-administered the GDS, with assistance as needed. All patients were also evaluated by one of three geriatric psychiatrists who were blinded to the results of the GDS. The diagnosis of major depression was based on *DSM-III-R* criteria and made after a team meeting in which medical information and patients' records' were reviewed. Measures of interrater reliability were not obtained, although a comparison of mean number of GDS symptoms reported by patients classified as depressed or not depressed showed no differences across psychiatrists.

Sample. From a target group of 194 patients, 6 were excluded because of severe dementia (CDR 3), and an additional 6 did not complete the GDS. The final sample of 182 subjects included 67 cognitively intact patients (MMSE > 23; mean = 26.8, $SD = 1.9$) and 115 impaired patients (MMSE < 24; mean = 17.1, $SD = 5.2$). This sample included 66% females in the intact group and 74% females in the impaired group, with a mean age of 77.2 years ($SD = 6.5$) and 78.6 years ($SD = 6.9$), respectively, for the intact and impaired groups. Overall, 21% of patients were given a diagnosis of major depression (24% and 20% for the intact and impaired groups, respectively).

Summary. Receiver-operating characteristic curves (ROCs) were used to compare the utility of the GDS in cognitively impaired versus intact groups. For the total group, the area under the curve (AUC) was 0.81 ($z = 5.2$, $p < 0.0001$). AUCs for the cognitively impaired group and the intact group, respectively, were similar (0.82, $z = 4.0$, $p < 0.0001$; 0.80, $z = 3.1$, $p < 0.0002$). A separate ROC curve was examined for subjects diagnosed with possible or probable Alzheimer's disease, with an AUC of 0.88 ($z = 3.9$, $p < 0.0001$). The optimal cutoff score for the total group was 14, with a sensitivity of 59% and a specificity of 77% (sensitivity and specificity for the impaired group and the intact group, respectively, were 74% and 66%, and 81% and 61%). Sensitivity and specificity for cutoffs of 14 and 17 are reported; sensitivity appeared to decrease more for intact versus impaired subjects at higher cutoff levels.

Discussion. The authors conclude that the GDS is as effective in screening for depression in cognitively impaired patients as in intact patients. They speculate that the high concordance between GDS scores and clinical diagnosis is related to the use of geriatric psychiatrists, who may be more sensitive to depression in older adults than are nongeriatric specialists. The authors also caution, however, that the methodology of this study—whereby patients are assessed using the GDS and by the psychiatrist on the same day—may provide more favorable results than when there is a greater test-retest interval.

Kafonek SD, Ettinger WH, Roca R, Kittner S, Taylor N, & German PS. (1989). Instruments for screening for depression and dementia in a long-term care facility. _J Am Geriatr Soc_, 37, 29–34.

Design. The sensitivity and specificity of the GDS and the MMSE were examined by comparing scores with clinical diagnoses of depression and cognitive impairment determined by psychiatric examination for patients newly admitted to an academic nursing home facility. Within 3 weeks of admission, subjects were given the GDS and MMSE by a trained interviewer blind to other evaluations. For the GDS, a cutoff of ≥ 14 was used to indicate clinical depression. Subjects were interviewed by a psychiatrist within 6 weeks of admission for determination of a *DSM-III* diagnosis of depression, dementia, or delirium. The psychiatrist was blinded to the results of other scores. Each patient was also given a social assessment and physical examination and was assessed on the New York ADL scale.

Sample. Subjects were new admissions, ages 65+, to the skilled or intermediate level of care. Chronic care patients were excluded. Of the 169 eligible patients, 70 completed all parts of the study. Reasons for exclusion were refusal to participate, death of patient, transfer of patient, patient's inability to respond to assessments, and others. Subjects were similar to nonparticipants in demographic and diagnostic characteristics. Of the 70 subjects, 41 were diagnosed as demented, 13 as delirious and 15 as depressed; 1 was undetermined.

Summary. Results are reported here for the GDS only. Sensitivity and specificity for the GDS were reported to be 47% and 75% for the total sample. For subjects who were cognitively impaired (MMSE ≤ 23) versus cognitively intact (MMSE ≥ 24), the sensitivity and specificity of the GDS was 25% and 75%, and 75% and 75%, respectively.

Discussion. The authors suggest that the GDS is not sensitive to depression in a nursing home population. This may be largely due to its inability to detect depression in cognitively impaired residents. Note the small sample of depressed patients ($n = 15$) and the lack of validation of the psychiatrist's diagnosis. This study may have also included subjects who were more cognitively impaired that those in studies showing more favorable results. In a later reply to a letter to the editor, the authors state that the cognitively impaired group included 9 subjects who were unable to answer most of the questions on the GDS; these 9 subjects had a mean MMSE score of 4.8. The reader is referred to two letters to the editor and the authors' reply (Brink, 1989; Kafonek & Roca, 1989; Snowdon, 1990).

Koenig HG, Meador KG, Cohen HJ, & Blazer DG. (1992). Screening for depression in hospitalized elderly medical patients: Taking a closer look. _J Am Geriatr Soc_, 40, 1013–1017.

Design. This study evaluated the GDS and the Brief Carroll Depression Rating Scale (BCDRS) in men who were inpatients at a Veterans Administration medical center, using procedures typically found in applied clinical use of these scales as screening instruments. In such cases, the screening instrument is used first, followed by a diagnostic workup on a subsequent day for patients who score above an identified cutoff point. The authors state that previous studies evaluating these scales have not appropriately simulated real medical practice, and diagnostic workups have either preceded or immediately followed screening. In the present study, consecutive admissions of men ages 70+ who scored 15 or higher on the MMSE were targeted. Within 48 hours of admission, a social worker administered the 30-item GDS (assisted self-administration) and 12-item BCDRS. The next day, a fellow in geriatric medicine conducted a structured psychiatric interview with patients using the affective disorders section of the NIMH Diagnostic Interview Schedule (DIS). Data from the DIS and other psychological and medical record information were reviewed by a geropsychiatrist who made a clinical diagnosis of major depression using *DSM-III-R* criteria.

Sample.   Seventy percent of potential participants were screened; most patients who were excluded had MMSE scores less than 15. The final sample of 109 patients had a mean age of 74 years ($SD = 4.1$), and 27.3% were African American.

Summary.   Sensitivity and specificity rates for the two tests are as follows: GDS cutoff 11+: 0.82 and 0.76; GDS cutoff 14+: 0.55 and 0.90; BCDRS cutoff 6+: 0.73 and 0.79; BCDRS cutoff 7+: 0.36 and 0.93. Posttest probabilities for major depression were calculated. For the GDS, the positive predictive values (PPV) were 27% and 40% for cutoffs of ≥ 11 and ≥ 14, respectively. The negative predictive values (NPV) were 97% and 95%, respectively, for these same cutoffs. For the BCDRS, the PPV was 28% and 36% for cutoffs of 6 and 7, respectively, and the NPV was 96% and 93% for these cutoffs. When cognitively impaired patients (MMSE < 26) were excluded, the sensitivity of the GDS increased to 89% and the specificity was similar at 75% for a cutoff of 11.

Discussion.   These authors state that in this simulation of actual medical screening procedures, the sensitivity and specificity of both the GDS and the BCDRS were lower than in previous studies using different procedures. Overall, the GDS performed somewhat better than the BCDRS, and the GDS performed better in cognitively intact patients than in impaired patients. Note that the reliability and validity of the clinical diagnoses of depression were not assessed in this study. Whether results generalize to women patients is also unknown.

McGivney SA, Mulvihill M, & Taylor B. (1994). Validating the GDS depression screen in the nursing home. *J Am Geriatr Soc*, *42*, 490–492.

Design.   This study examined the sensitivity and specificity of the GDS for nursing home patients, with a focus on identifying the lowest Mini-Mental State Exam (MMSE) score for which the GDS is valid. All admissions to two nursing homes in New York City were screened over a 4-month period. Appropriate subjects were given a psychiatric assessment, the MMSE, and the 30-item GDS (by interviewers). The psychiatric assessment evaluated patients on *DSM-III-R* criteria for major depression, depressive symptoms, and no depression. Two psychiatrists both evaluated a pilot group of 30 patients with a high level of interrater reliability ($\kappa = 0.93$); thereafter, all subsequent patients were assessed by only one psychiatrist. Psychiatrists and interviewers were blinded to each other's findings. Order of the GDS, MMSE, and psychiatric evaluations was randomized across patients. A cutoff of ≥ 10 was used on the GDS.

Sample.   Of the 166 patients screened, 66 were selected for participation. Criteria for exclusion were: (1) death of patient; (2) inability to complete all three assessments, including MMSE score of < 5, aphasia, severe hearing deficiency, or language deficiency; (3) failure to complete testing within 2 weeks to 2 months after admission; and (4) refusal to participate. The final sample included 47 women (71%), with an average age of 83 years (*SD* = 4; range, 66–97).

Summary. For the total sample, the sensitivity and specificity of the GDS were 63% and 83%, respectively. For the subgroup with MMSE scores ≥ 15 (*n* = 42), the sensitivity and specificity of the GDS were 84% and 91%, respectively. For the subgroup with MMSE scores ≤ 14 (*n* = 24), sensitivity and specificity were considerably lower (27% and 69%, respectively).

Discussion. This study appeared methodologically sound, with criteria for selecting subjects clearly identified and high reliability for diagnostic procedures. Results validated the GDS for nursing home residents who score ≥ 15 on the MMSE. The authors recommend a two-step screening of nursing home patients, first to select residents with MMSE scores ≥ 15 and then to administer the GDS to this group. The detection of depression in residents with severe dementia under this system remains challenging.

Parmelee PA, Lawton MP, & Katz IR. (1989). Psychometric properties of the Geriatric Depression Scale among the institutionalized aged. *Psychol Assess*, *1*, 331–338.

Design. This study examined the reliability and validity of the GDS in a large sample of residents of a nursing home and congregate housing. All new admissions to either facility were targeted over a 28-month period, and current residents were sampled over a 12-month period. Appropriate subjects were interviewed by trained research assistants using the following measures: (1) GDS (30 items), with up to 20% missing items allowed (6 items); (2) depressive symptomatology using a 35-item checklist drawn from the Schedule for Affective Disorders and Schizophrenia (SADS). Interrater reliability checks on 46 interviews yielded ≥ 86.7% interrater agreement and κ coefficients ranging from 0.43 to 0.86 (mean = 0.73) across scales; (3) cognitive status, using a modified Blessed test; and (4) functional status using the Physical Self-Maintenance Scale (PSMS). In addition, depression ratings were obtained by direct care staff using the Raskin Depression Scale, and physical health ratings were obtained using the Cumulative Illness Rating Scale (CIRS). Finally, residents identified by interviewers as suffering from cognitive impairment (Blessed score of ≥ 11 errors) or any dysphoria or psychopathology were referred for separate evaluation by the psychology and psychiatry departments. It should be noted that the determination of absence of depression was not systematically confirmed, although 130 of the 249 patients identified as nondepressed by the GDS and by clinical standards were evaluated by the psychology and psychiatry departments.

Sample. Of 1,327 residents targeted, 521 (38.4%) were excluded for reasons including refusal to participate, cognitive impairment that prevented response, and physical limitations (speech or hearing deficits or severe physical illness). The final sample of 806 subjects included 70% women and ranged in age from 61 to 99 years (mean = 83.8). Two subjects were African American; the others were white. Just over one third (38.5%) lived in the nursing home, and the remainder lived in the congregate housing, with an overall average length of stay of 25.2 months (*SD* = 42.2). Compared with nonparticipants, participants were more likely to be men, younger, more recently admitted, and living in the congregate housing, and to have less cognitive impairment and higher physical functioning.

Summary. Only 51.7% of subjects completed all GDS items. The two items omitted by more than 10% of residents were: "Do you think that most people are better off than you are?" (10.3%) and "Is it hard for you to get started on new projects?" (12.4%). The reliability of the GDS was examined for the 417 subjects who completed all items. The scale was internally consistent (standardized $\alpha = 0.91$) and had a high test-retest reliability ($r = 0.85$; $p < 0.001$). A principal components analysis showed that although the scale was essentially unidimensional, six rotated factors could be identified: (1) dysphoria (eigenvalue = 8.96, 29.9% of variance); (2) worry (1.85, 6.2%); (3) withdrawal and apathy (1.48, 4.9%); (4) vigor (1.22, 4.1%); (5) decreased concentration (1.15, 3.8%); and (6) anxiety (1.03, 3.4%). Concurrent validity of the GDS was examined in three ways. First, a significant, though moderate, correlation ($r = 0.27$–0.33) was found between GDS scores and subscales of the staff-rated Raskin Depression Scale. Second, GDS cutoffs of 17+ (possible major depression), minor depression (11–16.9), and < 11 (no depression) were used to compare GDS scores with *DSM-III-R* diagnoses based on the SADS checklist of symptoms. In 73% of cases, the two classifications were in agreement on level of depression (major, minor, or none; $\kappa = 0.42$), and in 79.9% of cases they agreed on presence versus absence of depression. Using the *DSM-III-R* diagnosis as the criterion, the GDS resulted in 6.8% false negatives overall and 36% for minor depression, and 13.4% false positives. Finally, GDS scores were compared with clinical diagnoses; results were similar to those obtained for *DSM-III-R* diagnoses. Overall agreement between the GDS and clinical diagnoses was 67.5% for level of depression and 78% for presence versus absence of depression, with 13.8% overall false negataives and 16.7% and 40.9% false negatives, respectively, for major and minor depression. The sensitivity and specificity for the GDS were (respectively) 0.69 and 0.86 for presence of any clinically diagnosed depression, and 0.54 and 0.91 for major depression. No differences were found in reliability and validity between subjects who were cognitively intact and those who were mildly to moderately impaired (Blessed scores of ≤ 10 and ≥ 11, respectively). Relationships among GDS subscales, determined from the principal components analysis, and other variables of demographics, mood, and health were calculated using multivariate analyses of variance and Hotelling F tests.

Discussion. Overall, results supported the reliability and validity of the GDS with institutionalized residents, although a problem with false negatives was found for the identification of minor depressions. In this study—unlike previous work (e.g., *Burke et al., 1989)—no differences were found in reliability and validity between residents who were cognitively intact and those who were mildly to moderately impaired. In a subsequent letter to the editor (Parmelee & Katz, 1990), the authors speculate that this difference in findings may be attributed to the mode of administration of the GDS, which was in an interview format for the study by Parmelee et al. (*1989) and in an assisted self-administered format in the report by Burke et al. (*1989). The present study provides the most thorough description of methods and findings, along with a large sample, of the psychometric studies of the GDS. Note, however, that about one half of the subjects were unable to complete the GDS. This is not uncommon for nursing home studies, and screening for depression in this group remains challenging.

Applications

Agrell B, & Dehlin O. (1989). Comparison of six depression rating scales in geriatric stroke patients. *Stroke, 20,* 1190–1194.

Design.   Three self-rating scales (GDS, Zung SDS, and CES-D) and three examiner-rating scales (Hamilton Rating Scale, Comprehensive Psychopathological Rating Scale-Depression, and Cornell Scale) were compared with each other and with clinical ratings of depression for elderly stroke patients. Patients were recruited from an outpatient day hospital, a geriatric rehabilitation clinic, and a nursing home. Subjects were assessed over a 2- to 3-day period on all measures by the same investigator (order of administration was unspecified). Patients self-administered the three self-rating scales with assistance as needed. A clinical evaluation was used to provide a global rating of depression (no depression; minimal depression not interfering with social functioning; unmistakable but moderate depression; and serious, disabling depression). The Bartel Index was used to provide an evaluation of ADLs.

Sample.   Subjects were 40 patients (18 men and 22 women), with a mean age of 80 years (range 61–93) and a mean period of 14 months (range, 4 months–2.5 years) since their stroke. The criteria for exclusion were MMSE < 20 (although a small unspecified number with lower scores were included if they were deemed able to complete the assessments) and dysphasia. Forty-three percent of patients were classified as depressed by the global ratings.

Summary.   Results are presented for the self-rating scales only. Assessment of internal consistency showed that some items were not significantly correlated with the sum of the scores for each scale. On the GDS, those were item 1 ("Are you basically satisfied with your life?"), item 2 ("Have you dropped many of your activities and interests?"), item 12 ("Do you prefer to stay at home, rather than going out and doing new things?"), and item 14 ("Do you feel you have more problems with memory than most?"). For the Zung SDS, they were item 4 ("I have trouble sleeping at night") and item 9 ("My heart beats faster than usual"). On the CES-D, item 10 ("I felt fearful"), item 15 ("People were unfriendly"), and item 19 ("I felt that people disliked me") lacked internal consistency. The three scales were highly correlated with each other ($r = 0.81$–0.88; $p < 0.001$) and significantly correlated with the global ratings ($r = 0.75$, 0.72, and 0.73 for the GDS, Zung SDS, and CES-D, respectively, $p < 0.001$). The sensitivity and specificity for the GDS (cutoff 10), Zung (cutoff 45), and CES-D (cutoff 20) were 88%/64%, 76%/96%, and 56%/91%, respectively. Corresponding positive predictive values (PPV) were 58%, 93%, and 82%, respectively; and negative predictive values (NPV) were 88%, 84%, and 75%, respectively.

Discussion.   The authors conclude that, in terms of internal consistency, sensitivity, and predictive value, the best self-rating scales for use in the geriatric stroke population are the GDS and the Zung SDS. Note the small sample, the lack of data on reliability and validity for global ratings, and the lack of clarity regarding methodology. This paper is notable, however, in that it extends the use of these screening instruments to a stroke population.

Bolla-Wilson K, & Bleecker ML. (1989). Absence of depression in elderly adults. *J Gerontol Psychol Sci, 44*, P53–P55.

Design.   This study examined differences in depression scores for older and younger community-dwelling volunteers enrolled in the Johns Hopkins Teaching Nursing Home Study of Normal Aging. Because of the increase in physical illness associated with aging, particular attention was given to differences by age in response to somatic (versus affective) items on depression scales. Subjects were sent a packet of questionnaires that included the 30-item GDS (self-administered), the Minnesota Multiphasic Personality Inventory (MMPI), and the Beck Depression Inventory (BDI). The MMPI and BDI include more somatic items than the GDS does. The following cutoffs were used to indicate depression: GDS: > 18, MMPI: > 70, BDI: > 10.

Sample.   Subjects were 212 healthy volunteers (91 men and 121 women), recruited through newspapers, who ranged in age from 40 to 89 years, with 7–22 years of education. Subjects were classified as "young" if $\leq$ 60 years old (n = 40 men, 51 women), and "old" if > 60 (n = 52 men and 70 women). Subjects were excluded if they had any of a range of medical conditions, including stroke, uncontrolled hypertension, sleep disorders, and psychiatric disorders.

Summary.   Older adults did not report significantly more depressive symptoms relative to younger (middle-aged) adults. The mean scores on the GDS were 6.95 (SD = 15.66) for younger men, 5.40 (SD = 3.66) for older men, 5.67 (SD = 3.97) for younger women, and 7.80 (SD = 12.11) for older women. The comparable scores for the BDI were 4.62 (SD = 4.92) for younger men, 4.25 (SD = 3.66) for older men, 4.65 (SD = 3.93) for younger women, and 5.88 (SD = 4.68) for older women. Women scored significantly higher on the MMPI than men overall and for symptoms of physical malfunctioning. There were no differences across gender in the overall BDI and GDS scores. On the BDI, older subjects reported more somatic symptoms than younger subjects but did not differ on psychological-affective symptoms.

Discussion.   The authors conclude that the higher rate of depressive symptoms among older versus younger adults reported in earlier studies may be due to the higher rate of endorsement of somatic symptoms among older adults. The authors recommend using a depression scale such as the GDS that focuses on affective (versus somatic) symptoms. Although the increase in scores on the somatic items of the BDI with age supports this conclusion, it is interesting that there was no association between age and the overall BDI score. Note that because this is part of a study of normal aging, subjects with a wide range of physical and psychiatric illnesses were excluded, and thus the sample may not be representative of the general older population. The age bias produced by somatic symptoms might be more severe in a less healthy population. In addition, the "young" comparison group was primarily middle-aged, and the results may differ from the findings of studies including younger groups as comparators.

Fulop G, Reinhardt J, Strain JJ, Paris B, Miller M, & Fillit H. (1993). Identification of alcoholism and depression in a geriatric medicine outpatient clinic. *J Am Geriatr Soc*, 41, 737–741.

Design.   This was a cross-sectional study to evaluate the utility of screening instruments for alcoholism and depression among older medical outpatients. Patients seen at a geriatric outpatient medical clinic were interviewed using two alcohol screening measures— Michigan Alcohol Screening Test (MAST) and the CAGE—and the 30-item GDS. For the GDS, the following cutoffs were used: 0–10, no depression; 11–20, mild depression; 21–30, moderate to severe depression.

Sample.   Subjects were selected from 328 older adults who visited the Mount Sinai Medical Center's Coffey Geriatric Outpatient Clinic during a 20-day period. Criteria for exclusion were speaking only Spanish (n = 73), being demented (n = 70), and administrative reasons and errors (e.g., not being asked to participate, not being on the first visit; 86). Of the 99 eligible patients, 15 refused. The final sample consisted of 84 patients with a mean age of 77 years ($SD = 6.8$). Seventy-six percent were women; 27.4% were white; 53.6% were African American; 19.0% were Hispanic; 54.8% lived alone; and 53.6% reported never using alcohol.

Summary. The alcohol screening instruments did not identify patients who had not previously been identified by the clinic staff as alcohol abusers. Conversely, 32% of patients scored in the depressed range on the GDS (26% mild depression, 6% moderate to severe depression), of whom only one-third had been identified by the clinic staff as depressed.

Discussion. The GDS may be a useful adjunct to clinicians in identifying patients with depressive symptoms in an outpatient geriatric population. The relation between GDS scores and clinical diagnoses of depression was not examined.

Koenig HG, Cohen HJ, Blazer DG, Pieper C, Meador KG, Shelp F, Goli V, & DiPasquale B. (1992). Religious coping and depression among elderly, hospitalized medically ill men. *Am J Psychiatry*, *149*, 1693–1700.

Design. Research on the role and effectiveness of "religious coping" in medical illness (that is, using religion as a means of coping) has been unclear. This study evaluated the frequency of religious coping and its relation to depression among older medical inpatients. Men ages 65+ who were admitted to the medical or neurological service of a Veterans Administration medical center over a 16-month period were screened for depression, using the 30-item GDS (interview format; score ≥ 11 indicating depression) and Hamilton Rating Scale for Depression (score ≥ 15 indicating depression). A number of functional and physical health and sociodemographic measures were also collected, along with a Mini-Mental State Examination (MMSE) and a measure of religious coping. Measures of internal consistency, test-retest reliability, and interrater reliability for the religious-coping index were adequate and ranged from 0.81 to 0.87. A subsample of subjects who were readmitted to the medical or neurological services during the study and in the 5 months afterward were reevaluated on the GDS and the religious-coping measure.

Sample. Criteria for inclusion were (among others): MMSE score of ≥ 15, being physically capable of undergoing a psychiatric evaluation, and not being a psychiatric patient. Of the 1,110 new patients during the study period, 260 did not participate, for reasons that included advanced dementia and delirium. Nonparticipants were more likely to be older, African American, and residents of nursing homes, and to have neurological or respiratory illnesses. The final sample of 850 men averaged 69.8 years of age, with 8.9 years of education, a mean annual income of $8,582, and a mean MMSE score of 26.4. Of these, 28.3% were African American, 67.9% were married, and 22.1% scored ≥ 11 on the GDS. A range of Christian religious groups were represented, with the largest group indicating conservative or African American Protestant affiliations (63%). A total of 202 subjects were screened at a second admission; these subjects differed from the total sample only in diagnosis (they were more likely to have cancer and less likely to have a neurologic disease).

Summary. On the first-religious coping question, regarding general coping strategies, 20% of subjects spontaneously mentioned religion. Mean ratings of the helpfulness or importance of religious coping were 6.5 ($SD = 3.1$) and 5.7 ($SD = 3.2$), respectively, for subjects' and interviewers' ratings. The mean religious-coping index score was 14.3 (*SD* = 8.7) out of a possible 30 points. Stepwise regression analysis indicated that variables associated with religious coping were race (African American), age (older), being retired, belonging to a fundamentalist Protestant denomination, having high social support, using little or no alcohol, a history of psychiatric problems, and higher cognitive status. Controlling for health and sociodemographic variables, religious coping was inversely and significantly related to depression for both the GDS and the Hamilton. Analyses of follow-up data for the 202 readmissions indicated that religious coping at time 1 was the only baseline predictor of follow-up coping; again, an inverse relationship was found.

Discussion.   Religious coping was inversely related to depression in older, hospitalized men. Causal relationships and the generalizability of these findings to other sociodemographic populations and non-Christian religions remain unknown.

Koenig HG, Ford SM, & Blazer DG. (1993). Should physicians screen for depression in elderly medical inpatients? Results of a decision analysis. *Int J Psychiatry Med*, 23, 239–263.

Design.   A decision analysis was used to determine the utility of three courses of action for clinicians treating older medical inpatients: (1) screen all patients for depression with a measure such as the GDS, (2) screen all patients for depression using clinical assessment, and (3) do not screen patients for depression. As is typical of this type of analysis, a number of assumptions (e.g., that tricyclic antidepressants—TCAs—are the only treatment for depression in this setting), probabilities, and utilities (i.e., value of various outcomes) were used in developing a decision tree and analyzing projected outcomes for each course of action.

Sample.   Results from a range of studies and consensus of the authors were used to generate the data entered into the decision analysis.

Summary.   Results indicated that, assuming that TCAs are the only modality of treatment, the best decision regarding screening for depression is to do nothing. However, there was a very small difference (0.04 units on a 0–100 scale) between this and the other two possible outcomes; thus the decision regarding screening is a virtual toss-up. These authors note, though, that even small modifications in clinical or test characteristics could give screening a higher utility. For example, screening with the GDS has the highest utility in settings where medical contraindications, spontaneous remissions, and side effects are low. Conversely, *not* screening has the highest utility when patients are physically sicker and less responsive to antidepressants. In addition, if psychotherapy is considered as the primary treatment, screening becomes the method of choice.

Discussion.   Decision analyses can be used to guide clinical decision making. The present study suggested that the utility of the decision to screen (and how to screen) is influenced by clinical and test characteristics, as well as by the intended treatment modality. Readers are encouraged to review the full report to evaluate the assumptions, probabilities, and utilities used in this analysis.

Koenig HG, Meador KG, Goli V, Shelp F, Cohen HJ, & Blazer DG. (1992). Self-rated depressive symptoms in medical inpatients: Age and racial differences. *Int J Psychiatry Med*, 22, 11–31.

Design. This study was part of the Durham Veterans Administration (VA) Mental Health Survey and provides a cross-sectional examination of age and racial differences in symptoms of depression in men who were medical inpatients. Over a 16-month period from September 1987 to January 1989, all men under age 40 and over age 65 who were admitted to medical or neurological services were screened for depression. Within 48 hours of admission, patients were interviewed by a social worker regarding sociodemographic and health data. Patients also self-administered the 30-item GDS, with assistance as needed; a cutoff of ≥ 11 was used to indicate depression. A subgroup of patients were also administered the Hamilton Depression Rating Scale (HDRS) by a fellow in geriatric medicine; order of administration of the HDRS and the GDS was varied across patients.

Sample. Of 1,303 new admissions over the 16-month period, 1,011 were included in the present analysis, and 438 completed both the GDS and the HDRS. Criteria for exclusion included admittance or transfer to other services, scoring less than 15 on the Mini-Mental State Exam, and inability to respond due to illness or other cause. The final sample consisted of 161 men under age 40 and 850 men 65 years and older, with a total age range of 20–102 years. African American patients were 52.2% of the < 40-year-old sample and 28.3% of the ≥ 65-year-old group. Relative to the younger group, older subjects were more likely to be married and retired and to have less education, lower functional and cognitive status, and more severe medical illness. Younger men more often had a history of psychiatric disorder and alcohol use.

Summary. Overall, 33.3% of young men and 22.1% of older men scored ≥ 11 on the GDS. This percentage was highest in younger whites (40.0%) and lowest in older African Americans (19.4%). Hierarchical regression analyses showed that age, race, retirement status, occupational status, psychiatric history, physical health, functional status, and cognitive status were related to depression; social support and moderate use of alcohol were inversely related to depression. When GDS was compared with observer-rated depression (HDRS), patients overall were more likely to score in the depressed range on the GDS. Correlations between the GDS and HDRS ranged from 0.60 (for older African Americans) to 0.84 (for younger whites).

Discussion. The authors conclude that self-rated depressive symptoms are common among medical inpatients and are linked with certain sociodemographic and health characteristics, and that the GDS may be a relatively insensitive measure of depression in older African Americans.

Lee MA, & Ganzini L. (1992). Depression in the elderly: Effect of patient attitudes toward life-sustaining therapy. *J Am Geriatr Soc*, *40*, 983–988.

Design. This study examined the effect of depression on decisions regarding life-sustaining therapy in older medical inpatients. Eligible subjects were given the Mini-Mental State Exam and the 30-item GDS. Other measures of function and medical condition were also used. A psychiatrist who was blinded to GDS results also conducted a structured interview with patients using the depression items from the Diagnostic Interview Schedule (DIS). Subjects were considered depressed if they scored > 14 on the GDS and were diagnosed as having major depression by the psychiatrist. The control group consisted of subjects who scored ≤ 14 on the GDS and who were assessed as being nondepressed by the psychiatrist. Subjects whose DIS and GDS scores were discrepant were excluded. To assess preferences regarding treatment, subjects were given a series of hypothetical scenarios of illness with varying prognoses and asked if they would want any of a list of seven invasive but lifesaving interventions if needed (e.g., intravenous fluids with medications, dialysis, mechanical ventilatory support, and cardiopulmonary resuscitation). Subjects were asked to respond yes or no to each procedure for each illness. Responses were scored, with a maximum total score of 23 if all possible interventions were chosen for all illnesses. The reliability and validity of this preference measure was tested and appeared adequate.

Sample.   Subjects were selected from among new patients ages 65+ at the Portland VA Medical Center over a 1-year period. Potential patients were drawn from (1) a random selection of new admissions and (2) medical inpatients referred to the psychiatry service for evaluation of depression. Criteria for exclusion were placement in an intensive care unit, inability to communicate, psychiatric disorders other than depression (e.g., dementia, psychosis, substance abuse) that could affect the patient's decision regarding medical treatment, terminal illness with a life expectancy less than 6 months, and scoring less than 24 on the MMSE. The final sample consisted of 50 depressed and 50 nondepressed subjects, with a mean age of 71 and a mean education level of 12 years. The sample were 95% men, 68% married, 96% white, and 64% Protestant; 92% of subjects lived in a private home or apartment.

Summary.   Depressed subjects chose fewer medical interventions than controls for their current health situation and for illnesses with good prognoses; no differences were found between depressed and control subjects for illnesses with poor prognoses. The GDS score accounted for ≤ 5% of the variance in decision making.

Discussion.   Depression may be a predictor (albeit the relationship is weak) of refusal of treatment for illnesses with good prognoses. This is consistent with at least one other report (Gerety et al., 1993) and may not reverse with treatment of depression (Lee & Ganzini, 1994).

Morley JE, & Kraenzle D. (1994). Causes of weight loss in a community nursing home. *J Am Geriatr Soc*, *42*, 583–585.

Design.   Causes of weight loss in a community nursing home were determined from a retrospective chart review of all weights over the prior 3 to 6 months. Current weight was determined by weighing in light clothing. Residents who had lost ≥ 5 pounds were interviewed using the GDS and Mini-Mental State Exam (MMSE) and assessed using a range of clinical observations and measures to determine the causes of the weight loss.

Sample.   A total of 156 residents who had been in the nursing home for at least 3 months were examined. The mean age was 80.1 years (range 51–105 years).

Summary.   A total of 30 residents had lost 5 or more pounds. Frequencies of clinically determined causes of weight loss were examined visually. The cause most frequently listed was "depression" (11 residents, 36% of sample), which was noted at least five times more often than any other cause.

Discussion.   These authors conclude that depression is the most common cause of weight loss in nursing homes. They cite the need for careful identification of reasons for weight loss, along with appropriate treatment for such causes as depression, although they note that many cases of depression in the current sample were unresponsive to treatment. If correct, these results could indicate the clinical value of weight loss as a marker for depression among nursing home residents. However, as noted in subsequent letters to the editor, this study was correlational and had a small sample, and the assertion of a causal relationship is not appropriate. In addition, cutoffs used for the GDS were not specified, and the GDS indicates depressive symptoms rather than clinical depression. The reader is referred to comments by Applegate (1995), Breuer (1995), Kahn (1995), Morley and Kraenzle (1995), and Retan (1995).

Parmelee PA, Katz IR, & Lawton MP. (1991). The relation of pain to depression among institutionalized aged. *J Gerontol Psychol Sci, 46,* P15–P21.

Design. This study provided a cross-sectional examination of the relationship between depression and pain. Residents of a multilevel care facility between December 1985 and April 1988 were assessed on the following variables: pain (McGill Pain Questionnaire); depression (checklist based on *DSM-III-R* criteria used to classify subjects as possible major depression, minor depression, and no depression); 30-item GDS (total score used and cutoffs used where *DSM* checklist was incomplete, with a score of 18+ indicating possible major depression, 11–18 indicating minor depression, and < 11 indicating no depressed); affect (Profile of Mood States, POMS); and health and functional status (Physical Self-Maintenance Scale; Cumulative Illness Rating Scale).

Sample. Of 1,302 possible subjects, the final sample consisted of 598 older adults living in a skilled or intermediate nursing home (*n* = 191) or a congregate apartment facility (*n* = 407). Criteria for exclusion were (among others) cognitive impairment, being too physically ill, speech or hearing deficits, and refusal to participate. The final sample were 70% women with a mean age of 83.6 years (*SD* = 5.9) and an average length of stay of 28.8 months (*SD* = 44.3).

Summary. A significant relationship was found between pain and *DSM-III-R* diagnosis of depression; reports of pain were highest among possible major depressives, intermediate among minor depressives, and lowest among nondepressives. Geriatric Depression Scale (GDS) scores were significantly correlated with pain for the total sample and for minor depressives and nondepressives, but not for possible major depressives. Corresponding results were found for the POMS. A similar relationship between pain and depression was found when the researchers controlled for functional and health status.

Discussion. Results indicate a significant association between pain and depression in institutionalized elderly people that is not wholly accounted for by physical and functional disability. Differences between higher-functioning and lower-functioning residents were not provided. The absence of a relationship between GDS and possible major depression may have been due to the restricted range in what may have been a fairly homogeneous population.

Woo J, Ho SC, Lau J, Yuen YK, Chiu H, Lee HC, & Chi I. (1994). The prevalence of depressive symptoms and predisposing factors in an elderly Chinese population. *Acta Psychiatr Scand, 89,* 8–13.

Design. This survey extended the use of the GDS to elderly Chinese in Hong Kong. Home interviews were conducted, assessing a range of variables, including socioeconomic factors, social support, physical health, and functional status. Cognitive function was assessed using the information and orientation section of the Clifton Procedure for the Elderly (CAPE I/O). Depression was measured using the 15-item Chinese version of the GDS. The authors report their own unpublished data indicating an optimum cutoff of ≥

8, yielding sensitivity and specificity rates of 96.3% and 87.5%, respectively, for detection of depression.

Sample.   Potential subjects were selected by stratified random sampling (by age and gender) from a list of all recipients of old age and disability allowances in Hong Kong ($\geq$ 90% of all persons ages 70+). Approximately 60% of potential subjects responded to a mailed request to participate; of these, subjects scoring $\leq$ 7 on the CAPE I/O were excluded. The final sample consisted of 877 men and 734 women.

Summary.   The adjusted overall prevalence of depression was 29.2% for men and 41.1% for women. Depression was significantly higher in women relative to men in the 70–79 age groups, and increased with age for men. Stepwise logistic regression identified the following factors predicting depression: socioeconomic characteristics (e.g., borderline financial stability); poor social support; functional disability; and poor physical health.

Discussion.   The authors note the relatively high prevalence of depression in this population; the extent to which these data generalize to the 40% nonresponders is unknown. Nevertheless, there appears to be a significant population with depressive symptoms, and regression analysis suggests that there are associated factors that may be modifiable. Note that the prevalence of depressive symptoms is higher than the 15% typically reported in American studies of community-dwelling elderly. It is not clear whether this represents true differences in depression prevalence in the two populations or cultural differences in responses to the GDS. Publication of data on the reliability and validity of the Chinese GDS would be helpful.

Beck Depression Inventory (BDI)

Development and Methods: Long Form of the BDI

Beck AT, Ward CH, Mendelson M, Mock J, & Erbaugh J. (1961). An inventory for measuring depression. *Arch Gen Psychiatr*, 4, 561–571.

Design.   This paper describes the development of the Beck Depression Inventory (BDI).

Sample.   The instrument was administered by a trained interviewer first to 226 patients and then to a replication sample of 183 patients. These patients were drawn from routine admissions to the psychiatric outpatient department of a university hospital and the outpatient plus inpatient admissions to a psychiatric service of a metropolitan hospital in the same city. The combined group were 60.9% women and 64.7% white; only 6.1% were 55 or older. Patients with organic brain damage and "mental deficiency" were excluded.

Summary.   Responses to the inventory were compared with experienced psychiatrists' clinical estimation of "depth of depression," rated on a four-point scale. Despite efforts to establish common criteria among the four participating psychiatrists before the interviews began, a preliminary assessment of 100 patients by two psychiatrists showed that they agreed completely only 56% of the time. The internal consistency of the BDI was assessed by (1) comparing the first 200 patients' scores for each of the 21 categories with their total scores and (2) determining the split-half reliability for 97 cases in the first sample. The first method showed that there was a significant relationship for all categories ($p <$ 0.001 for all but one); the second yielded a Pearson r between the odd and even categories of 0.86 (0.93 after the Spearman-Brown correction). No formal test-retest or interrater reliability tests were performed. However, the BDI was administered to 38 patients at two different times, and the change in their scores was compared with the change in the clinical rating of depth of depression; in 85% of the cases (28/33) where the clinical depth-of-depression rating changed, the two scales changed in the same direction. The scores obtained by each of the three interviewers were also plotted against the clinical ratings; there was a "very high degree of consistency" (p. 57) in mean scores for each interviewer at each level of depression. Several methods were used to measure the concordance between the BDI and the clinicians' ratings. For example, it was found that there were statistically significant differences in the means of the BDI for each category of depth of depression. After collapsing the clinicians' ratings from four categories to two, the Pearson biserial r was 0.65 in one sample and 0.67 in the other ($p < 0.01$ for both). A copy of the 94-item inventory is included in the article.

Discussion. The inventory (BDI) appears to discriminate effectively among groups of patients with differing degrees of depression and to measure change over time. However, it was developed using a sample of younger psychiatric patients, so its generalizability to other populations was not established in this study. Also, the weakness of the "gold standard" against which the BDI was judged (i.e., psychiatric interviews) makes it more difficult to assess the results of the tests of validity. However, many of these points were addressed in later studies using the BDI.

Gallagher D, Breckenridge J, Steinmetz J, & Thompson L. (1983). The Beck Depression Inventory and research diagnostic criteria: Congruence in an older population. *J Consult Clin Psychol, 51,* 945–946.

Design. The study examined the congruence between BDI scores, using conventional cutoff points, and Research Diagnostic Criteria (RDC; Spitzer et al., 1978) diagnoses of major and minor depressive disorders. The latter were derived from information from the Schedule for Affective Disorders and Schizophrenia (SADS; Endicott & Spitzer, 1978).

Sample. The sample consisted of 102 older adults who were seeking psychological treatment. There were 82 women; the mean age was 68.97 years ($SD = 5.92$).

Summary. With depression defined as a score of 11 or more on the BDI and the RDC diagnosis used as the "gold standard," false positives were 18.5% and false negatives were 6.7%, for sensitivity and specificity of 93.3% and 81.5%, respectively. False negatives were higher for minor depressives (according to the RDC) than for major depressives. The authors tried to confirm these results by administering the BDI to 128 individuals living in senior centers and residential complexes who were not seeking psychological treatment. They then administered the SADS to 13 of the 15 who scored 17 or higher on the BDI. Twelve were classified as depressed (2 minor depressives and 10 major depressives) and 1 as not depressed using the RDC.

Discussion. This study appears to supply further evidence of the reliability of the BDI in older populations. However, the generalizability of the results is limited by the fact that the original sample consisted of psychological patients. The results from the second sample, while suggestive, are not sufficiently thorough to provide evidence of the reliability of the BDI in a nonpatient, community-dwelling population.

Gallagher D, Nies G, & Thompson LW. (1982). Reliability of the Beck Depression Inventory with older adults. *J Consult Clin Psychol, 50,* 152–153.

Design. This article reports on a test-retest study of the reliability of the BDI in older adults. The BDI was administered twice, 6 to 21 days apart. All subjects were first given a mental status examination "to rule out organic impairment."

Sample. The first sample consisted of 77 patients who met the Research Diagnostic Criteria (RDC) for a current major depressive disorder. The second sample consisted of 82 community volunteers in Los Angeles, none of whom was receiving treatment for depression or "any other significant mental health problem." The groups were similar in terms of ratio of men to women, marital status, ethnic background, educational level, and perceived health status. The mean age of the patient group was 67.8 years (*SD* = 6.07); the volunteer group was slightly older, with a mean age of 69.9 years (*SD* = 4.08, *p* < 0.05).

Summary. The mean BDI score in the total sample was 14.40 (*SD* = 11.23) for the first test and 12.38 (*SD* = 10.04) for the second test. The comparable data for the volunteer group were 5.54 (*SD* = 4.67) and 4.61 (*SD* = 4.84); the comparable data for the patient group were 23.96 (*SD* = 7.21) and 20.96 (*SD* = 7.83). Three statistics were used to assess reliability: The Pearson product moment correlation coefficients for the total sample, volunteer group, and patient group were 0.90, 0.86, and 0.79, respectively. Similarly, the split-half statistics using the Spearman-Brown correction were 0.84, 0.74, and 0.58; the coefficient alphas were 0.91, 0.76, and 0.73. The smaller values for the two separate groups as compared with the total sample are expected, given the greater homogeneity within each group than across groups. Only the split-half estimate for the patient group was less than adequate, in the authors' opinion. They conclude that the results provide evidence of the relative adequacy of the BDI both for research purposes and as a clinical screening instrument.

Discussion. This study provides evidence of the adequate reliability of the BDI in older populations and is strengthened by the inclusion of both patient and nonpatient groups.

Gatewood-Colwell G, Kaczmarek M, & Ames MH. (1989). Reliability and validity of the Beck Depression Inventory for a white and Mexican-American gerontic population. *Psychol Rep*, *65*, 1163–1166.

Design. The objective of this study was to examine the reliability and validity of the BDI in a nonclinical older population while comparing responses by gender and ethnicity (whites versus bilingual Mexican Americans). Scores on the BDI were compared with the GDS. Both instruments were administered in English.

Sample. The sample consisted of 51 community-dwelling volunteers. The mean age was 70.2 years (range, 60–80). There were 15 white women, 11 white men, 13 Mexican American women, and 12 Mexican American men. None of the subjects was currently receiving psychotherapy or counseling.

Summary. Cronbach's α (alpha) for the group's response was 0.80. The Pearson product moment coefficient between the BDI and the GDS was 0.79 (*p* < 0.05). No significant differences were found across gender or ethnic groups. The mean BDI score was 9.41 (*SD* = 4.12); the mean GDS score was 8.98 (*SD* = 3.91). The authors questioned the use of the standard cutoff of 11 as indicating the presence of depression in this population. Use of that cutoff would have identified 46.7% of the white women, 35.4% of the white men, 38.6% of the Mexican American women, and 33.3% of the Mexican American men as depressed.

Discussion.   This study provides suggestive evidence that the BDI performs adequately in a different ethnic group from that for which it was developed. However, the small sample limits the generalizability of the results.

Norris JT, Gallagher D, Wilson A, & Winograd CH. (1987). Assessment of depression in geriatric medical outpatients: The validity of two screening measures. *J Am Geriatr Soc*, 35, 989–995.

Design.   This study evaluates the validity of the BDI and GDS in screening for depression among older, medically ill outpatients. Scores on both measures were compared with Research Diagnostic Criteria (RDC) and *DSM-III* diagnoses based on a SADS interview for a subsample of 31 individuals. Questions relating to somatic symptoms were eliminated in evaluating the SADS responses if it was clear that the somatic symptoms were directly attributable to physical problems. The patients' primary care physicians were also asked to indicate whether or not each patient was depressed.

Sample.   Patients from a Veterans Administration clinic for patients with complex medical problems were asked to participate in the study. Of 118 clinic patients, 68 were included (among those excluded were 25 who were too demented to complete the consent form). The mean age of the sample was 78 (range 60–95); 59% lived with their spouses and 16% lived alone; only 3 were female.

Summary.   According to both RDC and *DSM-III* criteria, 9 of the 31 patients completing the SADS were depressed. Both the BDI scores and the GDS scores were compared with the RDC and *DSM-III* diagnoses using two different cutoffs for each. The sensitivity of the BDI ranged from 0.89 (using a cutoff of 10 and RDC or *DSM-III*) to 0.50 (using a cutoff of 17 and *DSM-III*); the analogous range for the specificity is 0.82 to 0.92. The sensitivity of the GDS ranged from 0.89 (cutoff of 10 and RDC or *DSM-III*) to 0.78 (cutoff of 14 and *DSM-III*); the specificity ranged from 0.73 to 0.86. The correlation between the GDS and BDI was 0.854 ($p < 0.001$). No further data on the performance of the GDS and the BDI in the full sample were reported. Physicians' ratings of depression agreed with both the RDC and the *DSM-III* diagnoses in only 64% of the cases (14 of 22). Thus, it appears that physicians would benefit from using these screening tools to identify patients who are depressed. Furthermore, these authors point out that although the BDI seems slightly more consistent with the RDC and *DSM-III* diagnoses than the GDS, the GDS has two other advantages. First, its yes-no format may be easier to complete. Second, it has fewer questions regarding somatic symptoms; this is generally considered to be an advantage when working with older populations.

Discussion.   As the authors note, the generalizability of the results is limited by the low response (and therefore the possibility of self-selection bias among the respondents) and the fact that the sample consisted predominantly of men. Nevertheless, the article provides useful information both on the validity of the BDI itself and on its performance in comparison with the GDS. It is interesting that despite the concern about the somatic content of the BDI, the correspondence between the BDI and the RDC and the *DSM-III* was relatively good. The poor performance of the physicians' ratings—although it is not surprising, given the results of other studies—does show the need for aids in detecting depression. However, the relatively small samples for both sets of comparisons should be kept in mind.

Development and Methods: Short Form of the BDI

Beck AT, & Beck RW. (1972). Screening depressed patients in family practice: A rapid technic. *Postgrad Med*, *52*, 81–85.

Design. This is a general article encouraging the use of the BDI to identify depressed patients in family practice. It also includes a description of the development of the short form of the BDI.

Sample. The same sample was used as in the development of the long form of the BDI. (See *Beck et al., 1961.)

Summary. The data used to develop the long form were reanalyzed, and items from the short form were selected on the basis of correlations between each of the 21 items and the total BDI score and the psychiatrists' ratings of depth of depression. The final product includes 13 items. The order of the possible responses within each item was also reversed so that severity decreases as one reads down the list; this change was made to facilitate completion of the scale by the respondent. The correlation of the total score on the short form with that on the long form was 0.96; the correlation with the clinical depth-of-depression ratings was 0.61. Mean scores on the resulting short form were calculated for each of the categories of depth of depression; a one-way analysis of variance of the means was significant ($p < 0.001$). The recommended cutoff scores are 0–4 for no or minimal depression; 5–7, mild depression; 8–15, moderate depression, and 16+, severe depression. The maximum score is 39. The article includes a copy of the BDI short form.

Discussion. This is a preliminary description of the development of the short form of the BDI. The necessary cross-validation and reliability and validity studies were done later. It is also subject to the same limitations discussed in the annotation of *Beck et al., 1961.

Beck AT, Rial WY, & Rickels K. (1974). Short form of depression inventory: Cross-validation. *Psychol Rep*, *34*, 1184–1186.

Design. This study is a cross-validation of the short form of the BDI, which compares results in a new population to responses on the long form and to clinical evaluation by psychiatrists.

Sample. The short form was tested in five patient samples totaling 431 individuals. The samples were composed of randomly selected patients in a general practice ($n = 93$); patients hospitalized for attempted suicide (two samples with a combined total of 241 subjects); depressed patients with no previous suicide attempts ($n = 58$); and hospitalized schizophrenic patients ($n = 39$). Aggregating over all five groups, 58% were women; 59.9% were white and 39.7% African American; the mean age was 33.6 years.

Summary. The product-moment correlation coefficient between the long and short versions was reported for only two of the samples, and it ranged from 0.89 to 0.96 ($p < 0.01$). The correlation between the short form and physicians' rating of depression ranged from 0.55 in one group of suicide attempters (versus 0.49 for the long form) to 0.67 in the general medical sample ($p < 0.01$). "Correlations between scores on the short form and age, sex, and race were of zero-order magnitude and nonsignificant" (p. 1185).

Discussion. This study suggests that the short form correlates quite well with the long form, although data are not provided on all of the samples. The correlations with clinical judgment were not nearly as high but appeared to be in the same range as the correlations between the long form and psychiatrists' clinical evaluation (see also *Beck et al., 1961). As with the original sample, the mean age was quite young, and about three quarters of the sample had some type of mental illness.

Foelker GA Jr, Shewchuk RM, & Niederehe G. (1987). Confirmatory factor analysis of the short form Beck depression inventory in elderly community samples. *J Clin Psychol*, *43*, 111–118.

Design. This article relies on the confirmatory factor analysis method to examine the factor structure of the BDI short form (BDI-SF) in two samples of older individuals. The authors compared the first sample with four models previously described in the literature. After identifying the best-fitting model, they made several adjustments to improve the fit and then repeated the analyses on the cross-validation sample.

Sample. The first sample was composed of 199 older volunteers in several nonpsychiatric health agencies and social groups in Tampa, Florida. The average age was 70.1 years (range, 60–99; $SD = 7.6$); the sample was 91% white and 78% women. The cross-validation sample consisted of 113 community-dwelling, older individuals from Houston, TX, who participated in a broader study on vulnerability to late-life depression. Twenty percent of the sample were receiving outpatient psychiatric treatment. The average age was 73.0 years (range, 60–88; $SD = 7.0$). The sample was 89% white and 80% women.

Summary. The mean score on the BDI-SF was 3.04 ($SD = 3.24$) in the Tampa sample and 4.20 ($SD = 4.32$) in the Houston sample. The mean score was higher in men than in women in the Tampa sample, but the opposite was found in the Houston sample. In both groups, individuals in their seventies had lower scores than those either younger or older than them. Cronbach's α (alpha) was 0.74 for the Tampa sample and 0.80 for the Houston sample, providing evidence that the BDI-SF has "satisfactory reliability" in this population. The previously published factor analytic model by Reynolds and Gould (1981) was found to provide the best fit for the data. The 13 items of the BDI-SF were grouped into three factors: negative self-esteem, anergy, and dysphoria. Several indices of overall fit were examined; the χ^2 statistic divided by the degrees of freedom was 2.28 for the original Reynolds and Gould model in the Tampa sample and 1.81 for the modified model; the corresponding data for the Houston sample are 1.78 and 1.65. The analytic approach and results are discussed in considerable detail in the article.

Discussion. As the authors point out, this study provides strong evidence for the construct validity of the BDI-SF and also shows the generalizability of the Reynolds and Gould (1981) factor structure across a wide age range. Furthermore, the three factors identified correspond to current thinking about the construct of depression and, the authors argue, therefore suggest that the syndrome of depression is fairly consistent across age groups.

Knight RG. (1984). Some general population norms for the short form Beck Depression Inventory. *J Clin Psychol*, *40*, 751–753.

Design. This article uses data collected during a general health survey to develop general populations norms for the BDI-SF.

Sample. The original sample consisted of 1,127 people, or 78% of the population over 16 years old living in Milton, New Zealand, in 1981; 1,091 completed all items of the BDI-SF. Fifty-two percent of the sample were women; 16% of the men and 21% of the women were 60 or older.

Summary. The mean BDI-SF score for men was 2.29 (*SD* = 2.22) for 60–69-year-olds; 3.00 (*SD* = 1.75) for 70–79-year-olds; and 3.00 (*SD* = 2.12) for 80–89-year-olds. The corresponding figures for women were 2.89 (*SD* = 2.90), 2.83 (*SD* = 2.20), and 2.00 (*SD* = 1.69). The means for the entire population were 2.16 (*SD* = 2.77) for men and 2.82 (*SD* = 3.54) for women. Overall, women's scores were significantly higher than men's. (The trend does not seems to hold up in the oldest age groups, although the sample sizes for 80–89 are very small.) The internal consistency (coefficient α, alpha) was 0.81. On seven items, however, over 85% of the sample scored 0. The percentage scoring 0 ranged from 97.8% for suicide to 49.7% for fatigability.

Discussion. This article provides useful data on mean BDI scores in a general population. Of course, it provides no data to validate the BDI scores, so the true prevalence of depression in this population is unknown. In addition, care should be taken in extrapolating these results to the United States, because of possible cultural differences that might affect responses to this questionnaire. Other studies do suggest, however, that the results are quite robust across a variety of settings (e.g., *Gatewood-Colwell et al., 1989).

Scogin F, Beutler L, Corbishley A, & Hamblin D. (1988). Reliability and validity of the short form Beck Depression Inventory with older adults. *J Clin Psychol*, 44, 853–857.

Design. This study examines the reliability and validity of the BDI-SF in older adults.

Sample. The sample consisted of a depressed group of patients who met the criteria for major depressive disorder and who were participating in a study of medication and psychotherapy outcomes (*n* = 61) and community volunteers recruited from senior citizens' agencies (*n* = 57), none of whom was receiving psychiatric treatment. The two groups were similar with respect to age (71 versus 72 years; all were at least 60); ratio of men to women (26/35 versus 22/35), and years of education (13 versus 12).

Summary. Patients completed the BDI-SF and Hamilton Rating Scale for Depression before treatment and each week for 20 weeks during treatment; volunteers completed the BDI alone once. The mean BDI score was 2.92 (*SD* = 3.44) for the volunteers; for the patients, it was 11.01 (*SD* = 4.72) at the beginning of treatment and 9.27 (*SD* = 5.98) at the end of treatment. The Spearman-Brown split-half reliability coefficient was 0.84 for the entire sample; it was lower for patients than for volunteers (0.82), particularly before treatment (0.66 versus 0.81 after treatment). The α coefficient was 0.90 for the whole sample. For the patient group, the Pearson product-moment correlations between the BDI and the Hamilton were 0.42 ($p < 0.01$) before treatment and 0.54 ($p < 0.01$) after treatment; these were lower than expected. The difference in the total scores on the BDI-SF in the depressed and volunteer groups was statistically significant ($p < 0.01$), showing that the short form does discriminate reliably between the two groups. Using the traditional cutoff score of 4 as indicative of depression and comparing the depressed and volunteer groups, researchers found the sensitivity of the BDI-SF to be 98% and the specificity 65%; increasing the cutoff score to 5 improved specificity (77%) but had little impact on sensitivity (97%). The authors conclude that the BDI-SF is a reliable instrument for measuring depression in older adults but express concern about the relatively low correlations between the BDI and Hamilton scores; they call for further study of the convergent validity of the BDI.

Discussion. The results suggest that the BDI-SF is appropriate for use with older adults. Some of the results should be interpreted with caution, however. The calculations of sensitivity and specificity appear to be based on the assumption that none of the volunteer sample is depressed; this assumption is questionable, given the prevalence of depression found in samples of community-dwelling older adults. As the authors mention, the low correlation with another depression scale is also a cause for concern.

Applications

Artinian NT, Duggan C, & Miller P. (1993). Age differences in patient recovery patterns following coronary artery bypass surgery. *Am J Critical Care,* **2,** 453–461.

Design. This study compares physical, psychological, and social recovery within the first 3 weeks following coronary artery bypass surgery (CABS) across three age groups (less than 60, 60–70, and over 70 years). Patients were interviewed before discharge and at 1, 3, and 6 weeks after discharge. A number of instruments were administered by mail after discharge: six subscales of the Sickness Impact Profile, a 20-item inventory of symptoms, a Cantril Ladder Scale to obtain perceptions of both physical and psychological health, the BDI, and the Rosenberg Self-Esteem Scale.

Sample. A convenience sample was collected from patients in cardiac surgery recovery units at five teaching hospitals. Individuals who had a history of chronic mental illness or other physically disabling illness, had any indications of a possible postoperative cerebral vascular accident, had undergone valve repair surgery, or had undergone repeat CABS were excluded. A total of 258 patients participated in the study, 72.9% were men; 184 (71%) provided complete data. The mean age was 63 years (range, 39–79; *SD* = 9.15). Twenty-nine percent were under 60 years old; 49% were 60–70; and 21% were over 70. Ninety-two percent of the sample were white, and 83% were married.

Summary. The authors report that the three groups had similar characteristics with regard to cardiovascular health and surgery, but few details of cardiovascular health are reported by group. Patients over 70 did have significantly longer stays in the hospital than younger patients. Mixed design, repeated measures, and multivariate analyses of variance (MANOVA) were used to analyze the data. With regard to physical recovery, there were no significant differences across age groups, although there was an improvement over time within each of the age groups. With regard to depression, there was no evidence of significant depression in any of the age groups at any of the follow-up interviews. Within each age group, depression scores improved over time, but there were no differences across age groups. Cronbach's α for the BDI was 0.82. The mean score at 1 week was 9.53 for those under 60 years old, 8.50 for those 60–70, and 9.15 for those over 70. The corresponding data were 7.26, 7.13, and 7.33 at 3 weeks and 3.80, 4.88, and 5.67 at 6 weeks. (These data are apparently mislabeled "ambulation dysfunction" in figure 2 of the article.) No age-related effects were found on any of the other measures of psychological or social recovery, but for the majority of them scores improved over time for all three groups. Several of the measures had a low Cronbach's α.

Discussion. This study provides information on mean BDI scores among patients recovering from CABS and suggests that there is no change in incidence of depression with age. However, as the authors note, the attrition rate was quite high. Furthermore, the data reported do not provide a complete picture. It would be useful to know the following, for example: (1) What are the distributions of the BDI scores? (2) Do the distributions change with age or over time? (3) How many individuals would be categorized as depressed (according to BDI scores) at each point? It would also be interesting to explore the relationship among physical, psychological, and social recovery; each of these dimensions is analyzed separately in this article. Finally, although the authors report that the three age groups were similar in terms of cardiovascular disease, they do not provide any data on the burden of comorbid disease, which might well vary across the age groups.

House A, Dennis M, Mogridge L, Warlow C, Hawton K, & Jones L. (1991). Mood disorders in the year after first stroke. *Br J Psychiatry*, *158*, 83–92.
Design.   This study examines the range, frequency, severity, and course of psychiatric disorders experienced by patients after their first stroke. Psychiatric symptoms, as assessed by the BDI and a short version of the Present State Examination (PSE), were compared over the course of the first year among stroke patients and between patients and controls.
Sample.   Individuals reported to the Oxfordshire Community Stroke Project with a confirmed diagnosis of a first stroke between November 1985 and November 1986 were included. Ninety-five patients were seen at 1, 6, and 12 months, and 33 were seen at 6 and 12 months. The control group consisted of a "stratified random sample of the age-sex registers of four of the ten general practices from which the stroke patients were referred" (p. 84); 111 of the 128 selected (87%) were interviewed. The average age of the stroke patients was 71.2 years (range, 18–96; $SD = 13.7$); that of the controls was 69.6 years (range, 30–86; $SD = 11.4$). Forty-five percent of the stroke patients and 40% of the controls were men. Only 38% of the patients were admitted to the hospital for the stroke. Eight patients had definite psychiatric disorders in the year before their stroke. Individuals with "linguistic, praxic or other cognitive deficits" (p. 84) were not included.
Summary.   The BDI was completed by 77% to 88% of patients at each interview and by 97% of the controls. The mean score among patients was 7.4 ($SD = 6.4$) at 1 month, 7.2 ($SD = 5.6$) at 6 months, and 5.6 ($SD = 4.5$) at 12 months. The mean score among controls was approximately 6.7 (estimated from graph). Detailed information on responses to each BDI question is provided in the paper. The overall conclusions are as follows: (1) The mean scores for patients and controls were not significantly different at any of the follow-up interviews. (2) The decline in scores over time among patients was not significant ($p = 0.06$) for individuals who completed all three interviews (who also had lower initial scores) or for the cognitive affective symptoms; there was a significant decline, however, in the somatic symptoms. (3) Of 128 patients, 39% were identified as depressed at some time during the year using a cutoff of 10 or greater, and 20% using a cutoff of 13 or more. However, for the most part, the depression did not persist: The individuals identified as depressed at each period tended to be different people. (4) There was no bimodal distribution to the BDI scores, suggesting that any identification of a cutoff point for defining depression is somewhat arbitrary. The BDI, these results imply, is an inaccurate method of identifying individual cases. (5) Contrary to earlier reports, depression in these patients did not appear to be different from depression among other physically sick patients. (6) The results are unavoidably biased by attrition over time (i.e., the sickest people died before the end of the follow-up period). The results from the PSE are provided in the paper; a variety of other symptoms, such as irritability and social

withdrawal, were noted in the stroke patients. A comparison of the BDI and PSE results is found in *House et al., 1989.

Discussion. This study had a strong design that was deliberately intended to address some of the methodological weaknesses of earlier studies in this area. In extrapolating from this study to other populations, however, the patients' spectrum of disease should be kept in mind. It appears that many were not severely disabled by the stroke, although the low hospitalization rate may also in part be a product of differences in admission practices between Britain and the United States.

Morgan RE, Palinkas LA, Barrett-Connor EL, & Wingard DL. (1993). Plasma cholesterol and depressive symptoms in older men. *Lancet, 341*, 75–79.

Design. The objective of this study was to determine whether there is a relationship between depression and low plasma cholesterol concentrations in men 50 years and older. Such a relationship might help to explain the increase in deaths from nonmedical causes, including homicide, suicide, and accidents, seen in studies of men with low cholesterol levels and in cholesterol-reducing trials. Using data from the Rancho Bernardo, CA, cohort, the authors compared subjects' responses to an 18-item version of the BDI with plasma cholesterol levels. They examined the relationship for different age groups and also controlled for weight, change in weight, and change in cholesterol level (between the early 1970s and mid-1980s), number of coexisting chronic diseases, number of medications, perceived level of physical functioning, and perceived health status.

Sample. The sample consisted of 1,020 white men aged 50–80 years who remained in the Rancho Bernardo, CA, cohort in 1984–1987.

Summary. The reliability of the BDI was assessed using Cronbach's α, which was 0.75. Three items that covered guilt, expectation of punishment, and self-hate were deleted from the original BDI in an effort to reduce the length and to remove potentially threatening items. The cutoff point used to indicate depression was 13. There was a statistically significant increase in both mean depression levels and the number of depressed individuals with age. The mean scores ranged from 3.66 ($SD = 3.63$) for 50–59-year-olds to 6.80 ($SD = 4.46$) for 80–89-year-olds. The percentage with low plasma cholesterol levels (< 4.14 mmol/L) also increased with age, from 6.5% for 50–59-year-olds to 11.9% for 80–89-year-olds. In the oldest age group, the relative risk of depression associated with low cholesterol levels compared with normal cholesterol levels was 6.7. The BDI was also positively associated with the number of coexisting chronic diseases, number of medications, perceived level of physical functioning, and perceived health status; it was negatively associated with plasma cholesterol levels and weight. In a stepwise multiple regression model, low cholesterol levels were a significant independent predictor of depression, although they contributed less than age, perceived health status, and perceived level of physical functioning ($R^2 = 0.10$).

Discussion. The BDI is a measure of depressive symptoms and does not necessarily indicate the presence of clinical depression. Therefore, although the association between a relatively high BDI score and low plasma cholesterol levels is interesting, it does not necessarily account for the increase in nonmedical causes of death in individuals with low cholesterol. Furthermore, the relationship is evident only in individuals 70 or older; the authors do not provide any information on the age distributions of the individuals with the elevated mortality levels in the previous studies. If the elevated mortality is found across age groups, it would weaken the implications of this study.

This article is one of a number of studies from the Rancho Bernardo cohort on the relationship between depression (as measured by the BDI) and other diseases or symptoms. These studies include an examination of the relationship between type 2 diabetes and depressive symptoms in older adults (Palinkas et al., 1991), between estrogen use and depressive symptoms in postmenopausal women (Palinkas & Barrett-Connor, 1992), and between low blood pressure and depression in older men (Barrett-Connor & Palinkas, 1994).

Peck JR, Smith TW, Ward JR, & Milano R. (1989). Disability and depression in rheumatoid arthritis: A multitrait, multimethod investigation. *Arthritis Rheum*, 32, 1100–1106.

Design.   This study examines the relationship between disability and depression in patients with rheumatoid arthritis (RA) and assesses the accuracy of instruments intended to measure these two factors. There has been concern that estimates of the prevalence of depression have been confounded by the presence of somatic items on the BDI. The authors therefore compared the results of a variety of instruments and also performed a factor analysis of the BDI results to search for disease-related components. The instruments included the Disability Index of the Stanford Health Assessment Questionnaire (HAQ); visual analog scales for pain, impact of disease, and activity of disease; the BDI; and the Hamilton Rating Scale for Depression (HSRD). Self-reported responses to the Disability Index were compared with responses to the same index by interviewers and spouses or other close relatives; similarly, responses to the BDI were compared with the interviewer-administered HSRD. In administering the HSRD, the interviewers ignored any responses to somatic items that they believed were attributable to disability or disease. In addition, 20 rheumatologists were asked to indicate which items on the BDI were likely to be reported by RA patients that would be due to the impact of the disease; 15 of 20 responded.

Sample.   One hundred and forty-nine patients with definite or classic rheumatoid arthritis from the outpatient rheumatology clinics at a university and a VA medical center in Utah were asked to participate in the study; 107 (72%) agreed to do so. Of the 107 participants, 63% were women and all but 4 were white. The mean age was 59.3 years (range, 23–81). The majority (*n* = 70) were in functional class II; 9 were in class I; 28 were in class III.

Summary.   The mean BDI score was 11.81 (range, 0–63; *SD* = 7.71); the mean HSRD score was 5.1 (range, 0–50; *SD* = 4.45). The Pearson correlation coefficient for the two instruments was 0.69 ($p < 0.001$). This value was significantly larger than the association between the BDI and any of the measures of disability, whose correlations ranged from 0.31 to 0.50 (all *p* values < 0.05). The factor analysis indicated the presence of two factors, which the authors named dysphoric mood and somatic complaints; two of the items could not be assigned to a factor. The somatic factor included items 4 and 15–21. Items 15–21 have been defined as the somatic items in other studies as well; see *Bolla-Wilson and Bleecker, 1989. These factors were roughly consistent with the rheumatologists' ratings. When the correlations between the two subscales and the HSRD and disability measures were examined, it was found that (1) the dysphoric mood subscale was more highly correlated with the HSRD than the somatic complaints subscale (0.65 versus 0.49); (2) the somatic complaints subscale was more highly correlated with the disability measures than the dysphoric mood subscale (0.39–0.58 for the three disability measures versus 0.16–0.31); and (3) the dysphoric mood subscale was significantly more correlated with the HSRD scores than with the disability measures (all p values < 0.05), but the same was not true of the somatic complaints subscale. The pain measure was also significantly more highly correlated with the disability measures than with the depression measures; however, it was more closely related to the somatic complaints subscale than to the dysphoric mood subscale. The authors concluded that although there is strong evidence of the convergent and divergent validity of the BDI, the clear presence of a somatic component probably leads to overestimation of the prevalence of depression in patients with RA. They suggest that the dysphoric mood subscale may be a more valid measure of depression in these patients than the full BDI. Furthermore, they conclude that with the proper methods, valid estimates of both disability and depression measures can be derived.

Discussion. The data presented in this study on the levels of depressive symptoms in patients with RA are valuable. It is also important to recognize the potential confounding between disability and depression posed by the use of depression-screening instruments that include somatic items. To conclude, however, that the proper estimate of prevalence of depression should be derived from instruments with no somatic items seems to overlook the possibility that some responses to somatic items among patients with RA probably represent effects of disease and some probably reflect depression. We may need to recognize that it is difficult to disentangle the two completely.

Stewart RB, Blashfield R, Hale WE, Moore MT, May FE, & Marks RG. (1991). Correlates of Beck Depression Inventory scores in an ambulatory elderly population: Symptoms, diseases, laboratory values, and medications. *J Fam Practice*, *32*, 497–502.
Design. The objective of this study was to determine the correlates of depression in the elderly, so that clinicians can use this information to identify patients at high risk of depression. Individuals completed the BDI, as well as a detailed health questionnaire, and underwent several laboratory tests and a brief clinical evaluation. Information on 30 to 40 diseases, 30 to 40 symptoms, the 26 most commonly used medications, and some laboratory values were analyzed through four stepwise regressions to determine which ones were significant predictors of the BDI score. The significant factors were then combined into another stepwise regression to determine significant predictors of the BDI score when the other types of factors were present.

Sample. The sample consisted of 1,048 older residents of Dunedin, FL, who participated in the Florida Geriatric Research Program. Sixty-eight percent of the subjects were women. The women's average age was 80.0 years; the men's average age was 80.9. Most of the participants were upper-middle-class white retirees.

Summary. The mean BDI score was 6.9 ($SE = 0.21$) for women and 5.6 ($SE = 0.24$) for men. Fourteen percent of the men and 21% of the women scored above 10. Results from the four initial stepwise regressions showed that 10 signs and symptoms, 8 diseases, 6 drugs, and 4 laboratory values were correlated with the BDI scores. A combined stepwise regression was run with all of these factors, as well as the total number of reported symptoms, diseases, and drugs. The following 8 factors were significantly associated with the BDI score: (1) total number of signs or symptoms reported, (2) pain in the abdomen, (3) loss of memory, (4) lower red blood cell count, (5) loss of vision, (6) number of drugs used, (7) a feeling of awkwardness, and (8) complaints of shortness of breath. The total number of symptoms was the best predictor of the BDI score and had a much greater impact than any of the others (partial $R^2 = 0.2551$; next highest is 0.0089). None of the diseases or drugs were included in the final model.

Discussion. The authors were surprised by the relatively high levels of depression identified in this study and compared them with a recent review by Blazer (1989). Blazer reported a prevalence of major depression of 1%–2% among community-dwelling older adults, plus another 2% with dysthymia or neurotic depression. However, as noted above, the Beck screens for depressive symptoms, not for major depression. Furthermore, while the results of this study are interesting, they should be considered with caution. Although the sample was large, the data were analyzed extensively using stepwise regression procedures. The results should be considered tentative until they are tested in an independent sample. It would also be interesting to know whether similar results would occur if one ran the same regression using the short form of the BDI, from which most of the questions related to physiological symptoms were dropped. In other words, do the results actually reflect an association between depression and the eight factors described above, or are they in part due to the fact that the BDI includes a variety of questions on somatic symptoms? The answer has important implications for whether or not the results can be used by clinicians to identify high risk individuals, as the authors suggest.

REFERENCES

Abrams RC, Teresi JA, & Butin DN. (1992). Depression in nursing home residents. *Clin Ger Med, 8*, 309–322.

*Agrell B, & Dehlin O. (1989). Comparison of six depression rating scales in geriatric stroke patients. *Stroke, 20*, 1190–1194.

*Alden D, Austin C, & Sturgeon R. (1989). A correlation between the Geriatric Depression Scale long and short forms. *J Gerontol, 44*, P124–P125.

Alexopoulos GS, Abrams RC, Young RC, & Shamoian CA. (1988). Cornell scale for depression in dementia. *Biological Psychiatry, 23*, 271–284.

Allen-Burge R, Storandt M, Kinscherf DA, & Rubin EH. (1994). Sex differences in the sensitivity of two self-report depression scales in elder depressed inpatients. *Psychol Aging, 9*, 443–445.

Altamura AC, Mauri MC, Colacurcio F, Scapicchio PL, Hadjchristos C, Carucci G, Minervini M, Montanini R, Perini M, Rudas N, Carpiniello B, D'Aloise A, & Malinconico A. (1988). Trazodone in late life depressive states: A double-blind multicenter study versus amitriptyline and mianserin. *Psychopharmacology, 95*, S34–S36.

Ambrosio LA, Marchese G, Filippo A, Romano E, & Musacchio R. (1993). The effect of mesoglycan in patients with cerebrovascular disease: A psychometric evaluation. *J Int Med Res, 21*, 158–160.

American Psychiatric Association. (1994). *Diagnostic and statistical manual of mental disorders:* (4th ed.) (*DSM-IV*). Washington, DC: Author.

*Andresen EM, Malmgren JA, Carter WB, & Patrick DL. (1994). Screening for depression in well older adults: Evaluation of a short form of the CES-D. *Am J Prev Med, 10*, 77–84.

Applegate WB. (1995). Reply (Editor's Letter). *J Am Geriatr Soc*, *43*, 82–83.

*Artinian NT, Duggan C, & Miller P. (1993). Age differences in patient recovery patterns following coronary artery bypass surgery. *Am J Critical Care*, *2*, 453–461.

*Baker FM, & Miller CL. (1991). Screening of a skilled nursing home population for depression. *J Geriatr Psychiatry Neurol*, *4*, 218–221.

Barrett-Connor E, & Palinkas LA. (1994). Low blood pressure and depression in older men: A population based study. *BMJ*, *308*, 446–449.

Barsa J, Toner J, Gurland B, & Lantigua R. (1986). Ability of internists to recognize and manage depression in the elderly. *Int J Geriatr Psychiatry*, *1*, 57–62.

*Beck AT, & Beck RW. (1972). Screening depressed patients in family practice: A rapid technic. *Postgrad Med*, *52*, 81–85.

*Beck AT, Rial WY, & Rickels K. (1974). Short form of depression inventory: Cross-validation. *Psychol Rep*, *34*, 1184–1186.

*Beck AT, Ward CH, Mendelson M, Mock J, & Erbaugh J. (1961). An inventory for measuring depression. *Arch Gen Psychiatr*, *4*, 561–571.

Berkman LF, Berkman CS, Kasl S, Freeman DH, Leo L, Ostfeld AM, Cornoni-Huntley J, & Brody JA. (1986). Depressive symptoms in relation to physical health and functioning in the elderly. *Am J Epidemiol*, *124*, 372–388.

*Blalock SJ, DeVellis RF, Brown GK, & Wallston KA. (1989). Validity of the Center for Epidemiological Studies Depression Scale in arthritis populations. *Arthritis Rheum*, *32*, 991–997.

Blazer D. (1989). Depression in the elderly. *N Engl J Med*, *320*, 164–166.

*Blazer D, Burchett B, Service C, & George LK. (1991). The association of age and depression among the elderly: An epidemiologic exploration. *J Gerontol*, *46*, M210–M215.

Blazer DG. (1994). Is depression more frequent in late life? An honest look at the evidence. *Am J Geriatr Psychiatry*, *2*, 193–199.

Blazer DG, & Williams CD. (1980). The epidemiology of dysphoria and depression in an elderly population. *Am J Psychiatry*, *137*, 439–444.

Bojrab SL, Sipes GP, Weinberger M, Hendrie HC, Hayes JR, Darnell JC, & Martz BL. (1988). A model for predicting depression in elderly tenants of public housing. *Hosp Community Psychiatry*, *39*, 304–309.

*Bolla-Wilson K, & Bleecker ML. (1989). Absence of depression in elderly adults. *J Gerontol*, *44*, P53–P55.

Boyd JH, Weissman MM, Thompson WD, & Myers JK. (1982). Screening for depression in a community sample: Understanding the discrepancies between depression symptom and diagnostic scales. *Arch Gen Psychiatry*, *39*, 1195–1200.

Breuer B. (1995). Determination of causality. *J Am Geriatr Soc*, *43*, 82.

Brink TL. (1989). Proper scoring of the Geriatric Depression Scale. *J Am Geriatr Soc*, *37*, 819.

*Brink TL, Yesavage JA, Lum O, Heersema PH, Adey M, & Rose TL. (1982). Screening tests for geriatric depression. *Clin Gerontol*, *1*, 37–43.

*Burke WJ, Houston MJ, Boust SJ, & Roccaforte WH. (1989). Use of the Geriatric Depression Scale in dementia of the Alzheimer type. *J Am Geriatr Soc*, *37*, 856–860.

*Burke WJ, Nitcher RL, Roccaforte WH, & Wengel SP. (1992). A prospective evaluation of the Geriatric Depression Scale in an outpatient geriatric assessment center. *J Am Geriatr Soc*, *40*, 1227–1230.

Burke WJ, Roccaforte WH, & Boust SJ. (1990). Reply [to Christensen and Dysken, 1990]. *J Am Geriatr Soc, 38,* 725.
*Burke WJ, Roccaforte WH, & Wengel SP. (1991). The Short Form of the Geriatric Depression Scale: A comparison with the 30-item form. *J Geriatr Psychiatry Neurol, 4,* 173–178.
Burnam MA, Wells KB, Leake B, & Landsverk J. (1988). Development of a brief screening instrument for detecting depressive disorders. *Med Care, 26,* 775–789.
Callahan CM, Hui SL, Nienaber NA, Musick BS, & Tierney WM. (1994). Longitudinal study of depression and health services use among elderly primary care patients. *J Am Geriatr Soc, 42,* 833–838.
*Callahan CM, & Wolinsky FD. (1994). The effect of gender and race on the measurement properties of the CES-D in older adults. *Med Care, 32,* 341–356.
Cho MJ, Moscicki EK, Narrow WE, Rae DS, Locke BZ, & Regier DA. (1993). Concordance between two measures of depression in the Hispanic Health and Nutrition Examination Survey. *Soc Psychiatry Psychiatr Epidemiol, 28,* 156–163.
Christensen KJ, & Dysken MW. (1990). The Geriatric Depression Scale in Alzheimer's disease. *J Am Geriatr Soc, 38,* 724–725.
Cipolli C, Neri M, Andermarcher E, Pinelli M, & Lalla M. (1990). Self-rating and objective memory testing of normal and depressed elderly. *Aging, 2,* 39–48.
Cohen GD. (1990). Psychopathology and mental health in the mature and elderly adult. In JE Birren & KW Schaie (Eds.), *Handbook of the psychology of aging* (3rd ed., pp. 359–371). San Diego: Academic Press.
*Colantonio A, Kasl SV, & Ostfeld AM. (1992). Depressive symptoms and other psychosocial factors as predictors of stroke in the elderly. *Am J Epidemiol, 136,* 884–894.
Colantonio A, Kasl SV, Ostfeld AM, & Berkman LF. (1993). Psychosocial predictors of stroke outcomes in an elderly population. *J Gerontol, 48,* S261–S268.
Colsher PL, Wallace RB, Pomrehn PR, LaCroix AZ, Cornoni-Huntley J, Blazer D, Scherr PA, Berkman L, & Hennekens CH. (1990). Demographic and health characteristics of elderly smokers: Results from established populations for epidemiologic studies of the elderly. *Am J Prev Med, 6,* 61–70.
*Davidson H, Feldman PH, & Crawford S. (1994). Measuring depressive symptoms in the frail elderly. *J Gerontol, 49,* P159–P164.
Depression Guideline Panel. (1993). *Depression in primary care: Clinical practice guideline, number 5,* (2 Vols.) (AHCPR Publication No. 93-0550). Rockville, MD: U.S. Department of Health and Human Services, Public Health Service, Agency for Health Care Policy and Research.
DiPietro L, Anda RF, Williamson DF, & Stunkard AJ. (1992). Depressive symptoms and weight change in a national cohort of adults. *Int J Obes, 16,* 745–753.
Eaton WW, & Kessler LG. (1981). Rates of symptoms of depression in a national sample. *Am J Epidemiol, 114,* 528–538.
Endicott J, & Spitzer RL. (1978). A diagnostic interview: The Schedules for Affective Disorders and Schizophrenia. *Arch Gen Psychiatry, 35,* 837–844.
*Foelker GA, & Shewchuk RM. (1992). Somatic complaints and the CES-D. *J Am Geriatr Soc, 40,* 259–262.
*Foelker GA Jr, Shewchuk RM, & Niederehe G. (1987). Confirmatory factor analysis of the short form Beck Depression Inventory in elderly community samples. *J Clin Psychol, 43,* 111–118.

Frerichs RR, Aneshensel CS, & Clark VA. (1981). Prevalence of depression in Los Angeles County. *Am J Epidemiol, 113*, 691–699.

*Fulop G, Reinhardt J, Strain JJ, Paris B, Miller M, & Fillit H. (1993). Identification of alcoholism and depression in a geriatric medicine outpatient clinic. *J Am Geriatr Soc, 41*, 737–741.

Gallagher D. (1986). The Beck Depression Inventory and older adults: Review of its development and utility. *Clin Gerontol, 5*, 149–163.

*Gallagher D, Breckenridge J, Steinmetz J, & Thompson L. (1983). The Beck Depression Inventory and Research Diagnostic Criteria: Congruence in an older population. *J Consult Clin Psychol, 51*, 945–946.

*Gallagher D, Nies G, & Thompson LW. (1982). Reliability of the Beck Depression Inventory with older adults. *J Consult Clin Psychol, 50*, 152–153.

Garcia M, & Marks G. (1989). Depressive symptomatology among Mexican-American adults: An examination with the CES-D scale. *Psychiatry Res, 27*, 137–148.

*Gatewood-Colwell G, Kaczmarek M, & Ames MH. (1989). Reliability and validity of the Beck Depression Inventory for a white and Mexican-American gerontic population. *Psychol Rep, 65*, 1163–1166.

Gerety MB, Chiodo LK, Kanten DN, Tuley MR, & Cornell JE. (1993). Medical treatment preferences of nursing home residents: Relationship to function and concordance with surrogate decision-makers. *J Am Geriatr Soc, 41*, 953–960.

Gerety MB, Cornell JE, Mulrow CD, Tuley M, Hazuda HP, Lichtenstein M, Aguilar C, Kadri AA, & Rosenberg J. (1994). The Sickness Impact Profile for Nursing Homes (SIP-NH). *J Gerontol, 49*, M2–M8.

Golden RR, Teresi JA, & Gurland BJ. (1984). Development of indicator scales for the Comprehensive Assessment and Referral Evaluation Interview Schedule. *J Gerontol, 39*, 138–146.

*Goldstein MS, & Hurwicz ML. (1989). Psychosocial distress and perceived health status among elderly users of a health maintenance organization. *J Gerontol, 44*, P154–P156.

Gurland B. (1992). The impact of depression on quality of life of the elderly. *Clin Geriatr Med, 8*, 377–386.

Gurland BJ, Golden R, Teresi J, & Challop J. (1984). The SHORT-CARE: An efficient instrument for the assessment of depression, dementia and disability. *J Gerontol, 39*, 166–169.

Hamilton M. (1967). Development of a rating scale for primary depressive illness. *Br J Soc Clin Psychol, 6*, 278–296.

Hanninen T, Reinikainen KJ, Helkala EL, Koivisto K, Mykkanen L, Laakso M, Pyorala K, & Riekkinen PJ. (1994). Subjective memory complaints and personality traits in normal elderly subjects. *J Am Geriatr Soc, 42*, 1–4.

Harper RG, Kotik-Harper D, & Kirby H. (1990). Psychometric assessment of depression in an elderly general medical population: Over- or underassessment. *J Nerv Ment Dis, 178*, 113–119.

Harris RE, Mion LC, Patterson MB, & Frengley JD. (1988). Severe illness in older patients: The association between depressive disorders and functional dependency during the recovery phase. *J Am Geriatr Soc, 36*, 890–896.

Herr KA, Mobily PR, & Smith C. (1993). Depression and the experience of chronic back pain: A study of related variables and age differences. *Clin J Pain, 9*, 104–114.

Himmelfarb S, & Murrell SA. (1983). Reliability and validity of five mental health scales in older persons. *J Gerontol, 38*, 333–339.

*House A, Dennis M, Mogridge L, Warlow C, Hawton K, & Jones L. (1991). Mood disorders in the year after first stroke. *Br J Psychiatry, 158*, 83–92.

Hurwicz ML, & Berkanovic E. (1993). The stress process in rheumatoid arthritis. *J Rheumatol, 20*, 1836–1844.

Jacobs S, Hansen F, Berkman L, Kasl S, & Ostfeld A. (1989). Depressions of bereavement. *Comp Psychiatry, 30*, 218–224.

Jamison C, & Scogin F. (1992). Development of an interview-based Geriatric Depression Rating Scale. *Int J Aging Hum Dev, 35*, 193–204.

*Kafonek S, Ettinger WH, Roca R, Kittner S, Taylor N, & German PS. (1989). Instruments for screening for depression and dementia in a long-term care facility. *J Am Geriatr Soc, 37*, 29–34.

Kafonek SD, & Roca RP. (1989). Reply (Letter to the Editor). *J Am Geriatr Soc, 37*, 819–820.

Kahn R. (1995). Weight loss and depression in a community nursing home. *J Am Geriatr Soc, 43*, 83.

Kaszniak AW. (1990). Psychological assessment of the aging individual. In JE Birren & KW Schaie (Eds.), *Handbook of the psychology of aging* (3rd ed., pp. 427–445). San Diego: Academic Press.

Kaszniak AW, & Allender J. (1985). Psychological assessment of depression in older adults. In GM Chaisson-Stewart (Ed.), *Depression in the elderly: An interdisciplinary approach* (pp. 107–160). New York: Wiley.

Keele-Card G, Foxall MF, & Barron CR. (1993). Loneliness, depression, and social support of patients with COPD and their spouses. *Public Health Nurs, 10*, 245–251.

Kennedy GJ, Kelman HR, Thomas C, Wisniewski W, Metz H, & Bijur PE. (1989). Hierarchy of characteristics associated with depressive symptoms in an urban elderly sample. *Am J Psychiatry, 146*, 220–225.

*Kessler RC, Foster C, Webster PS, & House JS. (1992). The relationship between age and depressive symptoms in two national surveys. *Psychol Aging, 7*, 119–126.

*Knight RG. (1984). Some general population norms for the short form Beck Depression Inventory. *J Clin Psychol, 40*, 751–753.

Koenig HG, & Blazer DG. (1992). Epidemiology of geriatric affective disorders. *Clin Geriatr Med, 8*, 235–251.

Koenig HG, Cohen HJ, Blazer DG, Krishnan KRR, & Sibert TE. (1993). Profile of depressive symptoms in younger and older medical inpatients with major depression. *J Am Geriatr Soc, 41*, 1169–1176.

Koenig HG, Cohen HJ, Blazer DG, Meador KG, & Westlund R. (1992). A brief depression scale for use in the medically ill. *Int J Psychiatry Med, 22*, 183–195.

*Koenig HG, Cohen HJ, Blazer DG, Pieper C, Meador KG, Shelp F, Goli V, & DiPasquale B. (1992). Religious coping and depression among elderly, hospitalized medically ill men. *Am J Psychiatry, 149*, 1693–1700.

*Koenig HG, Ford SM, & Blazer DG. (1993). Should physicians screen for depression in elderly medical inpatients? Results of a decision analysis. *Int J Psychiatry Med, 23*, 239–263.

Koenig HG, Meador KG, Cohen HJ, & Blazer DG. (1988a). Depression in elderly hospitalized patients with medical illness. *Arch Intern Med, 148*, 1929–1936.

Koenig HG, Meador KG, Cohen HJ, & Blazer DG. (1988b). Self-rated depression scales and screening for major depression in the older hospitalized patient with medical illness. *J Am Geriatr Soc, 36*, 699–706.

*Koenig HG, Meador KG, Cohen HJ, & Blazer DG. (1992). Screening for depression in hospitalized elderly medical patients: Taking a closer look. *J Am Geriatr Soc, 40*, 1013–1017.

*Koenig HG, Meador KG, Goli V, Shelp F, Cohen HJ, & Blazer DG. (1992). Self-rated depressive symptoms in medical inpatients: Age and racial differences. *Int J Psychiatry Med, 22*, 11–31.

*Kohout FJ, Berkman LF, Evans DA, & Cornoni-Huntley J. (1993). Two shorter forms of the CES-D depression index. *J Aging Health, 5*, 179–193.

*Lee MA, & Ganzini L. (1992). Depression in the elderly: Effect of patient attitudes toward life-sustaining therapy. *J Am Geriatr Soc, 40*, 983–988.

Lee M, & Ganzini L. (1994). The effect of recovery from depression on preferences for life-sustaining therapy in older patients. *J Gerontol, 49*, M15–M21.

Lesher EL. (1986). Validation of the Geriatric Depression Scale among nursing home residents. *Clin Gerontol, 4*, 21–28.

*Lesher EL, & Berryhill JS. (1994). Validation of the Geriatric Depression Scale—Short Form among inpatients. *J Clin Psych, 50*, 256–260.

Liang J, Van Tran T, Krause N, & Markides KS. (1989). Generational differences in the structure of the CES-D Scale in Mexican Americans. *J Gerontol, 44*, S110–S120.

Logsdon RG, & Teri L. (1995). Depression in Alzheimer's disease patients: Caregivers as surrogate reporters. *J Am Geriatr Soc, 43*, 150–155.

Lubin B, & Rinck CM. (1986). Assessment of mood and affect in the elderly: The Depression Adjective Check List and the Multiple Adjective Check List. *Clin Gerontol, 5*, 187–191.

Lyness JM, Cox C, Curry J, Conwell Y, King DA, & Caine ED. (1995). Older age and the underreporting of depressive symptoms. *J Am Geriatr Soc, 43*, 216–221.

Mahard RE. (1988). The CES-D as a measure of depressive mood in the elderly Puerto Rican population. *J Gerontol, 43*, 24–25.

Mahoney J, Drinka TJK, Abler R, Gunter-Hunt G, Matthews C, Gravenstein S, & Carnes M. (1994). Screening for depression: Single question versus GDS. *J Am Geriatr Soc, 42*, 1006–1008.

Marottoli RA, Berkman LF, & Cooney LM. (1992). Decline in physical function following hip fracture. *J Am Geriatr Soc, 40*, 861–866.

*McGivney SA, Mulvihill M, & Taylor B. (1994). Validating the GDS depression screen in the nursing home. *J Am Geriatr Soc, 42*, 490–492.

Mendes de Leon CF, Rapp SS, & Kasl SV. (1994). Financial strain and symptoms of depression in a community sample of elderly men and women. *J Aging Health, 6*, 448–468.

*Morgan RE, Palinkas LA, Barrett-Connor EL, & Wingard DL. (1993). Plasma cholesterol and depressive symptoms in older men. *Lancet, 341*, 75–79.

*Morley JE, & Kraenzle D. (1994). Causes of weight loss in a community nursing home. *J Am Geriatr Soc, 42*, 583–585.

Morley JE, & Kraenzle D. (1995). Reply (Letter to the Editor). *J Am Geriatr Soc*, *43*, 84.
*Mossey JM, Knott K, & Craik R. (1990). The effects of persistent depressive symptoms on hip fracture recovery. *J Gerontol*, *45*, M163–M168.
Murrell SA, Himmelfarb S, & Wright K. (1983). Prevalence of depression and its correlates in older adults. *Am J Epidemiol*, *117*, 173–185.
Myers JK, Weissman MM, Tischler GL, Holzer CE 3d, Leaf PJ, Orvaschel M, Anthony JC, Boyd JH, Burke JD Jr, Kramer M, et al. (1984). Six-month prevalence of psychiatric disorders in three communities: 1980–1982. *Arch Gen Psychiatry*, *41*, 959–970.
Nicassio PM, & Wallston KA. (1992). Longitudinal relationships among pain, sleep problems, and depression in rheumatoid arthritis. *J Abnormal Psychol*, *101*, 514–520.
*Norris JT, Gallagher D, Wilson A, & Winograd CH. (1987). Assessment of depression in geriatric medical outpatients: The validity of two screening measures. *J Am Geriatr Soc*, *35*, 989–995.
O'Hara MW, Hinrichs JV, Kohout FJ, Wallace RB, & Lemke JH. (1986). Memory complaint and memory performance in the depressed elderly. *Psychol Ageing*, *1*, 208–214.
O'Hara MW, Kohout FJ, & Wallace RB. (1985). Depression among the rural elderly: A study of prevalence and correlates. *J Nerv Ment Dis*, *173*, 582–589.
O'Riordan TG, Hayes JP, O'Neill D, Shelley R, Walsh JB, & Coakley D. (1990). The effect of mild to moderate dementia on the Geriatric Depression Scale and on the General Health Questionnaire. *Age Ageing*, *19*, 57–61.
*Oxman TE, Berkman LF, Kasl S, Freeman DH, & Barrett J. (1992). Social support and depressive symptoms in the elderly. *Am J Epidemiol*, *135*, 356–368.
Pachana NA, Gallagher-Thompson D, & Thompson LW. (1994). Assessment of depression. In MP Lawton & JA Teresi (Eds.). *Annual review of gerontology and geriatrics*. Volume 14: *Focus on assessment techniques* (pp. 234–256). New York: Springer.
Palinkas LA, & Barrett-Connor E. (1992). Estrogen use and depressive symptoms in postmenopausal women. *Obstet Gynecol*, *80*, 30–36.
Palinkas LA, Barrett-Connor E, & Wingard DL. (1991). Type 2 diabetes and depressive symptoms in older adults: A population-based study. *Diabetic Med*, *8*, 532–539.
Parikh RM, Eden DT, Price TR, & Robinson RG. (1988). The sensitivity and specificity of the Center for Epidemiologic Studies Depression Scale in screening for post-stroke depression. *Int J Psychiatry Med*, *18*, 169–181.
Parmelee PA, & Katz IR. (1990). Geriatric Depression Scale. *J Am Geriatr Soc*, *38*, 1379.
*Parmelee PA, Katz IR, & Lawton MP. (1991). The relation of pain to depression among institutionalized aged. *J Gerontol*, *46*, P15–P21.
*Parmelee PA, Lawton MP, & Katz IR. (1989). Psychometric properties of the Geriatric Depression Scale among the institutionalized aged. *Psychol Assess*, *1*, 331–338.
*Peck JR, Smith TW, Ward JR, & Milano R. (1989). Disability and depression in rheumatoid arthritis: A multi-trait, multi-method investigation. *Arthritis Rheum*, *32*, 1100–1106.
Perez-Stable E, Miranda J, Munoz RF, & Ying YW. (1990). Depression in medical outpatients: Underrecognition and misdiagnosis. *Arch Intern Med*, *150*, 1083–1088.
Printz-Feddersen V. (1990). Group process effect on caregiver burden. *J Neurosci Nurs*, *22*, 164–167.

*Radloff LS. (1977). The CES-D Scale: A self-report depression scale for research in the general population. *Appl Psychol Meas, 1,* 385–401.

Radloff LS, & Teri L. (1986). Uses of the Center for Epidemiological Studies-Depression Scale with older adults. In TL Brink (Ed.), *Clinical gerontology: A guide to assessment and intervention.* New York: Haworth.

Rankin SH, Galbraith ME, & Johnson S. (1993). Reliability and validity data for a Chinese translation of the Center for Epidemiologic Studies-Depression. *Psychol Rep, 73,* 1291–1298.

Rapp SR, Parisi SA, Walsh DA, & Wallace CE. (1988). Detecting depression in elderly medical inpatients. *J Consult Clin Psychol, 56,* 509–513.

Retan JW. (1995). Causes of weight loss in a nursing home. *J Am Geriatr Soc, 43,* 83.

Reynolds WM, & Gould JW. (1981). A psychometric investigation of the standard and short form Beck Depression Inventory. *J Consult Clin Psychol, 49,* 306–307.

*Salive ME, & Blazer DG. (1993). Depression and smoking cessation in older adults: A longitudinal study. *J Am Geriatr Soc, 41,* 1313–1316.

Schonwetter RS, Teasdale TA, Taffet G, Robinson BE, & Luchi RJ. (1991). Educating the elderly: Cardiopulmonary resuscitation decisions before and after intervention. *J Am Geriatr Soc, 39,* 372–377.

*Scogin F, Beutler L, Corbishley A, & Hamblin D. (1988). Reliability and validity of the short form Beck Depression Inventory with older adults. *J Clin Psychol, 44,* 853–857.

Sheikh VI, & Yesavage VA. (1986). Geriatric Depression Scale (GDS): Recent evidence and development of a shorter version. In TL Brink (Ed.), *Clinical gerontology: A guide to assessment and intervention* (pp. 165–174). New York: Haworth.

Shinar D, Gross CR, Price TR, Banko M, Bolduc PL, & Robinson RG. (1986). Screening for depression in stroke patients: The reliability and validity of the Center for Epidemiologic Studies Depression Scale. *Stroke, 17,* 241–245.

Shrout PE, & Yager TJ. (1989). Reliability and validity of screening scales: Effect of reducing scale length. *J Clin Epidemiol, 42,* 69–78.

Snowdon J. (1990). Validity of the Geriatric Depression Scale. *J Am Geriatr Soc, 38,* 722–729.

Somervell PD, Beals J, Kinzie JD, Boehnlein J, Leung P, & Manson SM. (1993). Criterion validity of the Center for Epidemiologic Studies Depression Scale in a population sample from an American Indian village. *Psychiatry Res, 47,* 255–266.

Spitzer RL, Endicott J, & Robins E. (1978). Research diagnostic criteria: Rationale and reliability. *Arch Gen Psychiatry, 35,* 773–782.

*Stallones L, Marx MB, & Garrity TF. (1990). Prevalence and correlates of depressive symptoms among older U.S. adults. *Am J Prev Med, 6,* 295–303.

*Stewart RB, Blashfield R, Hale WE, Moore MT, May FE, & Marks RG. (1991). Correlates of Beck Depression Inventory scores in an ambulatory elderly population: Symptoms, diseases, laboratory values, and medications. *J Fam Practice, 32,* 497–502.

*Stommel M, Given BA, Given CW, Kalaian HA, Schulz R, & McCorkle R. (1993). Gender bias in the measurement properties of the Center for Epidemiologic Studies Depression Scale (CES-D). *Psychiatry Res, 49,* 239–250.

Sunderland T, Alterman IS, Yount D, Hill JL, Tariot PN, Newhouse PA, Mueller EA, Mellow AM, & Cohen RM. (1988). A new scale for the assessment of depressed mood in depressed patients. *Am J Psychiatry, 145,* 955–959.

Thapa PB, Meador KG, Gideon P, Fought RL, & Ray WA. (1994). Effects of antipsychotic withdrawal in elderly nursing home residents. *J Am Geriatr Soc, 42,* 280–286.

Toner J, Gurland B, & Teresi J. (1988). Comparison of self-administered and rater-administered methods of assessing levels of severity of depression in elderly patients. *J Gerontol, 43,* 136–140.

Tudiver F, Hilditch J, & Permaul JA. (1991). A comparison of psychosocial characteristics of new widowers and married men. *Fam Med, 23,* 501–505.

Vida S, Gauthier L, & Gauthier S. (1989). Canadian collaborative study of tetrahy-droaminoacridine (THA) and lecithin treatment of Alzheimer's disease: Effect on mood. *Can J Psychiatry, 34,* 165–170.

*Wallace J, & O'Hara MW. (1992). Increases in depressive symptomatology in the rural elderly: Results from a cross-sectional and longitudinal study. *J Abnorm Psychol, 101,* 398–404.

Ware JR, & Sherbourne CD. (1992). The MOS 36-item Short-Form Health Survey (SF-36): I. Conceptual framework and item selection. *Med Care, 30,* 473.

Weiss IK, Nagel CL, & Aronson MK. (1986). Applicability of depression scales to the old old person. *J Am Geriatr Soc, 34,* 215–218.

Wells KB, Stewart A, Hays RD, Burnam A, Rogers W, Daniels M, Berry S, Greenfield S, & Ware J. (1989). The functioning and well-being of depressed patients: Results from the Medical Outcomes Study. *JAMA, 262,* 914–919.

*Woo J, Ho SC, Lau J, Yuen YK, Chiu H, Lee HC, & Chi I. (1994). The prevalence of depressive symptoms and predisposing factors in an elderly Chinese population. *Acta Psychiatr Scand, 89,* 8–13.

*Yesavage JA, Brink TL, Rose TL, Lum O, Huang V, Adey M, & Leirer VO. (1983). Development and validation of a Geriatric Depression Screening Scale: A preliminary report. *J Psychiatr Res, 17,* 37–49.

Zung WWK, & Zung EM. (1986). Use of the Zung Self-Rating Depression Scale in the elderly. *Clin Gerontol, 5,* 137–148.

Author Index

Subject Index

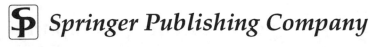
Springer Publishing Company

Geriatric Assessment Technology
The State of the Art

Laurence Z. Rubenstein, MD, MPH, **Darryl Wieland,** PhD, MPH, and **Roberto Bernabei,** Professor

The field of comprehensive geriatric assessment has been rapidly evolving worldwide as an effective methodology for improving care of increasing aging population. This book updates and synthesizes our current knowledge of comprehensive geriatric assessment (CGA). CGA includes the assessment of physical health, mental health, functional ability, and social and environmental parameters. The editors address both the technical and methodologic areas of how to perform the assessment as well as the programmic and clinical areas of how to organize services in a practical way within diverse health care systems. Contributors include Barry Gurland, Robert Kane, Rosalie Kane, Knight Steel, and Bruno Vellas.

Partial Contents: Comprehensive Geriatric Assessment: Meta-analysis of Main Effects and Elements Enhancing Effectiveness • Comprehensive Geriatric Assessment: Assessment Techniques • The Medical Evaluation • Assessment of Functional Status: Activities of Daily Living • Performance Measures of Physical Function in Comprehensive Geriatric Assessment • The Clinical Assessment of Gait, Balance, and Mobility in Older Adults • Assessment of Social Functioning: Recommendations for Comprehensive Geriatric Assessment • Detection and Assessment of Cognitive Impairment and Depressed Mood in Primary Care of Older Adults: A Systems Approach to the Uses of Brief Scales • Clinical Assessment of Physical Activity in Older Adults • Assessment of Lower Urinary Function • Nutritional Assessment as Part of the Geriatric Evaluation • Hospital Geriatric Assessment and Management Units • Hospital Consultation Teams • Special Hospital Geriatric Units • Preventive Home Visits to Elderly Persons; Status and Perspectives • Nursing Home Assessment • Evolving Methods for Comprehensive Assessment by General Practitioners: The UK Experience • Defining and Refining Targeting Criteria • Promoting the Effectiveness of CGA Programs Through Quality Improvement Approaches • The Role of Geriatric Assessment in Different Countries

1995   320pp   0-8261-9930-5   hard $65.95 (outside US $73.80)

536 Broadway, New York, NY 10012-3955 • (212) 431-4370 • Fax (212) 941-7842

⑤ *Springer Publishing Company*

Promoting Health and Mental Health in Children

David S. Glenwick, PhD
Leonard A. Jason, PhD, Editors

This book begins with a behavioral look at community health and mental health promotion. It then addresses a range of critical issues including school-based problems, physical and sexual abuse, childhood accidents, substance abuse, adolescent pregnancy, AIDS, and vehicular safety. It also provides three innovative strategies for health/mental health promotion.

Contents:

I. Introduction: Behavioral Approaches to Prevention in the Community: A Historical and Theoretical Overview, *D. S. Glenwick and L. A. Jason*

II. Targeting Specific Health and Mental Health Problems: School-Based Interventions for Promoting Social Competence, *J. Rhodes and S. Englund* • Prevention of Child Physical and Sexual Abuse, *S. K. Wurtele* • Childhood Injury Prevention, *L. Peterson, et al* • Prevention of Substance Abuse, *S. H. Kelder and C. L. Perry* • Preventing Teenage Pregnancy, *W. L. Robinson, et al* • Prevention of AIDS, *J. A. Kelly and D. A. Murphy* • Increasing Road Safety Behaviors, *E. S. Geller*

III. Innovative Strategies for Promoting Health: Media-Based Change Approaches for Prevention, *R. A. Winett* • Applications of Social Support to Preventive Interventions, *G. Anne Bogat, et al* • Promoting Health Through Community Development, *S. B. Fawcett, et al*

1993   280pp   0-8261-7310-1   hard $39.95 (outside US $44.80)

536 Broadway, New York, NY 10012-3955 • (212) 431-4370 • Fax (212) 941-7842

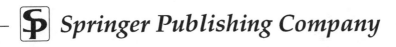

Springer Publishing Company

Health Promotion and Aging

David Haber, PhD

This informative and practical text fulfills the need for a broad and integrative perspective on health promotion for the elderly. Based on extensive research, the author emphasizes individual responsibility for healthy living in collaboration with professionals, as well as through social support.

By focusing on health rather than disease, this book provides useful guidelines for health professionals, educators, and students of gerontology. Includes extensive illustrations.

Health
Promotion
and Aging

David Haber

𝕊

Springer Publishing Company

Contents:

- Introduction
- Health Professionals and Older Clients: A Collaboration
- Medical Screenings and Health Assessments
- Health Education: Introduction and Exercise
- Health Education: Nutrition
- Health Education: Other Topics
- Social Support
- Behavior and Psychological Management
- Community Health
- Societal Reform

1994   296pp   0-8261-8460-X   hardcover

536 Broadway, New York, NY 10012-3955 • (212) 431-4370 • Fax (212) 941-7842